1017

REACHING HEALTH FOR ALL

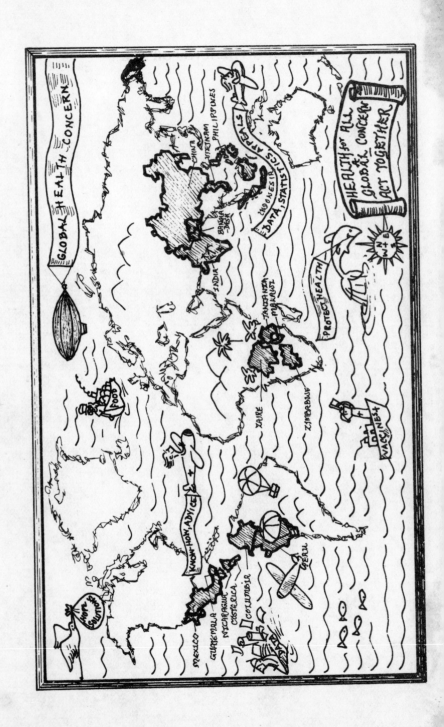

Reaching Health for All

Edited by
JON ROHDE
MEERA CHATTERJEE
DAVID MORLEY

Illustrated by
STEPHEN MARAZZI

DELHI
OXFORD UNIVERSITY PRESS
BOMBAY   CALCUTTA   MADRAS
1993

Oxford University Press, Walton Street, Oxford OX2 6DP

New York Toronto
Delhi Bombay Calcutta Madras Karachi
Kuala Lumpur Singapore Hong Kong Tokyo
Nairobi Dar es Salaam
Melbourne Auckland

and associates in
Berlin Ibadan

First published March 1993
Second impression June 1993

ISBN 0 19 563236 2

Printed in India
Typeset by Vibrant, Rohini, Delhi 110085
Printed at Crescent Printing Works Pvt. Ltd., New Delhi 110001
Published by Neil O'Brien, Oxford University Press
YMCA Library Building, Jai Singh Road, New Delhi 110001

Ah, but a man's reach should
exceed his grasp,
Or what's a heaven for?

—ROBERT BROWNING
Andrea del Sarto

Contents

Foreword

Many greeted the call for 'Health for All by the Year 2000', first enunciated at the WHO/UNICEF meeting at Alma Ata in 1978, as unrealistic development rhetoric. Experience in the 1970s had shown that primary health care based in the community and relevant to the most common and pressing needs of the poor was indeed possible. The 1980s saw an accelerating pace, with an expansion of community activities, larger-scale national projects, nation-wide programmes which reoriented priorities to emphasize primary health care, and the emergence of global programmes focused on the most pressing needs of immunization, diarrhoeal disease, family planning and nutrition. These have amply demonstrated both the need to involve the community and the potential for achievement when social action and mobilization actually occur.

The success of these expanded efforts in health led, in the year 1990, to the Global Summit for Children, the largest-ever gathering of world leaders. These leaders committed themselves to a decade of hard work and ambitious goals that provide both the formula and a recommitment to the achievement of 'Health for All' by the end of this decade. These ambitious goals form a development agenda on human issues unprecedented in world history. The global challenges of the 1980s, culminating in unforseen and unprecedented economic and political changes in 1990–91, have led to an even greater need than ever for the establishment of social safety nets in countries and populations where structural adjustment and failure of socialist political systems have left large populations vulnerable. While market forces may be acknowledged as the best guidelines to economic activities, it is well recognized that public programmes are required to protect the most vulnerable members of society and to ensure the basic investments in people required for a truly equitable and healthy development.

This book provides an in-depth view of the strategic and operational issues underlying the quest for 'Health for All'. Through more than 20 case studies it illustrates the tensions and trade-offs between the array of options that face any decision-maker attempting to efficiently allocate limited resources to improve the health of millions. The choices are difficult but critical, for it is the balance of these choices faced daily by decision-makers that will determine both the efficiency and equity of the outcome. These case studies are relevant to practitioners and students of public health, to managers, workers and teachers who wish to understand, design and run the programmes of the 1990s.

. Above all, this book shows the hope and promise that 'Health for All' can indeed be met. The cases amply demonstrate the power of community action, the potential of low-level health workers and their relevance and acceptance by the communities they serve. They show how countries can afford essential primary health services which are effective, efficient and equitable. They describe how global efforts amply supported by mobilization of modern communication, political will and socially-committed people and organizations can accomplish far more than even those things the sceptics said could never be done. This book details the issues and the means by which *reaching* 'Health for All' could become a possible dream in our time.

JAMES P. GRANT
Executive Director
UNICEF

Preface

In 1983 the book *Practising Health for All* (*PHFA*) presented 18 studies of programmes ranging from village-level developments in health to national efforts to implement the substance and spirit of the 1978 Alma Ata Declaration. A 'case study approach' was used to describe specific village, community, non-governmental and national government programmes, leaving to the reader the task of drawing lessons and principles, with only limited guidance from the editors. The series of studies revolved around the political nature of primary health care and emphasized community involvement and the political will required for large-scale health activities. The book as a whole was testimony to the philosophy that many roads lead towards 'Health for All' and that experience is the best teacher in this quest.

PHFA proved to be useful to practitioners and teachers of public health throughout the world, selling over 23 000 copies which required five reprintings. It was used in schools of public health and medicine in both developed and developing countries, a particularly popular tool for discussion groups and open-ended learning techniques. Many readers began to express interest in an update of the book.

However, during the 1980s a vast amount of experience accumulated throughout the world in the thematic areas explored by *PHFA*. Indeed, 'Health for All' had grown into a movement in new areas, with considerably diverse paths and varying outcomes. It became apparent that the cases described in *PHFA* itself had evolved in substantial ways. Clearly what was called for was a new book describing critical experiences during the decade, the challenges faced by and issues emerging in the quest for 'Health for All'. Thus, *Reaching Health for All* (*RHFA*) has been prepared to present a new set of studies embracing the extensive efforts in Primary Health Care in the 1980s.

To build on earlier experience, authors who had contributed to *PHFA* were invited to prepare articles on the progress of their programmes through the decade. In addition, new experiences were identified and articles on them sought. Thus, *RHFA* includes case studies from Latin America, Africa and Asia, reflecting health care efforts in the community, in large multi-community projects, at national and international levels. We hope that this new collection of studies will prove stimulating to practitioners and students of health throughout the world, encouraging them to renew their efforts to reaching 'Health for All' in the decade ahead.

The preparation of a multi-authored book requires considerable co-ordination and patience. Many authors produced their articles in record time, while others took considerably longer. All, however, approached their task with expertise and dedication, and have graciously accepted both the intensive editorial scrutiny and delay caused by the editors' involvement in other full-time work. All have generously donated their work free of cost or royalty in order to ensure a publication affordable to community health workers and students throughout the world. We are grateful for the enthusiasm and commitment shown by all who have participated.

We have been saddened by the deaths of two of our colleagues, shortly after completing their case studies. Mary Johnston had only recently returned to her native Australia from years of working in Indonesia. Progressive illness claimed her life in October 1991. Catherine Lovell was able to put the finishing touches on her book about the Bangladesh Rural Advancement Committee only days before she succumbed to chronic illness. The publication of this book, and particularly of their articles, is a small testimony to the many contributions they made to 'Health for All' in their life-times.

This book could not have been prepared for publication without the careful, tireless and dedicated efforts of Uma Shanker. She not only typed numerous revisions of all the manuscripts but also carried on extensive correspondence, eventually exceeding in number of pages those of the book itself!

Stephen Marazzi carefully studied the articles before preparing the line-drawings which so richly illustrate the important lessons of each story. His imagination and talent have substantially enhanced the value of this effort.

Oxford University Press, New Delhi, have encouraged us and been supportive throughout the process of producing this book.

We are grateful to these friends and colleagues and all others who have given of their time and energy so generously.

JER
MC
DM

Contributors

Mr F. H. Abed
Bangladesh Rural Advancement
 Committee (BRAC)
66 Mohakhali CA
Dhaka 1212
Bangladesh

Dr James Allman
17 rue de l'Alouette
94160 Saint Mande
France

Ms Jayshree Balachander
2 Poes Garden
Madras 600086
India

Dr Rolando O. Borrinaga
Assistant Professor
University of Philippines
Institute of Health Sciences
Palo, Leyte
Philippines

Dr Meera Chatterjee
E-6/14 Vasant Vihar
New Delhi 110057
India

Dr Richard Garfield
Columbia University
School of Nursing
630 West 168th Street
New York, NY 10032
USA

Dr Lukas Hendrata
Yayasan Indonesia Sejahtera
Kramat 6/11
Jakarta
Indonesia

Dr Terrel Hill
UNICEF
3 UN Plaza
New York, NY 10017
USA

Dr Urban Jonsson
Senior Advisor (Nutrition)
UNICEF
3 UN Plaza
New York, NY 10017
USA

Dr Robert Kim-Farley
Expanded Programme on
 Immunization
World Health Organization
1211 Geneva 27
Switzerland

Dr Anthony Klouda
International Planned
 Parenthood Federation
Regent's College
Inner Circle
Regent's Park
London, NW1 4NS
UK

Dr Björn Ljungqvist
UNICEF
P.O. Box 7047
Kampala
Republic of Uganda

Dr Halfdan Mahler
Secretory General
International Planned
   Parenthood Federation
Regent's College, Inner Circle
Regent's Park
London, NW1 4NS
UK

Dr Edgar Mohs
Professor of Paediatrics
National Children's Hospital
Apartado 1654, 1000
San Jose
Costa Rica

Dr David Morley
Professor Emeritus
TALC
P.O. Box 49, St Albens
Herts AL1 4AX
UK

Dr Frits Muller
Public Health Consultant
Suderein 40
9255 LC Tietjerk
Holland

Dr Patricia J. Nickson
IPASC Nyankunde
P.B. 21285
Nairobi
Kenya

Dr Robert S. Northrup
Director
Primary Care and Health Services
International Health Institute
Brown University
Box G
Providence
Rhode Island 02912
USA

Dr Susan Rifkin
SAI Institute for Tropen Hygiene
   im Neuenheimer Felo 330
D-6900 Heidelberg
Germany

Dr Jon E. Rohde
Special Adviser
UNICEF
73 Lodi Estate
New Delhi 110003
India

Mr John Rowley
International Planned
   Parenthood Federation
Regent's College
Inner Circle
Regent's Park
London, NW1 4NS
UK

Dr David Sanders
Department of Community
   Medicine
Faculty of Medicine
University of Zimbabwe
P.O. Box A178
Avondale, Harare
Zimbabwe

Dr Alfred Sommer
Dean
Johns Hopkins University School
  of Hygiene and Public Health
615 North Wolfe Street
Baltimore
Maryland 21205
USA

Dr Carl E. Taylor
Institute for International Programs
Johns Hopkins University School
  of Hygiene and Public Health
103 East Mount Royal Avenue
Baltimore
Maryland 21202
USA

Dr Haryono Suyono
Director
National Family Planning
  Coordinating Board (*BKKBN*)
P.O. Box 186
Jakarta 10002
Indonesia

Dr David Werner
Director
The Hesperian Foundation
P.O. Box 1692
Palo Alto
California
USA

Dr Isabel Tantuico-Koh
Director
University of Philippines
Institute of Health Sciences
Palo, Leyte
Philippines

Dr Olivia Yambi
Project Officer
UNICEF
73 Lodi Estate
New Delhi 110003
India

THE EDITORS

Jon Rohde, M.D., is a paediatrician who taught community health in the medical faculty at Yogjakarta, Indonesia, in the 1970s. Based in New Delhi since 1986, he is currently Special Adviser to the Executive Director of UNICEF, dealing with programmes for children throughout the world.

Meera Chatterjee, Ph.D., a nutrition scientist and health planner, has worked extensively researching for, designing the technical aspects of, and evaluating several of India's major health programmes. She is the author of a seminal book, *Implementing Health Policy*.

David Morley, M.D., was Professor of Tropical Child Health at the University of London for two decades. He set up the charitable organization TALC to distribute teaching-aids at low-cost. He is the author of several widely acclaimed books including *Pediatric Priorities in the Developing World*.

Towards Health for All

Reaching Health for All looks back at experiences in health care during the decade of the 1980s and forward toward the year 2000. It continues some of the stories that chronicled the enthusiastic quest for equitable health care in the early 1980s. Nine chapters in this series describe a further decade of progress in experiences reported in *Practising Health for All*.* They point to the continued evolution of both thought and action and innovation within these maturing programmes. Community involvement and people's active control of programmes are a recurring theme. The results are often dramatic, sometimes surprising, always interesting and informative.

In addition, many new programmes developed and began to demonstrate their effectiveness in contributing toward 'Health for All' in the 1980s. Nine of these, some community-level projects and other national efforts on a much larger scale, are described here.** As commitment to providing universal health care began to be taken seriously by countries throughout the world, attempts were made to create or readjust health systems to meet the goals and strategies suggested at Alma Ata. However, as many of these

---

*These are the chapters by Klouda on prevention; Johnston, Rohde and Suyono *et al.* on different aspects of primary health care in Indonesia; Borrinaga and Koh on the Philippines; Muller on Colombia, Peru and Guatemala; Chatterjee on India and Rifkin and Taylor on China.

**These are the chapters by Nickson on Zaire; Werner on Project Piaxtla in Mexico; Balachander on the Tamil Nadu Integrated Nutrition Project; Jonsson *et al.* on Iringa, Tanzania; Lovell and Abed on the Bangladesh Rural Advancement Committee; Garfield on Nicaragua; Mohs on Costa Rica; Sanders on Zimbabwe and Allman on Vietnam.

cases demonstrate, social concern for equity and efforts to fulfil the promise of 'Health for All' have been plagued by the financial woes of the decade.

The 1980s also saw the emergence of coordinated efforts to provide specific health care interventions globally. *Reaching Health for All* includes four chapters concerned with this truly 'universal' approach to health.* These transnational efforts arose from the enthusiasm for the Child Survival and Development Revolution. They contributed to increasing political involvement in health issues throughout the decade, which culminated in the largest ever gathering of world leaders at the Global Summit for Children in September 1990. The Summit's Declaration of Goals for the 1990s established a wide range of global targets in health, nutrition, education and environment. Far more specific than the original call for 'Health for All by the Year 2000', these Goals established an ambitious yet precise global agenda of activities which must be undertaken. Yet some observers find that global goals and programmes are incompatible with the principles of primary health care which are based in community action. Many of the studies in this book address the compromises and benefits inherent in these differing approaches—both of which may be necessary.

FROM COMMUNITY EFFORTS TO GLOBAL PROGRAMMES

The cases in this book are grouped into four sections: community efforts, larger-scale community-based programmes, national approaches to health, and international initiatives. The community projects stress approaches to health and development in which communities examine their problems, prioritize their needs, make their own decisions and formulate their programme actions. These efforts are decentralized and participatory. They depend entirely on community initiative and consensus-building, emphasizing process rather than outcomes.

The larger-scale community-based programmes focus—not coincidentally—on nutrition which is recognized by communities as underlying many of their health problems and involving a host of social issues. While the problem to be tackled is specifically identified as 'malnutrition', the solutions developed are multiple and complex but limited in scope. These programmes are larger and have higher coverage than the community projects in the first section, and their inputs are more substantive and outcome-

---

*These are the chapters on immunization by Hill *et al.*, on oral rehydration therapy by Northrup, on Vitamin A by Sommer and on birth spacing by Rowley and Mahler.

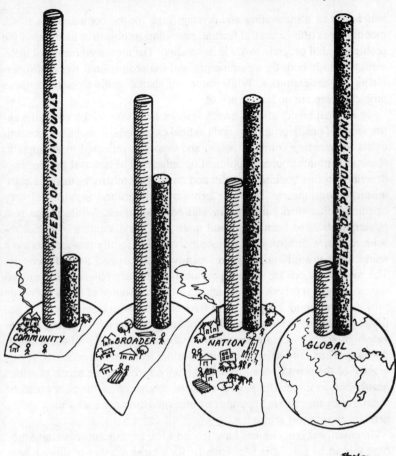

This book is organized in four sections, reflecting a progression from small community projects to global programmes. As health efforts grow in scale, their design is tailored less to differences between individuals and communities, and more to the common needs of large populations.

oriented. Nevertheless, activities happen in the community and are conducted by the community. They may, however, follow certain standards and norms developed outside the community. Analogous to the smaller community projects, these programmes have recognized and attempted to address the inter-relationships between nutrition, health and the wider arena of development. Common to all these programmes is an information system which acts as a motivating and driving force for the community. Growth monitoring is often a central feature, providing an objective measure of the problem and of progress towards its solution. The measured results of interventions guide both the communities and the professional workers supervising the programmes. While there are shared goals throughout these projects, there are no targets *per se*.

In national health efforts, health systems must take into account the entire range of health promotion and medical care needs. A socialistic concern exists for meeting common needs, and equity is reflected in attempts to reach all within a country's political boundaries. The national programmes described in this book are broader and more comprehensive than the community programmes. They are professionalized and service-delivery oriented rather than participatory and demand-driven. While in the past governments have been concerned more with the allocation of public resources than with harnessing private individual or family finance, there is a rising trend towards utilizing community resources and to cost-recovery. The role of the private sector in national health care has been recognized increasingly as it is both popular and an important source of finance. Private providers are being coopted more frequently to participate in priority national programmes. However, all too often, public monies continue to provide high-visibility curative medical services for politically-articulate urban dwellers. Thus, it remains to be seen whether and how the increased involvement of the private sector promotes equity. If the private sector provides health care to those with paying capacity, the health of the poor could be improved by the release of public resources and their use to establish 'safety nets' for those most in need.

International programmes have tended to be technocentric because they have had to be carried out 'efficiently' for a large number of diverse peoples. They have tended to over-ride social, political and economic considerations because their interventions have been uniformly applied across boundaries of culture, political systems and levels of development. The health problems they have addressed are common to all. But, one might ask, why these problems—e.g. the immunizable diseases, diarrhoeas—alone? Why not others such as tuberculosis or leprosy? These may take too long or have no easy technological solutions. Why then a problem such as guinea-worm which is so narrow in focus and afflicts so few? Because it is eradicable. Why not malaria or kala azar? These affect only some populations and do not have definitive end-points. Why not worms? The overall impact of deworming on health is far from evident or proven. Thus, the choices of interventions for global programmes have been made on the basis of the universality of the problem being addressed and of the availability of affordable, effective solutions.

In the long run these standardized technological approaches can support the development of primary health care by organizing and strengthening the capacity of health systems to do far more than carry out the specific, isolated interventions. Appropriate application of existing technology helps to improve the administrative, managerial and organizational capacity of the systems, making them better able to adopt other technologies and apply them on a wide scale. While the setting of targets or goals can reduce attention to 'process', which is certainly important to the achievement of universal primary health care, and can obfuscate actual achievement because of the pressure placed on health systems to meet pre-set levels and deadlines, such goals can also spur on action within otherwise unmotivated or disorganized contexts. They can create a sense of purpose and confidence within the systems that 'Health for All' is, indeed, achievable.

UNDERSTANDING 'HEALTH FOR ALL'

What understanding of 'Health for All' has emerged during the decade of the 1980s? How does it differ from Alma Ata? How likely are we to reach it? What are the methods and approaches? What are the trade-offs that will be necessary? This book raises questions about the real meaning of 'Health for All' based on actual experiences of the past decade. While primary health care and other basic services for everyone are essential elements, is it enough to provide this set of services and reach a given array of targets or goals? *Reaching Health for All* entails an examination of issues at the community level regarding the control of resources and decision-making processes. There is great diversity in the resulting activities—even a lack of focus. But the inspired leadership that is required to nurture and guide the development process can have profound impact.

At the level of nations, governments have recognized their responsibility for entire populations. Programmes have had to operate on a scale commensurate with this need, resulting in standardized approaches and diminished local control. The important issue of equity is often compromised by national and local politics, and by the fierce competition for resources between the health sector and other areas of government activity. As resources have become even more limited during the economic crises of the decade and structural adjustment policies have been forced on needy countries, health and equity have often lost out.

The epidemiological similarities among poor countries have provided opportunities at a global level which have been largely addressed with technological solutions. The framing of global goals and targets has led to a further move away from community control, but yet has politicized health care in other positive ways. While technology and target-setting have served to advance specific activities, reaching new levels in the provision of some essential health services, the issue of whether they facilitate or stultify the achievement of overall health goals remains to be resolved.

A BALANCE BETWEEN NATIONAL AND COMMUNITY ACTION

A basic-question which emerges from several of the case studies concerns the appropriate balance between equity and efficiency. While community involvement and control over decisions and local resources are of the utmost importance, do they ensure equitable and efficient actions for health? National responsibility for universal health care of a minimum standard is too often in conflict with strong political forces, financial realities and the ever-present demand for high-technology medical care. At the global level, the effectiveness of concerted world-wide action has been amply demonstrated in the successful quest for universal immunization by 1990. Yet international pressure has also claimed its toll by over-riding local decision-making and priority-setting processes, reducing the responsibility of nations, communities and families, and creating dependency.

A careful reading of the experiences described here and discussion of the issues will contribute to appropriate choices for and a better understanding of the trade-offs involved in reaching the ambitious goal of 'Health for All'. This book is best used as a source-book of case material, for comparisons of ideas and approaches. It is recommended for use as a starting-point for discussions among persons concerned with development and health. It raises many questions, providing direction—not answers—through the specific experiences of some. If it generates debate, productive thinking and action towards alternative approaches to reaching Health for All, its objectives would have been served.

I

Community Health and Development

COMMUNITY INVOLVEMENT IN CHANGE

Community involvement in health is one of the precepts of 'Health for All'. And yet, throughout the decade of the 1980s, experience of community-generated, community-led and community-implemented health care has been limited. Even when examples have been found, it has been difficult to document and understand the essential ingredients of these experiences which have wider applicability and use in accelerating community participation in health care. The six chapters in this section describe the roles which various communities have played in their own health development, and the innovative approaches which have been evolved for dealing with problems of ill-health and underdevelopment at the community level. They demonstrate the power of community initiatives in implementing activities to reach a maximum number of people, particularly those most in need. They raise a large number of questions, among them:

— To what extent can a community identify its precise health needs? To what extent can it implement the solutions which are necessary?
— How do community initiative, consensus-building and ownership fit in with 'getting the job done'? What is the role of the outsider—catalyst, adviser, leader, doer?
— How does community leadership develop? How can it be developed and used? Can community health workers be trained for a catalytic/leadership role in the community? How?
— Is community-controlled health development (including community

health workers) a threat to existing health systems, existing political systems?

— Can 'Health for All' be achieved without true community development—development across all sectors? Is overall development necessary before health, or can health be an entry-point, a basis for initiating self-help and development?

FROM PREVENTION TO POLITICAL DEVELOPMENT

In the chapter entitled 'Prevention is *Still* More Costly than Cure' Anthony Klouda opens these issues by asking again, as he did in *Practising Health for All*, whether a community focus can really work. Does a health system actually address the basic issues of health? Or are health problems inherently mired in factors requiring social revolution and political upheaval for their solution, and thereby beyond the scope of health systems? The role of the health worker in going beyond technological solutions to exploring community dynamics is highlighted, and the potential of community action to bring about real change is illustrated.

In Mary Johnston's contribution on Indonesia we learn about an approach, *mawas diri* or 'community self-introspection', which involves the community in identifying its needs, deciding for itself what will be done about them, and measuring its own progress. A follow-up of the description in *Practising Health for All* of Banjanegara in Indonesia, the evolution of this approach demonstrates the power of community action and the wide range of interventions that a community can decide on and do for itself.

As far away as Boga, Zaire, a similar approach to community health and development was implemented through village health committees, as Patricia Nickson describes. The tremendous level of individual effort involved in mobilizing these communities and the wide array of actions they chose to implement are testimony to the dedicated leadership required for true community participation. The activities are diverse and often not directly related to the predominant health needs of the people. Nonetheless, the effort is deemed worthwhile as the results are truly responsive, independent and sustainable.

Describing the experience of the Institute for Health Sciences (IHS) in Tacloban, Philippines, Rolando Borrinaga and Isabel Tantuico-Koh address the important issue of what type of health worker is needed to assist in true community health and development. What training is necessary to prepare the 'health team' to undertake community development activities? The IHS has evolved an entirely new approach to training health workers. All workers in the team understand and appreciate the skills and contributions of others because they have passed through the same training themselves. Throughout training, experience in their own communities is the major source of learning and the site for application of new knowledge and skills. The resulting health manpower is uniquely suited to directing and facilitating a community-based approach to primary health care. But can these workers function effectively within the broader health care system? Or are they suppressed and moulded by the existing paradigms and expectations of health care as it has always been practised?

David Werner describes how a focus on a visible problem can mobilize an entire community to support primary health care. At Project Piaxtla in Mexico, the comprehensive action that resulted from community collaboration with disabled people demonstrates both the capacity of handicapped people and the empowerment which their involvement can bring to an entire community. The role played by disabled persons as prime implementors —not recipients—of a village primary health care movement, demonstrates the self-help concept dramatically. Here is the means by which primary health care can elevate an entire community to meet its own developmental and humanitarian needs.

The experiences of six other Latin American communities in Peru, Colombia and Guatemala which show how community action can initiate progress in health care are related by Frits Muller. He strikes a sobering note with the recognition that politics, finance and even well-meaning outside forces emphasizing primary health care activities such as EPI, can stifle or even kill initiative and result in a decline of community involvement. External factors, especially political and economic, can overwhelm the best intentions of communities and diminish their innovative efforts in primary health care.

These six chapters together reveal the wide range of approaches that communities can take to improving their health situations in recognition of the complexity of factors underlying poor health. They illustrate activities and the roles of community members, workers and outsiders. They describe varying dynamics between people, ideas, technology and resources which bring about change. They examine how forces within communities can develop and sustain health action and equally how external forces can facilitate or disrupt community initiatives. Thus, they have lessons for the design, processes, sustainability, replicability and expansion of primary health care.

CHAPTER 1

Prevention is *Still* More Costly than Cure

ANTHONY KLOUDA

The author contends that addressing the underlying causes of ill-health in the developing world, though desirable, is beyond the means of most poor countries and that a realistic approach to both preventive and curative health care is essential.

Anthony Klouda, M.D., lived in Tanzania from 1978 to 1982 and later in Malawi. Since 1987 he has been Coordinator of the AIDS Prevention Unit of the International Planned Parenthood Federation with responsibility for integrating AIDS and family planning activities in 132 member associations throughout the world.

INTRODUCTION

The central thesis of 'Prevention is more costly than cure: health problems for Tanzania, 1971–81', the original chapter in *Practising Health for All*,[1] was that health is maintained through a complex series of social and service interactions. With particular reference to Tanzania, it was shown that development strategies of the time were not using such interactions to prevent the ill-health of the poorest people and that to do so would be very costly indeed. The implication was that the cost of prevention would be too expensive for most governments in the world—if not all. Indeed, most governments evidently preferred to invest in the solid manifestations of health care—clinics and curative services—as these were acceptable signs that they were doing something for health.

The intention of that chapter was to underline the simplistic nature of most approaches to the prevention of ill-health, especially in the perception of those who provide health services. The point is not merely a financial one: it is also a political one. This update does not change that thesis or that intention. Instead, it reinforces the theme in broader and more worrying ways. At the same time it looks at what has been done in the name of Primary Health Care and suggests ways of improving it so that aims are more realistic and services more relevant to a broader range of people.

The experience of Primary Health Care development since the original chapter was written has shown that most governmental and non-governmental agencies have continued to build service-based delivery systems (or to attempt naive political change), rather than try to tackle the complex political, social and environmental issues that determine health. There are several possible reasons for this. It may result partly from a lack of allocation of time to working through issues with people in a fully participatory way; or partly from a lack of relevant training of service personnel or from a lack of appropriate intersectoral management. Whatever the reasons, and even if the situations result from the lack of money for their support, there is a clear lack of political interest at local, national and international levels in looking at health in a broader way.

The lack of interest can be illustrated best by three examples:

— the use of 'risk analysis' in PHC without appropriate measures to reduce that risk;

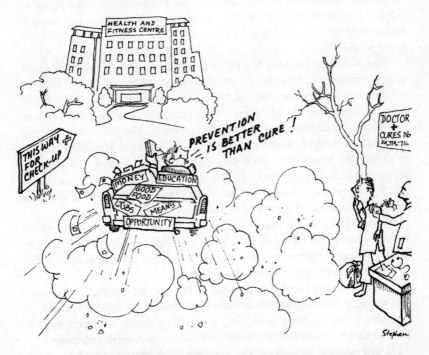

Prevention of ill-health requires elimination of underlying social and economic inequalities.

— the experience of the Primary Health Care programme in Malawi which shows the lack of interest amongst the government and donors;
— the development of the debate on 'comprehensive' versus 'selective' PHC, both of which avoid fundamental issues facing any service-based delivery system.

'RISK' APPROACHES

Risk approaches to health care have been with us for a long time—notably since a more thorough epidemiological approach to public health was established in the mid-nineteenth century. In these approaches, analysis of a population is used to show that those people who have a particular characteristic or 'risk factor', also have a particular pattern of ill-health. Interventions are then designed either to change the risk factor so that ill-health no longer results, or to focus particular attention on those with the factor in order to better care for the associated ill-health. This is alright when risk factors can simply be removed, such as when you identify a water pump as being linked to cholera and can then stop its use. However, when the risk factors themselves result from complex societal influences, their usefulness is not so clear.

Thus it is very tempting to look at mortality and morbidity distribution in any community and draw the conclusion that all efforts should be concentrated on serving the needs of those suffering the most mortality. Problems arise when the identification of such groups does not take into account the broader social realities underlying the mortality. The illustration on page 13 shows the pattern of under-five mortality in a typical Malawian village. It shows 100 households, each with only one child-bearing woman, observed over a four-year period. Deaths among children under-five occurred in 29 of these (less than one-third of the total). However, nine of these households accounted for over half the deaths.

These figures are not unusual. They are almost identical to those found by Meegama in Sri Lanka in 1978 when looking at patterns of infant mortality.[2] Whenever mortality rates are high it is likely that a few households will suffer a large proportion of deaths.

There are many interesting parallels to this skewed distribution. Income and resource distributions follow similar patterns; so do the distributions of pregnancy-spacing. Most interesting of all (though equally unsurprising) is the fact that the same families suffer in all of the skewed distributions.

If one wanted to analyse the possible 'risk factors' faced by these families, there are a huge number available, depending on the level and the

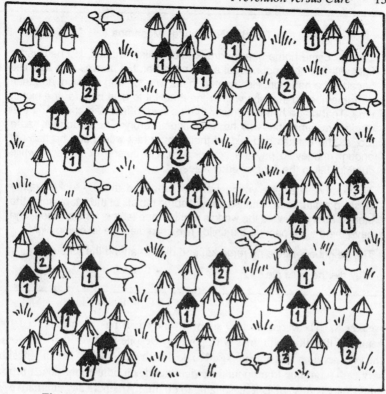

There is one house with 4 deaths, two houses with 3 deaths, six houses with 2 deaths, twenty houses with 1 death each and seventy-one houses with no deaths.

situation. There are individual, family, group, community, societal, economic, legal, political, biomedical, physical, chance and climatic forces involved, amongst many others. In Primary Health Care training there have been a number of orientation games that highlight this multiplicity of causes, giving to health workers and the communities they serve the choice of which risk factors to target.

The story of Charles Masamba (see box on p. 14) points to the obvious set of factors that lie behind the mortality distribution seen in the above figure. The set comprises poverty, lack of resources or lack of support (social, political, economic or individual). Robert Chambers has described people in such situations as suffering from a cluster of interrelated disadvantages: powerlessness, isolation, poverty, vulnerability and physical

Ths Story of Charles Masamba

Charles came home heavily drunk and feeling irritated. He had had a fight with his neighbour about a girl in the bar, but he was also satisfied because he had won. He shouted to his wife to bring his food, and then he remembered that she was in the hospital to give birth for the eighth time. That made him remember that he had to feed the child. And that made him remember why he had become drunk—he no longer had a job, as the estates had laid off their labour last week, and he had not enough money to pay the school fees. He cursed briefly and, while cursing, fell to the floor, already asleep.

Three days later, the youngest child, who had already looked rather sickly, got diarrhoea. Charles bought some tablets at the shop, which the storekeeper said were the world's number one tablets for diarrhoea, and gave them all at once to the child. The child died the following night.

The neighbour made no remarks, and did not attend the funeral.

Why did the child die?

weakness.[3] These risk factors are well known. It has been remarked for centuries that ill-health goes with poverty. Despite this wealth of wisdom, the very services that are supposed to deal with the issues of health—health services—continue to propound service-based solutions to the social problems. Why is this so? Is it reasonable to do this? Are there any alternatives?

When faced with the social realities that determine health, many health workers react with frustration and often with naive political viewpoints that can lead to their own destruction. Others ignore the issues quite happily. But if they ignore the issues and continue to look at risk factors to define those with highest risk, how do they hope to remove the factors?

THE EXPERIENCE OF MALAWI

In Malawi between 1982 and 1986, a serious attempt was made to develop an approach to Primary Health Care that recognized the fact that although under-five and maternal mortality were amongst the highest in the world, only a minority of the population suffered the bulk of this mortality, and that this was because of their cluster of disadvantages. The attempt was an interesting one, not only because of the issues that were addressed, but also because the initiative was driven by a small team of four people, three from the government and one from a mission hospital, based in the Malawi Ministry of Health. The team, known as the PHC Core Group, was set up after the government reviewed its pilot scheme in Primary Health Care with assistance from UNICEF.

The pilot PHC programme had been developed around the use of PHC workers (PHWs) who were trained by district workers, issued with a basic kit of medicines, and left to work in villages. The review revealed that this approach (as was the case in many other countries with similar approaches) had been totally unsuccessful in altering patterns of ill-health or in promoting healthier behaviour. As has been the experience in so many places, the faults in the system were many: domination by the health services, simplistic approaches to health problems, reliance on messages and drugs, lack of technical support of the PHWs, lack of clear objectives, lack of involvement of people, dependence of the PHWs on a system of payment, heavy top-down planning, the inability of local managers to reveal flaws to their superiors, the irrelevance of the training curriculum to local conditions, and the lack of resources in backing the system. All these factors will be readily recognized by those experienced in such work.

Since the Core Group recognized that most of the ill-health was suffered by those who were disadvantaged, the first problem to overcome was to talk about disadvantage in ways that did not imply that national politics or developmental strategies were in any way causing the disadvantages. To do so would have caused the immediate cancellation of the programme and would have put the careers of several people at risk. In addition it was clear that a basic problem with the pilot scheme was that it required a radically different approach to management in order to be both participatory and intersectoral.

The opportunity was therefore seized to tackle the real problems by dismantling the old PHC system entirely and building up a new one. The crucial arguments were:

— there was no way of sustaining the existing system and improving the relevance of the PHWs for the health of people;
— there were no resources to allow such a system to be utilized for the whole country;
— there were already a large number of workers potentially available for the support of communities.

It is interesting to reflect on this last point. When district managers from the various social support areas (health, agriculture, water, social services, education) were asked about the personnel available to them, it was found that there were, on an average, 17 workers for every 10 000 population.

However, it was obvious that their work was not having any impact on health as the health of local people was essentially unchanging in its pattern. If the PHC jargon of the time were to be believed, then health was dependent on the integrated involvement of all these sectors with the communities they were supposed to serve. The chapter about Tanzania in *Practising Health for All* highlighted this very issue.[1]

FOCUSING ON THE DISADVANTAGED

This situation led the Core Group to consider the solution of talking about the disadvantaged. The trick was not to begin with this but to find a way, using a simple set of questions asked of the district programme managers. These questions were:

— 'Which people are currently benefiting from your development efforts?'
— 'Which people are not benefiting from your development efforts?'

Each manager highlighted the poor, the disabled, the isolated, the people with few resources and the people with little land as not benefiting from their development efforts. It was then agreed that these were the same people who were in ill-health. The final question set the management tone of the new approach, avoiding implications about the political system:

— 'Given that your efforts for the majority of people have been so good, how will you now make your services relevant to the remainder who are currently not benefiting from your services?'

Perhaps a little more should be said about this key issue. It is to be appreciated that the services and advice offered by most health, water, agricultural and educational services are of benefit. They are of benefit to those who are comfortable with the methods of communication adopted by the service providers, who have the resources to utilize the services and to follow the advice proffered, and who are treated as equals by the service providers. It is equally to be appreciated that this group of people are just as likely to survive in reasonable health without the provision of the services.

There remains the large but minority group, identified by the Malawi managers, for whom the services are not relevant. This group is caught in the vicious cycle that develops between lack of access and lack of relevance. Lack of access does not refer only to *geographical* access: it refers to the lack of *real* access experienced by those who feel that the services provided are somehow not for them. Such people may have suffered humiliation or rejection by service providers who believe they are in some way better than the people they are serving. Or the service providers may not have found the means to communicate with these people as a result of lack of time or interest. These excluded people are found on the very doorsteps of clinics or the homes of PHC workers. Only a few programmes have tried to ensure that they are relevant in the cultural sense to the entire population in their immediate area. Most services tend to fall into the pattern either of setting-up shop and being happy with serving those who come, or of targeting particular groups in a community. When the objectives of such projects have been met, there is a tendency to extend the projects further afield.

By concentrating on relevance, access and coverage, the Malawi approach to PHC was centered on basic management principles and couched in language that, at first glance, was not political in nature. It led naturally to the idea of multisectoral teams working together at local, district and regional levels—not for health but for a focus on ensuring their services were of benefit to all in a community rather than just for some.

An important note here is that during the development of this approach

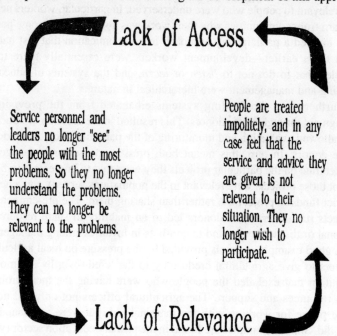

Lack of Access

Service personnel and leaders no longer "see" the people with the most problems. So they no longer understand the problems. They can no longer be relevant to the problems.

People are treated impolitely, and in any case feel that the service and advice they are given is not relevant to their situation. They no longer wish to participate.

Lack of Relevance

The vicious cycle by which services become progressively less responsive to the very people they are meant to serve.

an attempt had been made to concentrate the provision of services only on those families found to have children failing to grow. On the whole, this failed because the families did not like being singled out, the service personnel did not really know how to work with them in isolation, and the rest of the community disliked the shift of attention away from themselves. As a result, the programme was refocused on the provision of services to all groups, with orientation of the community and service providers to the fact that there were inadequacies in community and service structures for support to some families, those most 'at risk'. The strategy was not, however, to single them *out* but rather to ensure that they were included with the rest.

A further benefit from the use of teams of existing workers was that no new workers needed to be employed and existing resources could be used in new ways.

Although a difficult step to attain, forming teams was relatively easy compared with the task of making the new system work. A major difficulty that had been glossed over in the first stage of developing a new system was that some very sensitive issues had to be tackled in order to make the system relevant to people who were underserved. In particular, workers needed to learn from communities why their work was not relevant to some people. This implied a participatory approach to communication that just had not been there earlier—development workers were essentially there to *tell* people what to do, not to *listen* or *learn*, and the systems of education, training and management were hierarchical in nature.

Furthermore, the funding systems emanated from the provision of foreign aid through major donors. This resulted in the creation of structures that allowed evaluation and monitoring of the particular projects funded by these donors. In turn, this meant both pressure on sectoral managers to concentrate on the particular projects they were told to implement (whether or not those projects were relevant to the populations served), and a need to restrict funds to project use rather than sharing them. The pre-eminence of projects run under major donors led to an inability to share resources at national or district levels, and to conflicts in loyalties among managers.

A good example of this is provided by the pressure on local agricultural officers to give agricultural credit only to the 'credit-worthy'. Almost by definition that excluded the people who were having the most problems with resources and support. The agricultural officers not only did not receive praise for working with the marginalized, but were reprimanded if they did. Similar examples are found in the primary education sector (where donors enforced strict curricula for 'relevant' nutrition education) and even in other programmes run by the Ministry of Health.

Nevertheless, intersectoral teams were trained, and they were trained using a participatory approach that allowed them to develop their own methods of learning with communities. They were encouraged to establish an objective along with a community and seek to meet it with the community. In the light of experience they could modify objectives and strategies until a solution was found to the problem being addressed.

It took two or three years of intensive support and visiting from the national support team (the PHC Core Group) to see real change among the district teams. In two districts that achieved the most significant changes there was a stable district team, good leadership and more frequent support from the national team. The remaining districts suffered from very rapid turnover of staff, poor leadership and infrequent support from the national team.

MEASURING SUCCESS

Was this successful? It is usual to evaluate projects by determining the extent to which objectives are achieved. The Core Group was aiming at a fundamental shift in patterns of interaction between service providers and the communities they served. They believed that this itself would lead to improved health either through improved service-provision from all sectors or through pressure for political change that was generated locally. The Core Group had to generate enough enthusiasm to get teams to work together in integrated and harmonious ways within the context of a rigid, hierarchical system. The question was: Where to hit first?

The Group decided early in its existence to get things working at the district and local area levels first in the hope that the practical demonstration of success would have an impact on those making decisions in the various ministries at national level. It was thought that a lot of time would be wasted if the group was to try to influence uninterested ministries without that practical experience.

There is no doubt that the Core Group eventually failed in their ambition of persuading the national structures to pursue the establishment of the new approach to PHC. The Group never successfully included a member from a Ministry other than Health (except fleetingly from the Ministries of Agriculture and Social Development); and the Ministry of Health never showed any inclination to relinquish its 'hold' on the National Intersectoral PHC Committee to which the Core Group reported. Furthermore, although the Core Group demonstrated the success of participatory training techniques for local service personnel from all sectors, none of the sectors (including the Ministry of Health) adopted this methodology for any training outside the PHC programme.

None of the teams within the three or four years of life of the Core Group achieved any statistically significant changes in patterns of health in urban or rural communities. To achieve such change probably would have required a further four years of work. None the less, there was definite success at the intermediate level, showing that intersectoral teams could work together, that they could learn from the communities they served, and that they could set their own objectives in the light of what they had learned.

Two simple examples demonstrate the change that was achieved at least in management terms:

— In one district, the district managers actually *walked* together to villages around their headquarters for regular monthly meetings. Anyone acquainted with the syndrome of district managers not prepared to do anything without a four-wheel-drive vehicle would be aware of the significance of this event.

— In another district the head of the multi-sectoral PHC team wrote a letter to the Ministry of Health saying that they wanted less interference from the Ministry as they understood their local problems better than people from the capital. Interestingly, another district team had worked with villagers who expressed the same independence from the district. Those aware of the rigid hierarchy in Malawi will pause to take breath!

There were also more subjective measurements. The local and district teams were often 'friendlier' with the communities they served—members of the communities and the teams were often heard to comment on this aspect of their working more closely together. This was seen particularly in two districts. Where teams were friendlier, the coverage of services increased as people began to feel they might be receiving a more *relevant* service. In addition the staff began to feel better about the services they were providing—they would say that they felt more respected, were working in ways that had more interest than the mere repetition of mindless tasks, and that they felt they were being listened to by their bosses.

As this had to remain essentially a service-based model, it was recognized that more radical social change would not be attainable, and that success would always be useful but limited. What had been achieved, though, was a break in the vicious cycle between lack of access and lack of relevance.

Despite (or perhaps because of) the limited success, the approach was dismantled after four years. This was partly a result of the dispersal of the core team that had been responsible for the development and follow-through of the concept (the individual members had to return to their posts in the ministries). It was also partly the result of pressure from outside forces. In particular, some donors grew very impatient with the slow progress and wanted more rapid expansion (although the donor that had provided funding for the core programme remained supportive, it was unable to provide a level of funding to match that of the major donors). In addition the formation of intersectoral teams involved joint funding and this was unattainable, given the vertical nature of most donor funding. The loss of the core team proved most critical—there was no one left (apart from a coordinator who was sent for a two-year training course in the UK) to keep up the drive, vision and support that were necessary to ensure that the regional and district teams questioned what they were doing or achieving.

All these reasons only reflect the fundamental lack of interest on the part of the government. Although the new approach was essentially low cost in

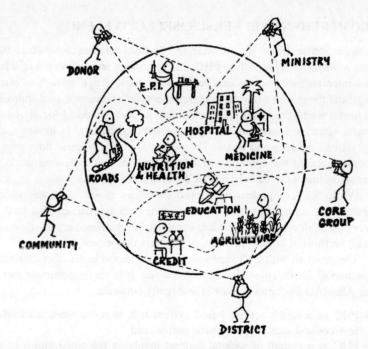

Each participant group views a comprehensive project from a different perspective, making success hard to define.

that it concentrated on using existing resources in new ways, the changes required of the system may have been too great in terms of shifts in management and funding practice and in terms of political goals. Malawi (and other countries) may well see it as a priority to concentrate development efforts on those who are already able to 'contribute' economically and politically, and those whose demands for education and service-provision are paramount. The services are indeed relevant to the bulk of those who are not marginalized. Many who are in power or who are already comfortable have no fundamental interest in the poor and disaffected. Efforts such as this in Malawi and among some non-governmental organizations may just be tolerated and forever kept to the sidelines.

The main lesson from Malawi was that, perhaps contrary to expectations, change in government systems for the benefit of those who are marginalized is possible, but may not be sustainable. 'Sustainability' has nothing to do with finance, as was shown in Malawi; rather, it has to do with political commitment.

'COMPREHENSIVE' VERSUS 'SELECTIVE' PHC

A rather sterile debate has grown in recent years between those who advocate a 'selective' approach to PHC—the provision and promotion of a few key interventions (such as oral rehydration, basic drugs, growth monitoring), and those who advocate a 'comprehensive' and coordinated approach to health which harnesses all development sectors, including locally-based health services, water, education, appropriate agricultural technology, cooperative financing and so on. The debate is sterile because both groups seem to accept the centrality of health services in the determination of health, in line with the WHO/UNICEF statement at Alma Ata.

While the 'comprehensive' approach comes closer to understanding health as a complex societal phenomenon, both approaches also tend to accept that 'development' services currently being offered are of relevance to all sections of any community, particularly the poorest.

The problem with both views may be understood better after closer inspection of the statements made at Alma Ata. It is very unfortunate that in the Alma Ata Declaration there is ambiguity between:

— PHC as a health service-based system that is coordinated with other services and uses people's participation, and
— PHC as a system of societal support involving the equal inputs of all development services, organizations and people.

Although there is considerable rhetoric emanating from policy-makers and service providers on the importance of the political and social environments which hint at an understanding of the second interpretation of PHC, most seem to view the first as the model for PHC. This view is reinforced by the fact that there are very few people *outside* the health services who promote Primary Health Care, although many are willing to pay lip service to 'cooperation with' a PHC programme. Supporters of both the 'comprehensive' and 'selective' approaches espouse this service-based model regardless of the level of participation of the communities being served.

The main trouble with this model as we have seen is that it is limited and does not tackle the root causes of ill-health. Despite this problem it may be the only option realistically available in most current political climates. However, if this option is chosen it would be useful if those promoting it talk clearly of its limited use. Thus, an imaginary briefing of trainers of health-service providers (or community health workers) might run as follows:

We are going to brief you fully on the political and environmental determinants of poor health. In this briefing it will be apparent that the prime cause of poor health for a large number of people is political and economic inequality. However, to attempt to change this may expose you or members of the community you serve to danger or even to death. You may be able to achieve a better understanding of the forces involved as you work, and it may be that as members of the community you may want to participate in action for social change. This is a decision you can take only after you have been able to ascertain that you are not imposing your own political views on a community you do not yet understand, and when you become an equal in that community with the same risks and consequences. While working with the community you have to ensure that you are not merely raising to people's attention problems of which they are already fully aware and for which they have achieved their own balances.

While you are working to understand this situation there is much you can do to ensure that your work is of immediate relevance. Look at the patterns of illness, disease and health in the community and discuss with people how your practical skills may be modified to be of relevance wherever possible. It may be that you will never overcome the fundamental problems, and it may be that you never achieve relevance for all people in a community, but keeping all this in your mind is an important first step.

There remains a further grave problem with a 'service-based' model for PHC. While it is certainly possible to improve the way in which services support the communities they serve, most of those advocating 'comprehensive' or 'selective' PHC do so without questioning the current orientation or practice of the service providers. In fact, as has been suggested

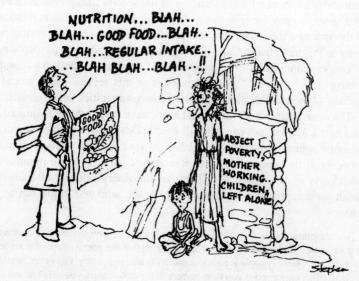

Health education often takes no recognition of the real causes of malnutrition or ill-health.

above, most service providers are still not geared to service all sections of their communities; rather, they are geared to 'service' the managers and donors of the systems of which they are part.

Let us look at a few practical examples taken from real field experiences between 1987 and 1990 of projects which variously ally themselves either to the 'comprehensive' or 'selective' model.

— At an MCH clinic in rural Africa, a group of mothers has been selected for special lectures on nutrition as their children are not putting on weight and are well below the desired weight-for-age. A glance at the growth cards shows that most of the children have been failing to grow for several months or, in some cases, years. On being questioned, the mothers say they have been attending the clinic regularly for two years (the growth cards bear testimony to this). They answer questions concerning the preparation of locally-obtainable foods perfectly. They know how to feed their children. The staff are asked whether the children continued to grow well after the nutrition intervention. They say that very few or none continued to grow well. Yet they continue to provide these talks and demonstrations knowing full well that they are not answering the problems faced by the mothers.

— In another clinic, weighing of children is done weekly. It is pointed out that children can only put on about 80 g a week at best, and that the Salter scales measure only in 100 g increments.

— At another clinic, staff give regular talks about oral rehydration using salt and sugar. They have been doing this for some years. Yet children still come to the clinic severely dehydrated. The staff do not even reflect on this or ask what might be wrong.

— In a programme with PHC workers in a village, none of the workers had a clear idea of their coverage of the community.

An article by Ashish Bose[4] on India's family planning programme says:

The states, in turn, feel that the Centre is being too dictatorial and trying to run the programme from New Delhi. At the district level, blame is put on the Primary Health Centre doctors and the ANMs (Auxiliary Nurse Midwives) at the sub-centres for neglecting their work. But if one talks to the doctors at the PHCs they tell you 'We are trained as doctors, and not as social workers. We cannot go with folded hands to the villagers in order to get family planning cases. What health work can we do? We are judged only by the number of sterilization cases.'

Then we move on to the sub-centres. The ANM will tell you, 'Has anybody cared to look into our problems? What about our physical security? We are constantly bullied and pressurized by all—*panchayat* (village government committee) members, youth leaders, doctors, bureaucrats . . . We have dozens of registers to fill up. We never get the registers on time and then we are accused of not doing our work. As if all this is not enough, we have to fulfil the family planning targets set for us by our bosses and if these are not fulfilled, we will be transferred to the worst places.

Finally, talk to the people themselves. They complain that there are not enough medicines at the PHCs; the doctors and nurses are not available; they are treated rudely; nobody cares once the sterilization operation is over; they do not know what to do if there are post-operative complications; the failure rate of the laparoscopic method is high . . . the *sarkar* (government) is not bothered about the plight of the people. Ask them what they want. Quick will come the answer, 'We want a hospital, good doctors, free medicines . . . Don't you get all these in the cities?'

All these examples are painfully familiar to those who do field work. What is so painful is that workers are forced to undertake mindless work as a result of the nature of the system and of their management. It is not the fault of the workers. They are not supported to develop meaningful or relevant programmes locally as to do so would subvert the system imposed by planners who remain essentially remote.

A common criticism is that workers trained 'at a certain level' are incapable of undertaking such exploratory work with communities and it requires training to the level of a PhD to even enter into such dialogue. In fact, the only training required is to help the workers become ordinary people again and to recognize the problems for what they are. While it takes considerable time to undo the training health workers have already received, there is no reason why community workers should not be prepared from the start to question and to probe, starting from their own knowledge and understanding of their community.

During supervision, I have often deliberately approached a health worker and asked him or her why people are not doing what the worker has told them to do in talks. Very often the reply runs along the lines, *'Oh, because they are too ignorant, or they don't listen.'* The worker thinks he/she has provided me with the answer I want. It is framed within their view of what a health service should do: tell the people what to do by delivering messages.

If instead I approach the same worker with a different question, such as *'Why do people have difficulty in doing what you ask them to do?'* the worker often gives an accurate answer, such as *'Oh, this family is too poor to afford sugar'* or *'That family has tried it and it didn't work'* or *'That mother has to work all day in the fields and cannot look after the children.'* The paradox is that the worker does not realize that he/she is answering the question in an entirely different way, and that the latter set of answers are the ones that should be guiding him or her to modify his/her approach to teaching.

Once workers are supported to recognize that their human perceptions are correct, they are often the best persons to modify their work to be of relevance to local problems. In fact it is often the highly-trained professionals who blunder and mess things up.

Making a distinction between 'comprehensive' and 'selective' PHC will do nothing to improve this situation. If a service is mindless, it is irrelevant.

CONCLUSIONS

Perhaps we cannot aim realistically for fundamental improvements in society to improve health. Opportunities for the type of legislation that changed so much in the UK at the turn of the century are unlikely to be found in poor countries because effective enforcement of legislation costs too much. This thesis lay at the heart of the original chapter, 'Prevention is more costly than cure', in *Practising Health for All.*[1]

Service-based systems are severely limited in their ability to achieve an integrated approach because of the 'vertical' demands made by donors and governments. But much can be improved if they are helped to adopt flexible responses to local situations in a friendly manner and in cooperation with other workers. New workers are generally not needed. This chapter has shown that given a sustained approach to supportive management and training, local workers can adopt flexible, responsive approaches. At the very least morale in health units can be boosted by good management. With a little more effort, coverage of a community by a service can increase. And if all this occurs, it may well turn out that some health benefits are seen!

There is no denying the patience and persistence required of any manager trying to organize such a system. Not only are there innumerable battles to fight, but the manager has to support workers through the inevitable frustrations and failures they experience when trying to respond to reality. The managers themselves require support. They also have to contend with objectives that may be shifting constantly as the perception of a problem changes. However, if managers and workers can be shown the rewards and excitement of this constant search with people for answers to problems—if we can help develop this model of active critical analysis—then we will find solutions to more of the problems for more of the people more often. A constant cycle of development can be achieved.

This chapter has not addressed the question of the real cost of prevention. In a way there is no answer: the cost can be as high as you please. The point is that we can (if we choose) do better with the resources at our disposal if we try to be a bit more realistic about our goals and objectives. The experiences described show what can be done with services already in existence. Each one of us can help donors, governments, trainers and service providers support such change.

References

1. Klouda, A. (1983). 'Prevention' is more costly than 'cure': health problems for Tanzania, 1971–81. In: *Practising Health for All*, (eds. D. Morley, J. Rohde and G. Williams), Oxford University Press, Oxford.
2. Meegama, S.A. (1980). Socio-economic determinants of infant and child mortality in Sri Lanka: An analysis of post-war experience. *WFS Scientific Report No. 8*, World Fertility Survey, London.
3. Chambers, R. (1983). *Rural development: Putting the last first*. Longman, London.
4. Bose, A. (1988). *From population to people, Vol. I*. B.R. Publishing Corporation, Delhi.

CHAPTER 2

Community Participation through Self-introspection

MARY JOHNSTON

The author describes innovative efforts in Indonesia to enhance community involvement through a self-survey technique. **Mawas diri** *is the basis for community action to improve the environment and health, and a tool for overall community development.*

Mary Johnston worked with a non-governmental agency, Yayasan Indonesia Sejahtera, in Central Java for 25 years, developing training programmes and community-based health care systems. She remained at work in the community until illness forced her to return to Australia, where she died in October 1991.

A STORY OF GANTI VILLAGE

For over three years the health worker from the local Community Health Centre had been informing the people of Ganti village in Central Lombok about the importance of healthy living. Ganti was a poor village with little water but the health worker believed that, if they wanted to, the people could live healthier lives. Each monthly visit she coaxed them to build toilets, to plant vegetables and fruit trees, to boil their water, cover their food, immunize their children. So many hints and yet it all seemed to no avail. Despite the installation of some water pumps, life with all its inadequacies went on much the same as it had always done. Maybe the pessimists were right. Being in a famine area Ganti had received rice assistance for many years. Community initiative appeared to be dead and people waited for things to happen to them.

But then there was the workshop—with amazing consequences. The health worker attended together with several Volunteer Health Workers (VHW), the village head, the chairperson of the Women's Movement, an active youth, the religious leader and the chairperson of Ganti's planning committee. They were confused when they heard that the workshop was about a planning and monitoring approach called *mawas diri* ('self-intro-spection'). However, for three days they listened, discussed, designed and practised *mawas diri*. Enthusiastically they made plans to collect data just one week later.

One month later on her routine visit to Ganti village the health worker was amazed to see the changes. Two VHWs told her of the plans to con-struct three public pit toilets in their part of the village. They showed her the bamboo and stones which had already been collected. Families had already dug rubbish pits in their backyards. In a more distant section of the village, families had begun the construction of a road and there were ambi-tious plans to move their scattered homes to face the road. At the same time they would add improvements, including windows and cement-sealed floors. Their yards would be fenced and planted with fruit trees.

When questioned why he had mended a hole in his roof, an old man replied: 'I felt embarrassed. No one has ever asked me before about my roof. I thought that if someone else takes an interest in my roof, surely I too should take an interest.' In another part of Ganti, families had begun to dig a drain—it would eventually stretch some 300 metres. The people's inge-nuity and enthusiasm staggered the health worker. To think that these 'apa-thetic' people had such ambitious plans and all on their own initiative, using their own resources!

Within six months the face of many parts of Ganti village had changed markedly. Home renovation activities were well under way, toilets were 'in fashion', yards fenced and planted with fruit trees which had been donated by a local non-governmental organization, and roads repaired. Family plan-ning and immunization figures had gone up and drains had been built in several water-logged areas. A *mawas diri* day, on which everyone worked on village improvement activities had been introduced. One group had set up a *mawas ekonomi* (economic innovation) programme—a rice bank from which members could take loans in times of trouble. The community had taken the initiative for village improvement into their own hands.

HOW *MAWAS DIRI* BEGAN

Eight years ago in 1984, *Yayasan Indonesia Sejahtera* (YIS), a non-govern-mental organization (NGO) which was involved in community health and development, was requested by the Indonesian Department of Health to design a monitoring tool which would enable greater community involve-ment in the process of solving health problems. A YIS task-force examined numerous existing monitoring tools and found that they were, almost without exception, geared to the needs of programme managers who came from outside the village communities. The concepts and language used were complicated; and sophisticated statistical analysis was required to draw conclusions from the data collected. Even if a village community understood the relevance of such tools to their situation and wished to use them, the method would most likely be beyond their grasp. There was the additional danger that the complexity of the tools would reinforce village people's feelings of inferiority and powerlessness and isolate them further from control over their own lives. Such tools enabled policy-makers to use the people's supposed 'lack of skills' to justify the continued imposition of 'top-down' programmes on the communities, even though they advocated 'lower level-upward' strategies and greater community participation.

Years of working with village communities had convinced the staff of YIS that people can become involved in all stages of a programme which affects their lives, provided they have the motivation, skills and appropriate tools.[1] To encourage and measure community participation, the YIS team was determined to design a tool which was:

— easily comprehensible;
— applicable to local conditions; and,
— most important of all, usable by the people.

Interested 'outsiders' would have to work out for themselves how they could obtain the required information. The result was an approach which was given the name *mawas diri*, self-correction through introspection.

THE APPROACH

The *mawas diri* approach is based on a problem-solving cycle which begins with the detection of a problem by the people themselves and goes through the steps of identifying solutions, taking action and evaluating effects on the problem.

To facilitate the process of detecting problems, the people develop a simple self-survey form which lists various aspects of life which are closely related to family and community health and welfare. These could include, for example, a healthy environment, a healthy way of life, family planning or socio-economic conditions. Each of these aspects is further sub divided. For example, a 'healthy environment' may cover the home and outside yard which could include:

Home: light, floor, ventilation, roof, cleanliness;
Yard: drainage, rubbish disposal, animal pens, plants, cleanliness.

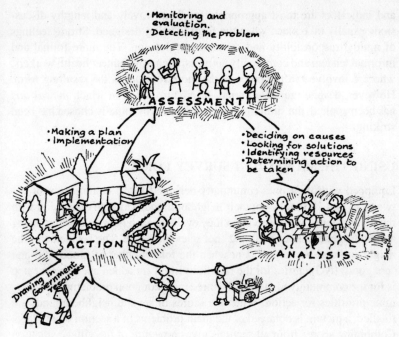

* Monitoring and
  evaluation.
* Detecting the problem

ASSESSMENT

* Making a plan
* Implementation

* Deciding on causes
* Looking for solutions
* Identifying resources
* Determining action to
  be taken

ACTION

Drawing in Government Resources

ANALYSIS

Mawas Diri—self-introspection is a problem-solving cycle run by the community.

Next, they identify indicators to determine acceptable standards for each component. For example:

Ventilation: a house has at least two windows which are opened every
                  day;

Rubbish
disposal: the yard has a rubbish hole;

Drainage: no stagnant water in the yard.

They choose indicators which are:

— related to local problems;
— as concrete as possible;
— measurable using 'good' and 'not good';
— challenging to correct or improve and yet feasible.

The unique feature of the *mawas diri* survey form is that it is designed by each individual community in cooperation with a health or community worker. It is the community that decides which aspects of life, components and indicators are most appropriate for them. Lively and lengthy discussions usually take place when the form is being designed. Strong feelings of mutual responsibility and commitment develop. The more formal and informal leaders and community activists, such as volunteer health workers, who are involved in the process, the more relevant is the resulting form. However, despite the wide variety of circumstances in which *mawas diri* has been applied, the similarity in the indicators eventually chosen has been striking.

USING THE *MAWAS DIRI* SURVEY FORM

Equipped with their own community-designed form, volunteers visit between 15 and 20 families in their neighbourhood. Through discussion with the home-keeper and observation they evaluate each item on the form using a simple 'good', 'not good' and 'not relevant' score. The problems in the neighbourhood become evident when the total number of 'good' (G) and 'not good' (NG) entries for the families visited are added up. The next step is for the community to discuss the three most common problems and determine priorities for action. When the scores of several neighbourhoods are totalled, a picture is obtained of the main problems in a section of a village. Combining scores from all sections gives a picture of the village situation overall. The three top priority problems are determined at the neighbourhood, section and village levels using data from as many families as possible. To decide which of the three problems to tackle first, the communities use two main considerations: the seriousness of the problem and their capacity to solve it using local resources. Discussions aimed at producing plans for specific actions are held with individual families, community groups and village leaders and planning bodies. Decisions resulting from these discussions are the basis for action.

Collective action to carry out the improvements identified in the survey is an important element of *mawas diri*. Working together, the village can gradually and visibly transform its situation according to the criteria and goals they have set for themselves. Starting initially with simple actions like providing drainage, planting flowers or a general village-wide clean-up, the community gathers confidence that they can change their situation. This leads gradually to more ambitious projects with more significant results for the community at large.

The final stage in the *mawas diri* approach is monitoring and evaluation. The *mawas diri* form is useful here too. Questionnaires are repeated every three or four months and compared with previous results. If the number of 'not good' responses has decreased it is apparent that some progress has been achieved. It is then time to move on to planning action to decrease other high 'NG' responses—the problem-solving cycle beginning all over again.

Development is a dynamic process and as circumstances change the community can adjust the items and indicators on the *mawas diri* form. New aspects can be added as a programme becomes more comprehensive including, for example, agriculture, animal husbandry or education. The indicators can be made more difficult to challenge people when conditions are improving. Aspirations can be raised, for example, from a 'dry floor' to a 'cement-covered floor', or from 'at least one useful plant in the yard' to 'growing at least three varieties of vegetables'. Communities using the form have been resourceful in adapting it to their changing needs and expanding their capacity for action.

THE BOYOLALI EXPERIMENT

Prior to developing *mawas diri*, YIS had been working for several years in four of the poorer districts of Boyolali Regency, Central Java, in cooperation with the Regency Department of Health Service. Boyolali is one of the poorest areas of Central Java. Low rainfall, infertile land and population pressure are the major causes of widespread poverty. The area is hilly; some villages are difficult to reach and virtually inaccessible in the rainy season. Nevertheless, there are natural resources such as fresh-water springs, under-utilized government resources, and a willingness to change among communities.

For these reasons it was decided to introduce the *mawas diri* approach in Mojosongo District of Boyolali in 1986. Starting with the district and village-level government officials and the people of Karangnongko village, a workshop was held. Their response to the new approach was enthusiastic. Between 1986 and 1989, 13 villages in Mojosongo and 15 in nearby Sambi adopted the approach. Some of the physical improvements which have been achieved are recorded in Table 1. These extensive improvements in village infrastructure are the outward manifestations of a transformed village mentality. A simple listing obscures the initiative, enthusiasm, creativity and contributions of time, labour and materials which characterized the activities of the village communities. A few materials which were not available locally, such as cement, were the only small infusions of resources required from outside. The people of Butuh village displayed exemplary courage and persistence in the construction of a one-and-a-half kilometre water pipeline

Table 1. Physical results of the *Mawas Diri* programme, Boyolali, 1986–89

Activity	Mojosongo district	Sambi district
Total beneficiaries	9495	9969
Toilets	3087	3849
Wells	88	1135
Glass roof tiles	1933	3360
Water disposal	763	—
Flooring/Chimneys	48	326
Fencing	209	—
Windows	10	102
Productive trees	3050	1197

through difficult terrain to bring clean water to their homes. There was also the growing willingness of government technical services to gear their programmes to meet needs detected through the village data collection. These important dimensions of human development cannot be portrayed in tables!

In 1991, YIS expanded the *mawas diri* approach to yet another district of Boyolali Regency. It continued to introduce *mawas diri* to other NGOs in the hope of extending its use to other provinces. News was received recently from an NGO in Padang, West Sumatra, of the positive reception of *mawas diri* by communities in that area.

MAWAS DIRI IN A WATER SUPPLY AND SANITATION PROJECT

In 1988 an invitation was received by YIS to introduce *mawas diri* in the Rural Water Supply and Sanitation Project (RWSS) implemented by the Department of Health and funded by the Australian International Development Assistance Bureau (AIDAB) in Central Lombok, Indonesia. The aim was to increase community participation in the utilization and maintenance of newly-installed clean water facilities. Over three years the project has worked in cooperation with community organizers, village facilitators and a local NGO, and has promoted community participation in the installation and renovation of water facilities significantly.

Central Lombok is a densely-populated, dry area which has suffered periodic famines in the past. The people's socio-economic conditions are depressed and emergency rice distributions have saved lives during these famines. Community initiative has been weak and little change has occurred in village life apart from programmes initiated by outside agencies. The situation is exacerbated by the distance between Lombok and Jakarta, the hub of national government.

The RWSS project and a local NGO cooperated with the local government to introduce *mawas diri* into four villages, each having a population between 5000 and 8000, in two districts. It was hoped that demonstrating a successful programme in strategically-situated villages would have maximum impact. After preparing the communities, two three-day workshops were held, each with 15 key people from two villages attending. After mastering the idea, the participants designed the tool and discussed steps for implementation. They each then tried out their form with five families who lived close to the training hall. This was the turning point. Enthusiasm increased as they added up the scores and told others of their experiences. Based on this feedback, some minor adjustments were made to the form. Next, simulated meetings were held to demonstrate how results could be fed back and discussed in hamlet and village meetings. Following a discussion on whom they would need to involve in the implementation of *mawas diri*, each of the teams from the two villages drew up plans for data collection in the hamlets (of 50 to 100 families) which they represented. They planned to begin immediately after rice-planting was completed.

A year later impressive changes had occurred in three of the four villages. Ganti village, described at the beginning of this article, was typical of the progress which was achieved. In the fourth village, however, action after data collection was negligible. Leadership schisms and the poor organizational skills of the VHW were the major causes for the lack of response. In the final analysis, development will always depend upon people and the quality of their social interactions. However, results in the three successful villages were sufficient to justify the expansion of the *mawas diri* approach to more villages.

In cooperation with the Regional Planning Board, YIS subsequently held a *mawas diri* Training for Trainers. The aim was to prepare teams to facilitate district and village workshops. Four three-person district teams participated, together with a six-person regional team selected from appropriate government departments, including Health, Community Development and the Planning Board, and four NGO workers. The facilitators designed this workshop on the village model. They aimed to introduce *mawas diri* by familiarizing the participants with the village workshop which they would be running eventually. Discussions were held also on the role of the regency and district teams in providing technical and moral support to the implementation of *mawas diri*-stimulated activities. It was the visit to villages

already implementing *mawas diri* on the second day that convinced participants that it was worthwhile being involved in the expansion of *mawas diri*.

Immediately following this Training of Trainers, four workshops were
run by the newly-trained district teams with back-up from the regency team.
They used the Trainers' Manual with which they had become familiar during their own workshop. A post-training session with the regency and district trainers revealed their deep satisfaction with the results. They claimed
they were committed to follow-up the activities in the eight villages which
participated (two villages per workshop), and to the expansion of the
mawas diri approach to other villages in their districts in the future. The
regency team's task was to train other district teams in preparation for expansion to more districts. The head of the Planning Board indicated his
intention to mobilize government funds to enable the expansion of *mawas
diri* eventually to cover all villages in the regency, over 300 in number.
More recently, two NGOs have begun the introduction of *mawas diri* into
the neighbouring regency of East Lombok, a similarly disadvantaged area.

Table 2 lists some of the physical results achieved in 13 villages in Central Lombok. As with all development programmes, it is difficult to isolate
one factor, in this case the introduction of *mawas diri*, as solely responsible
for these results. There is no doubt, however, that *mawas diri* has played a
key motivational role and given direction to the type of activities selected
by the community.

In addition to the activities whose results are shown in the table, a health

Table 2. Hamlet activities conducted

Village	Hamlets	Rubbish removal	Drains	Roads	Fences	Fruit trees	Toilets	Houses renovated
Marong	3	1	3	1	3	3	3	2
Ganti	3	-	3	1	2	3	3	3
Sengkareng	3	-	2	2	1	1	1	-
Semoyang	2	1	1	2	-	1	1	1
Mujar	2	1	1	2	1	2	1	1
Nyerot	3	-	-	-	-	1	2	-
Barejulat	7	5	1	-	2	2	-	-
Rambitan	4	4	4	1	3	4	3	-
Kuta	3	3	3	2	3	1	-	-
Janapria	2	2	-	-	-	1	2	-
Gaba	2	2	1	1	-	-	-	-
Pedem	3	3	-	-	-	1	3	-
Durian	4	2	1	1	3	3	2	1

insurance scheme, a rice bank to help people over difficult times, a weekly cleanliness campaign and a 'lottery' to assist the financing of development activities were established. Also, demand for and participation in health services has increased, with greater utilization of immunization and the monthly village-based weighing programme at the *posyandus* run by the women's organizations (see Chapter 7). Participation becomes a way of life, affecting all facets of development at the village level. And the human development dimension is strikingly evident where one meets the people involved in planning and organization.

A number of factors have contributed to the successful implementation of *mawas diri* at the micro-level. They revolve around the people—their motivation, skills, resources and willingness to be involved.

— *Mawas diri* functions most effectively as an integral part of an ongoing development programme by increasing the level of community participation. The village or unit where it is to be implemented is 'prepared'. Preferably, the community is involved actively in group activities; the leadership is concerned about village development; and potential implementors such as VHWs, teachers or other literate, motivated people are available.

— *Mawas diri* requires thorough social preparation of the people to stimulate their interest and curiosity and ensure that their best representatives attend the preparatory workshop. It is important to explain *mawas diri* approaches to all who will influence its outcome, including key government officials involved with development, the village head and representatives of the major groups in the community.

— *Mawas diri* is introduced into the community through a participatory workshop attended by those who will determine whether or not the approach 'takes off' and becomes a part of village development. These include village leaders, key informal leaders, VHWs and other prospective implementors. Women have proved keen and effective supporters of *mawas diri*. It is important to give particular attention to special groups such as racial minorities.

It is important to ensure that:

— there is an understanding and interest in *mawas diri* amongst as many 'influential' people as possible in the village and at higher levels of government;

— technical, material and moral support are provided from local government field-workers, administrators and NGOs in an imaginative and sensitive way when needed to sustain and increase community self-help;

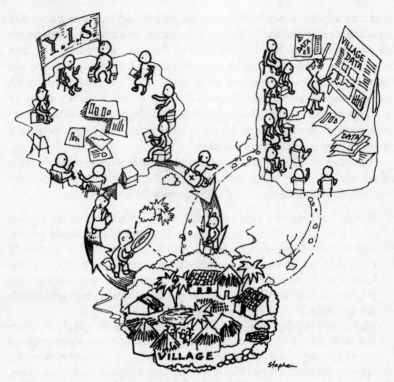

Mawas Diri is a participatory process.

— the data collected through *mawas diri* are fed into the village planning
   process so that the approach is incorporated into village development
   programmes and the data are utilized for planning activities at a higher
   level;
— the *mawas diri* tool stimulates initiative and creativity and is revised
   from time to time so that it remains a challenge to the implementors and
   families involved.

PROBLEMS ENCOUNTERED

The *mawas diri* approach has demonstrated its great potential to stimulate
meaningful community participation in development. Nevertheless it faces
a number of challenges which may hinder its effective use in a given situation; occasionally, they may lead to its failure.

An obvious limitation is the method's reliance on literate people who can fill in the form, and on people who are used to working with figures and can add and compare the data. Pairing data collectors has helped to 'increase' the skill-level of individuals as the two can assist and complement each other in information collection and recording. Illiterate people could be involved in the process if the forms are adapted for their use. A coordinator is usually selected—e.g. a teacher or community leader—to assist several data collectors with analysis. This is a case where 'several heads are better than one'.

An apparently small but, in fact, key logistical requirement is the provision of forms to ensure that they are available on a quarterly or four-monthly basis. In some cases sponsors such as the NGO or funding agency have taken on this responsibility. However, this encourages dependency and runs the risk of creating the impression that *mawas diri* is conducted in the interests of the sponsor. As *mawas diri* has expanded, provision of enough stencilled forms has become increasingly impractical. Hence, more recently, logistical matters such as this have been discussed during the initial workshop, and a commitment obtained from the village committees that they will assume responsibility for providing the forms when needed.

Another more serious challenge is that of 'routinism'. An Indonesian expression graphically describes the phenomenon of quickly-dying enthusiasm as 'the heat of hen's droppings'! The first experience with data collection, community meetings and activities has been sustained in most cases with a high level of enthusiasm, but four to six months later the situation may change. There have been cases where initial activities have stimulated new ideas and the process has gained its own momentum. 'Why,' the people ask, 'repeat the survey when there is so much activity going on?' If they fail to collect information subsequently, both the monitoring of success and future *mawas diri* cycles are jeopardised. In other cases, data has been collected religiously but stored away, often at the village office or, even worse, by the NGO or the health service, without being discussed by the community. Possibly, in such cases, the relevance of monitoring by the people themselves has not been grasped, or the simple skills required for analysis not mastered. However, a question arises as to whether it is necessary to continue regular data collection if an intuitive process has become part of a community's problem-solving ability following implementation of several cycles of the *mawas diri* process.

In programmes where data collection has been carried out several times, there have been cases where the VHWs have become 'behind the desk' data-recorders. They have failed to appreciate the significance of the contact and discussion with families when the form is being filled out in people's homes. Their routine behaviour suggests that they have made no effort to adjust the indicators on the form to the changing conditions in their community.

Support from YIS staff who come from outside the village communities has been a key factor in the implementation of *mawas diri* and an important component of its success. External interest is important to maintain community enthusiasm, assist with problems, possibly provide materials which are not available locally. It also has a role in giving feedback to higher authorities and reminding them of the need for expansion to other areas. In all areas where *mawas diri* has been introduced on a wide scale, the involvement of an NGO has been crucial to ensure that the momentum is sustained. Too often, government officials bound by top-heavy bureaucracy have been slow to take action, waiting for directions from above. Flexibility is not their strong suit either!

There have also been instances where an over-dose of support to a community has been detrimental. Insensitive encouragement can lead people to plan activities with the specific purpose of receiving outside assistance. For example, toilets are often proposed without thought to community needs or feelings. If constructed, they may not be used. Another effect may be to kill local initiative and voluntary contributions from the people.

Expansion of *mawas diri* activities within a village has been variable. It has proved impossible to train enough implementors in one workshop to cover a whole village. Trained implementors have been encouraged to train others by eliciting their participation in data collection. In some cases this has happened. In others, neighbours have observed and copied activities being implemented in a *mawas diri* section of the village. However, this has sometimes been done without the data collection step, thus negating the possibility of structured monitoring. Other villages have failed to expand at all despite very encouraging developments in the *mawas diri* sections.

NEWER FRONTIERS

1990 saw the introduction of *mawas diri* into two cities in Indonesia. The people of several *kampungs* (wards) in Surabaya, the third largest Indonesian city, and those of four *kampungs* in the coastal town of Cirebon have reacted enthusiastically to *mawas diri*. In both places increased community participation has helped already to improve environmental health, including the disposal of rubbish.

Mawas diri was extended to the Philippines also in 1990. The Philippines Department of Health introduced the approach into the Bohol Acute Respiratory Infections Research (BARIR) programme, renaming it *Pagpanamin Alang sa Kauswagan* (PAK). While the response in Indonesia had been most encouraging, it was to be seen how the *mawas diri* approach would be received in another country, another culture.

Two *barangays* (villages) in the poor dry island of Bohol were selected for the 'demonstration'. The Totulan community was coastal and semi-urban while Bangwalog was rural and isolated in the mountainous hinterland. The first workshop was held in Totulan where the socio-economic situation of most families was minimal and the environment unhealthy. Community activities were almost non-existent and village leadership was passive, responding only to government instructions. The community consisted of three heterogeneous sub-communities, the Moslem Badjao people, 'newcomers' who earn their living from fishing, the Catholic Bais people, also fisher-folk, and the Catholic Boholano people who are farmers and better-off fisherfolk. With their diverse backgrounds and traditions, there is very limited daily contact between these groups.

The preparation of the people for PAK was carried out on several visits to Totulan and included discussions with municipal authorities. Contact was made with *barangay* officials, *Barangay* Health Workers (BHW) and informal leaders of the three ethnic groups. The Badjao leader commented that it was the first time his people had been included in a *barangay* activity. Lengthy discussions resulted in the 'neutral' *Barangay* Health Station being selected for the workshop.

Despite the heat and cramped, noisy conditions, there was full attendance and enthusiastic participation. By the third day the three groups had integrated well. On the final day, plans of action were presented proudly. The Bais people planned a meeting immediately which was to be followed by data collection; the Badjao team planned a similar procedure for the following month; and the Boholano BHW planned to recruit and train survey assistants to cover approximately 100 families. The biggest surprise was the plan of the *barangay* captain and his councillors. They undertook to assist the implementation and monitoring of PAK and promised to hold a meeting with the Badjao and Bais people the very next day. The seeds for closer cooperation between the three groups, and with *barangay* officials had begun to grow.

The second *barangay*, Bangwalog, was quite inaccessible, making frequent contact impossible. However, this difficulty was eased by the homogeneity of its farming community, strong leadership and the people's on-going involvement in several community programmes. The participants' plan of action included immediate data collection. Everyone was enthusiastic to begin programme activities as soon as possible after the workshop.

Two months after the workshops in these different communities, the people of Totulan had not got beyond data collection. In Bangwalog, people were busy fencing their yards and constructing pig-pens. In both villages, there had been virtually no follow up by outside officials.

Reflecting on these two experiences, the community workers felt it was important to strengthen the weak organization of the community. Plans for expansion of PAK include organizing the sub-sections of a village *(puroks)* into cells of five families to facilitate effective planning and action. Each cell will elect a health representative to the *purok* health committee. In order to increase participation in the PAK process it is also planned to conduct two workshops for community leaders and for household heads.

MAWAS DIRI AND THE OUTLOOK FOR HEALTH FOR ALL

The *mawas diri* approach has proved attractive to a diverse group of people including middle-level policy-makers, village officials, government technical services and VHWs. The Indonesian Department of Health has renewed its interest in *mawas diri* and is in the process of incorporating this approach into its environmental health programme which covers all provinces of Indonesia.

Policy-makers comment on its potential for increasing community planning skills, an essential component in any 'lower level-upwards' planning procedure. A village can collect its own data and use it to draw up realistic plans for development. This can help overcome a major problem in the Indonesian planning process in which villages are encouraged to submit their own plans for funding. Too often these are drawn up 'on impulse' and do not reflect priority problems. The process also motivates the community to tackle creatively the problems which they themselves detect. Self-reliance is enhanced. The approach also has possibilities for promoting institution-building by strengthening the functions of local planning bodies.

Government technical services say that *mawas diri* can assist them in a number of ways. The data and prioritization of problems provides them with specific information on the location and extent of problems in a certain area. It can assist them in their planning activities and it enables them to make more effective allocation of funds and facilities in government programmes. Another positive result has been the stimulation of VHWs by the new activities. VHWs are keen because they have a tool which enables focused contact with families. Their role is clearly defined and the prioritization of problems provides them specific directions for family and group activities.

The *mawas diri* approach has proved that community participation is not only possible in all stages of a development programme, but also increases the quality of activities and contributes significantly to human development. By providing appropriate skills and tools to a community, organizers can have faith in the people's decisions for change. They can trust that programme preferences will be appropriate, a significant investment for the achievement of Health for All.

Greater participation can also have an impact on the quality of people's lives. Self-confidence and dignity are a product of gaining significant control over one's life. This only occurs through participation, not by programmes imposed from above. Through the *mawas diri* approach people gain skill in looking critically at their environment, in detecting problems and prioritizing them, in planning, implementing and monitoring improvements. In the process they develop initiative and creativity. Most important of all, by working in programmes which are of their choice, people gain greater confidence in their right and ability to control their lives.

Reference

1. Johnston, M. (1983). The ant and the elephant: voluntary agencies and government health programmes in Indonesia. In: *Practising Health for All*, (eds. D. Morley, J. Rohde and G. Williams), Oxford University Press, Oxford.

CHAPTER 3

Community-determined Health Development in Zaire

PATRICIA NICKSON

The author describes the transformation of health services delivered by a rural church-related hospital to a community-based 'self-help' initiative. In the latter, health was defined in its broadest sense and was sought actively by community action encompassing a wide-range of community improvements.

Patricia J. Nickson, Ph.D., has spent many years working in a mission hospital in Boga, Zaire. She is presently on the community health staff of the Liverpool School of Tropical Medicine, U.K., and Director of the Pan African Institute of Community Health, Zaire.

A LOSS OF PEACE

By 1987 the Rural Health Zone of Boga in north-western Zaire was able to boast of substantial improvement in standard health indices (immunization coverage of infants—76 per cent—well above the national average—about 36 per cent), a full range of primary health care (PHC) activities, and self-sufficiency in recurrent health care costs of pharmaceuticals, supplies, salaries and maintenance. However, there was no apparent improvement in living conditions. Malnutrition was still evident, severe in 2 per cent and moderate in 22 per cent of pre-school children, and too many people were still dying of diseases that were easily preventable or curable.

The paradox of continuing poor health despite the high utilization of PHC services was explored during 1988 within the Collectivité of Bahema Boga.* Two senior nurses (one national and one expatriate—the author) were challenged by a comment made by a mother following the death from kwashiorkor of her three year-old child. Asked why she had not brought the

---

*The collectivité of Bahema Boga has a population of 10 000, about one-third of the Boga health zone. A collectivité is the lowest level of civic administration and is headed by a Chief. The organization of the collectivité is traditional and remains largely autonomous, although its authority cannot surpass that of the state.

child to the hospital when he had become ill, the mother replied that the child had not been ill but had 'lost his peace'. 'Foreign doctors can heal foreign diseases,' she said, 'but when someone's peace has been lost even local doctors can seldom help.' The nurses shared their concern for this cultural gap in perception of health with other members of the health staff, the local chief and some village leaders. Together they decided to form a 'study team' comprising the two nurses, a secretary, a community health worker, the Chief and a village leader. This team catalysed community action that built on the resilience of village social structures which could overcome even the set-backs of recession, inflation, bribery and corruption that characterize post-independence Zaire.

THE COLLECTIVITÉ OF BOGA

The people of Boga are mostly of the Bahema tribe which has two distinct ethnic groups, cattle-owners of Nilotic origin and Bantu cultivators. While the isolation of Boga shelters it from the massive economic and administrative problems that beset Zaire, life in this area is constrained by tribal and clan relationships and structures and by the limited resources available to villagers.

Development efforts have been sponsored in a number of sectors: education, adult literacy, health, women's development, agriculture, water programmes and veterinary services. The Rural Health Zone (RHZ) of Boga* has a 75-bedded hospital and seven health centres, each serving a population of 5000 to 10 000, and staffed with at least one midwife and one community health nurse. The health centres have a full range of PHC activities including maternal and child health care, control of endemic diseases, health education, domiciliary visits and basic curative care. In late 1982 a development committee was established in each of the 15 villages of Boga RHZ, and the training of village health workers (VHWs) and traditional birth attendants (TBAs) commenced.** At first the work of the VHW was on a voluntary basis although he or she was able to make a small profit from medicines sold. This principle was revised in 1983 when it was decided that the health zone, the Collectivité and the respective village would each pay one-third of a given amount as remuneration for the services of the VHW. This system brought substantial improvement in the use of basic PHC ser-

*Population nearly 30 000 covering an area of 1800 sq. km.
**There was one VHW per 500 population, and TBAs only in villages more than 10 km from the nearest health centre.

vices through the 1980s, yet the cultural isolation of villages persisted. While the community was familiar with Western health care facilities, the traditional systems were still popular. These included herbal therapies, spiritual healing and the use of 'fetishes'.

The health team played a key role in facilitating the villages of Boga to undertake the self-study and community action that led to a broader achievement of health for all.

In 1988 the Chief of the Collectivité created a tradition reform committee, a group of elders charged with examining traditions in the light of contemporary development issues. The Chief has held weekly meetings with the Collectivité Action Group comprising community-elected village leaders (about 20 in all) as well as the leaders of development resource groups such as the headmaster, medical director, water engineer and the small health-study team to discuss political directives and community development. The meetings are open to leaders of non-governmental institutions such as the churches, schools, health programmes and development projects. They provide a forum for announcement of activities or discussion of problems. Those who attend the meetings are expected to express the needs and concerns of their respective groups as well as to relay information back to them.

EXAMINING THE PARADOX

Puzzling over the 'paradox', members of the health-study team realized that the existing socio-cultural environment had not been considered in the design of the health care structure. Alternative strategies that truly reflected the needs of the community were necessary. However, before these could be established it was vital to study the concept and cultural characteristics of health in Boga. It was also important to explore how community members could define their own health needs and identify strategies to meet their priority needs.

There had been no baseline studies of the health status of Boga. However, traditional health practices and illness-related decision-making processes as well as the everyday life of the community were already well-known to the team. Members of the team spent a considerable amount of time with groups of people in the villages—women's church groups, senior school classes, village development committees, even men drinking beer together—encouraging them to express their ideas. Over three months they examined the people's concepts of health, illness and health care. These were interrelated and included bereavement, the loss of or damage to property, misfortune and other cultural concepts such as those involved in decision-making processes and death rites.

It was felt that asking community members direct questions would not elicit truthful responses about local health concepts but only those that reflected the respondents' perceptions of the team's interests. Thus a novel approach was used to enable the groups to understand how they might express their 'felt needs' and to stimulate people to articulate local health-related problems. Groups were told a local version of 'Rakku's Story'[1] which vividly portrays a poor rural family and the cultural and socio-economic factors surrounding the death of their infant from diarrhoea (see box). The story demonstrates the gap between the health facilities available and their reaching, or being reached by, the needy. Group members identified with the situation, recounted and discussed the negative issues raised by the story, to eventually formulate positive criteria for a healthy family.

THE RESPONSE OF THE VILLAGE DEVELOPMENT COMMITTEES

Long, involved discussions occurred in which the local word *obusinge* (literally, health) was repeated frequently. *Obusinge* was seen as the right of and

---

A *RAKKU'S STORY* FOR BOGA

A resumé of *Rakku's Story*[1] was read in French to a group of student community health nurses, and each was asked to write a case study from her own field experience which highlighted a similar problem. Of the 13 studies written, the students chose the one which they felt depicted a typical Boga 'Rakku' tragedy. The story chosen was then translated into Swahili, the area language, and Kihema, the tribal language.

The Students' Story

Mugisa and his wife Tabu had seven children, of whom two had died. They lived in a small grass hut which always had a leaking roof. There was no kitchen or latrine but there was plenty of water as they were near the River Semliki. The small wage that Mugisa earned working in the fields was usually spent on alcohol, and so it was up to Tabu to find cash for salt, oil and daily needs. She collected fire-wood which she sold to neighbours, then used the money to buy plantains with which she brewed beer to sell to coffee merchants passing through the village. She grew cassava on a small patch of land, but it was difficult to find beans or vegetables.

continued

The eldest child was eight years old, but was not at school. The primary school at Boga was 40 kilometres away and enroling him would mean that he would have to live with relatives. Then he could not look after the smaller children during the day when both parents were out. Anyway there was no money for school fees.

One day the baby developed diarrhoea and vomiting and rapidly became weak. Mugisa went off to find a healer who demanded a chicken, saying that any lesser payment would reduce the power of the medicine he would give. The family only had one chicken but thought that the treatment would be worth the price. However, even though the child had been given the medicine, his condition deteriorated. A sorcerer was sought and he said that the price of seeking the cause of the disease was a goat. Since they had no goat Tabu offered two nearly-new pieces of cloth instead which were accepted by the sorcerer. He told them that jealous neighbours had planted evil bones at the side of the house, which he had removed and had replaced with special stones which would bring good luck.

The following day there was still no improvement in the child's condition. Mugisa decided to leave him to fate but Tabu climbed 20 kilometres up the escarpment to where a spiritual healer lived. His prayers brought no immediate relief, nor did the two-coloured capsules bought from a private nurse. The spiritual healer had recommended that Tabu take the child to the village health worker. This she did and was surprised by his concern and urgent care. He made up a solution of sugar and salt and gave half of it to the baby. The rest he gave to her to give to the child later. He sent her with a note to the hospital at Boga. But that was 20 kilometres further and she was dressed in rags. The children were at home without any food and if Mugisa drank he would become violent. The hospital charged for treatment and she had nothing left. But in desperation she pressed on.

At the hospital the child was attended to immediately while Tabu was given a meal. Within a few days the child recovered and was discharged. The staff decided that Tabu was really very poor and so should not be asked to pay the bill. When she arrived home, her husband, drunk but delighted to see his baby alive, remembered the treatment his mother had advised—a herbal enema—and gave it to the child to prevent the diarrhoea recurring. Soon the baby became sick again with a high fever. Now even his mother would not agree to return to the hospital, knowing that she had not paid the first bill. The child died. Mugisa had now lost three sons and was distraught in his bereavement. There were funeral rites to arrange and he would have to borrow money from his employers for the feast after the burial.

the norm for everyone. But beyond the Western concept of health, *obusinge* embodies a progressive expectation that the *obusinge* of today will be bettered by the *obusinge* of tomorrow. Furthermore, *obusinge* is seen in the context of social relationships: it cannot be present in the face of misfortune or the breaking of cultural norms (including prostitution, drunkenness, theft, laziness or lack of respect for the clan). *Obusinge* can be lost through the fault of another party.* The cultural context called for a focus on the health of the family rather than the individual. The attributes of a family that has *obusinge* were compiled from discussions with the various groups:

— peace within the family and between the family and its neighbours;
— two to six children with at least two years between each birth;
— both parents alive and free from serious chronic disease or disability, living together and capable of caring for their dependent children;
— education up to primary level for all children with the possibility for some to continue to secondary level;
— resourcefulness in domestic finances and in educational and health care development;
— cultivation of at least half a hectare of land per family member;
— two or more cooked meals a day, each consisting of at least one staple food and one or more other foods;
— an adequate standard of hygiene in and around the home, involving the use of a deep-pit latrine with cover, the control of vegetation in the compound, an outside kitchen, and maintenance of the house;
— access to water within 200 metres of the home;
— affordable health care within reach of the village.

The exercise of formulating a definition of family health proved important. Not only did it enable committee members to see that the health team was open to local concepts of health and to the communities' responsibility for health care, but it also helped the communities to understand that they could use the definition to assess their own health needs. Thus began a process of community-determined health development which progressed through the following steps:

— defining health;
— surveying health needs;
— selecting achievable goals;
— establishing strategies by which the goals would be met;

*Those who have contravened cultural mores or have caused others to lose their *obusinge* are not extended the normal clan sympathy or given practical help. They may be called before the clan tribunal where elders will give advice.

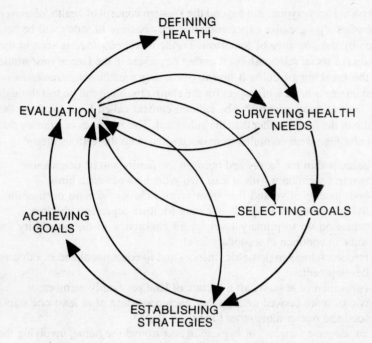

DEFINING
HEALTH

EVALUATION

SURVEYING HEALTH
NEEDS

ACHIEVING
GOALS

SELECTING GOALS

ESTABLISHING
STRATEGIES

The critical steps of the community-determined health development process.

— working towards achieving the goals; and
— regular evaluation.

Defining Health

Each village development committee modified the definition of a healthy family to suit its own concepts. This specification was the beginning of a commitment by each committee to rectify situations below local standards. A most important result of having the committees detail their own definition was their ownership of the process which became a 'trade-mark' or a 'banner' to march proudly under.

Surveying Health Needs

Village committee members then conducted surveys with technical guidance from the health team. Every family in each of the 15 villages was visited. This enabled the committees to measure the extent to which each criterion of their definition of *obusinge* was agreed upon and achieved within their communities. Reasons for shortcomings were recorded. The survey also served the important function of taking the committee members into the community and demonstrating to them the problems in their villages. As the committee members were at a higher socio-economic level than most of their fellow-villagers, they were clearly enlightened (if also embarrassed) when confronted with certain situations.

Selecting Achievable Goals

Following the survey, a wealth of information was available to each committee. Meeting all health needs would have been overwhelming, especially

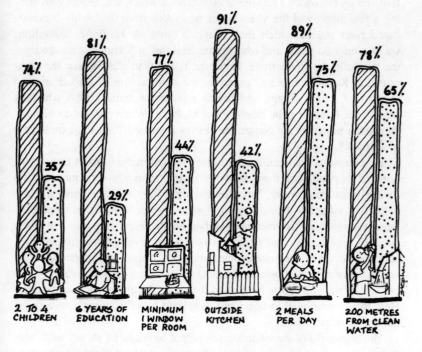

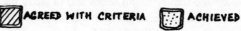

Perceived health needs of families and the extent to which these were achieved.

as the resources available to address those needs were slender. However, the committees could cope with the needs of the community by selecting goals or priorities and strategies by which these would be met. The 'priorities' themselves were not ranked nor were they necessarily the most urgent needs of the villages. Rather, achievable goals were selected. By having specific priorities the committees would be in a position to harness community support toward the goals. The cyclical nature of the community-determined health development process would enable other priorities to be considered in the future. Indeed, the results of the survey did not always have a major influence on the committees' selection of priorities. Other factors influenced their choices and priorities varied substantially between communities. For example, Kasingo, situated 40 kilometres from Boga centre, had no reasonable routes or communications. There was a footpath up the rocky 1220-metre escarpment, which was usable only during a few months of the year. Water was taken from the highly-contaminated river beside which the village is situated. Hygiene, sanitation, socio-economic status and educational facilities at Kasingo were amongst the lowest in the Collectivité. However, rather than clean water, the committee at Kasingo chose as priorities the construction of a road and the training of a new village midwife to replace the trained TBA who had moved out following the death of her husband. When pressed to identify their other priorities the committee always answered, 'Not until we have a road [track].'

In contrast to Kasingo, Kanisa village is right in the heart of Boga, with none of its population more than 100 metres from a water source or 500 metres from clean water. Nevertheless, the committee at Kanisa still decided that villagers should have a protected water source (i.e. tapped filtered water) within five metres of all households. Forty-nine per cent of the population of Kanisa had already achieved that level yet the protection of water sources remained one of their priorities. Kanisa had immediate road and radio communications; the hospital was situated in their village and 12 per cent of the population lived at or above the 'luxury' economic standard. Here the geographical location and its related benefits strongly influenced the choice of priorities.

The objectives of the village development committees' survey were both to identify individual and family health needs and to study the community as a whole. Some of these individual needs were identified as 'priorities', while others were acted upon unobtrusively by the committee.

For example, in Kinyanjojo a family had three children who were under-nourished and had received no health care. They were of a different tribe and had recently moved into the area. Their culture believed that if infants were taken into a different tribal group, the 'evil eye' of that tribe would detect and kill the strangers. The health worker responded sensitively, arranging for weighing and immunizations as well as health education to be carried out in the home. Within three months the mother was attending the village clinic regularly. While it might not have seemed necessary for this situation to be identified as a village 'priority', the health worker demonstrated the importance of responding to individual needs.

A few priorities affected more than one village. The best example of this was the need for a road to be cut between the commercial centre and Kasingo, 40 kilometres down the escarpment of the Rift Valley. Mugwanga was situated about mid-way between the two points and the only other village which the road would pass was Badundu, only a few kilometres from the main route with easy access to the commercial centre. Kasingo and Mugwanga both included the road in their priorities while Badundu did not. All three villages and especially the proximal one, Bandundu, needed to collaborate as each had to be responsible for a section of the road. This situation was resolved by the intervention of the Chief of Boga Collectivité who insisted on Badundu's collaboration.

The Chief was involved totally in each step of the process and selected the three most commonly-occurring priorities for his 1988–90 Plan of Action. These included: group cultivation, the protection of water sources and education for young children. Villages with these priorities were absolved from some of the other *solongo* (community work sessions) so that they could work towards their priorities. It could be argued that the Chief's selection of three priorities for the Collectivité as a whole detracted from the central idea of community determination, but he had established these from the discussions of the Collectivité Action Group.

Establishing Strategies to Meet The Goals

Having selected their priorities, the village development committees were responsible for planning strategies and organizing their communities to work towards meeting their goals. The committees tackled the problems in very different ways, reflecting specific committee and community characteristics.

The village of Malaya discussed at length how they were going to meet their priority of overcoming malnutrition among young children. The committee understood that the health and particularly the nutritional status of a family was related to the mother having had at least basic education. They analysed the problem as follows:

The village is on the road but at a distance of seven kilometres from the nearest primary school. This is too far for the younger children to walk. It is, therefore, not until a child is nine or ten years old that he or she starts school. The first task for any new school entrant is to learn Swahili since most children speak only Kihema (the local language) at home. This inevitably means repeating the first grade. By the time a child is 12 years old, he or she may be entering the second grade. But many Zairian girls of twelve are past menarche and are thus considered young ladies. They do not want to attend class with younger children from the immediate village and therefore drop out of school before they can do much more than write their names. These girls are at risk of losing their first and maybe subsequent children from malnutrition or related diseases because they have not benefited from a full primary education.

To address the problem the village development committee constructed three mud-and-wattle school-rooms in the village. They decided at the same time that a forest area of about five acres should be cleared and planted with coffee, and the income from this used to pay the salaries of three teachers. Coffee was chosen because its export price was less affected by inflation than certain other crops. The committee started without any money even for the seedlings. But rather than miss a growing season they constructed a nursery to grow the seedlings from beans. However, since the coffee plants would take two years to yield their first harvest, there would be a cash problem in the short-term. So either the villagers would have to delay the start of the new classes or find financial resources to bridge the gap. Once the coffee plantation had been established, the village development committee approached the Collectivité authorities for help. No funding was available immediately but the initiative taken by Malaya's community prompted the Collectivité to establish a loan fund from which Malaya was the first to benefit. Now, two years later, all boys and girls of primary school age are attending school. The plan worked because there was sufficient community support and determination.

In another village, Kinyanjojo, the committee decided to improve cultivation by establishing groups of about 12 families to work collectively. Nobody was to be allowed to seek work as a labourer until his own plot had been dug and even then he would be expected to take his turn on the night rota to prevent vandalism of the group's plots by thieves or monkeys. This was an original if not radical idea. The community's determination was strong and their initiative was supported by the Chief.

The committee of Kyabwohe, a cattle-rearing village in the plains, insisted that each member of the community should have a piece of land for the cultivation of vegetables. A major problem among cattle-herders is that cultivation is often neglected. Kyabwohe accepted that vegetables were important, but there was no more than a verbal commitment from families that they would increase their cultivation. It was likely that several growing seasons would be lost before any major progress was seen. Nevertheless, most families started planting groundnuts and soya beans between their cassava.

The strategy chosen by the committee of Badundu to reduce some of the risks of AIDS was an example of the confidence of the committee in its own authority. The members insisted upon a total ban on the sale of alcohol (but not the domestic consumption of alcohol) within the village. Concerned about AIDS, the committee had assessed that the most serious risk was from coffee traders who often spent the night in the village after selling their coffee. The traders' habit was to drink late into the evening and then take a local girl as a partner for the night. A ban on the sale of alcohol would dissuade the traders from staying in the village. At the same time, the committee was not unaware of the village's own promiscuity problems and so planned a series of educational meetings.

Only three villages (Bandundu, Buhurani and Kanisa) addressed peace as a separate priority although all had agreed that peace and health were essentially the same concept (*obusinge*). The committee of Buhurani was concerned that much of the indiscipline in the village was caused by youths who, because of their pride in being 'educated', were reluctant to help in the fields, preferring to depend upon their parents while leading their own lives. The committee decided that all youths over the age of 18 years who were not in full-time education, regardless of their marital status, should build their own homes. It was felt that this would force them into a sense of responsibility and would reduce drunkenness and anti-social behaviour. However, this rule was only enforced in a very few families and the objective has not been achieved.

Kanisa did not blame its own youths for problems in public order but rather those from other villages. This village has a cosmopolitan population and its committee is composed of members from many tribes. The advantages of this were demonstrated in their dealing with indiscipline. Examples of how each tribe dealt with public order were discussed and eventually a mixture of the suitable suggestions was adopted. The community would be responsible for informing the village leader of anyone behaving suspiciously. A drum would be used to summon community help if there was disorder.

Working towards Achieving their Goals

Interesting differences developed among villages as the committees motivated their respective communities to act. In some cases individuals resisted having to conform to village priorities, such as the construction of pit latrines, while in other villages radical edicts made by the committee were readily accepted by the community (e.g. no alcohol to be sold, every family to join the group cultivation scheme, all members of the community to help plant coffee or build a school).

The tribal community structure explains how priorities and strategies formulated by the committee elicited full community involvement. Traditionally, leaders within the community are respected. A lack of respect reflects the failure of a leader to conduct himself properly rather than a failure of community members to conform. Under colonial rule, fines or prison sentences had been imposed for the slightest contravention of public order. This habit of imposing fines has been continued by the village chiefs as well as other authorities. Where the system is abused, the effect is minimal since the whole population risks fines; but where it is carefully used, the system is honoured and the community respects the authority of the leader. Finally, clan or peer pressure can be persuasive. If one member of a clan is letting a village down, others will demand conformity. Some committees included the whole community in the decision-making process.

Regular Evaluation

The health study team encouraged regular village development committee meetings so that progress could be discussed and necessary modifications made. It was noticed by the committees that when they met irregularly there was less progress. One village asked the team to meet with them although their strategies were well-established and the community was working towards meeting them. However, they had found themselves becoming too casual and had lost some of their direction and incentive. Having a representative of the team present occasionally and able to give technical advice enabled them to think through what was happening.

The progress of the villages was discussed at the weekly meeting of the Collectivité Action Group, as was the support structure for the process. The Chief of the Collectivité encouraged village leaders to take advantage of all the information available to them and to use the development resource groups within the Collectivité.

Two seminars organized for the village committees were a further occasion for evaluation. Each village was able to give a report of its activities and to hear some of the other villages' progress. There was some cross-fertilization of ideas, some self-examination when committees were conscious of falling behind, and an opportunity for the resource groups to explain the different technologies and ideas available and how these could be implemented.

It had been decided by the Collectivité Action Group that an annual census, incorporating parts of the original surveys, would be conducted, enabling each committee to assess its progress and make necessary adjustments. It was hoped that this would be an occasion to review the definition of health; but rather than using a story to prompt discussions as had been done earlier, actual case studies from the villages would be considered. The first major review was to be held in July 1991, two years after the completion of the original study.

OVERCOMING CONSTRAINTS TO ACHIEVING DEVELOPMENT

Villages which chose several priorities found that the greater assortment of tasks made it possible for communities to work on different aspects, depending upon their interest and the time available. Often, priorities depended on technical help from resource groups (veterinary assistants, water engineers, agriculturists, health personnel), which occasionally was difficult to arrange. For example, many villages selected improvement of water supplies yet only one water technician served the entire area. Additionally there were delays as committees took a longer time than expected to collect necessary funds and construction materials. Often communities solved problems for themselves, such as Nyakabale where almost 20 per cent of the population began to raise small animals (guinea pigs, chicken, ducks and rabbits) to increase meat supply. While agricultural and animal husbandry expertise might have made this work more efficient, if 'outsiders' had assumed responsibility for changing and improving these practices, the community's sense of ownership might have been lost.

The village development committees tended to call upon the few technical resources available in an uncoordinated, *ad hoc* fashion. The Chief soon decided that a structure was necessary to coordinate assistance and maintain adequate encouragement and supervision. The team served to connect village committees with the appropriate development resource personnel ensuring optimal use of these limited resources as well as maximal inputs to village activities. The support structure built upon the structure of the Col-

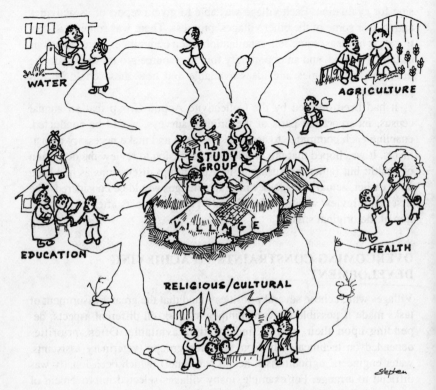

WATER

AGRICULTURE

STUDY GROUP

VILLAGE

EDUCATION

HEALTH

RELIGIOUS/CULTURAL

Stephen

The health study team helped to facilitate communities' access to technical resources available in the district.

lectivité. Traditional authority patterns and the charismatic leadership of the Chief were vital to success. Communities needed support and encouragement while having the autonomy to act on their own and being responsible for their accomplishments and outcomes.

The community-determined health development process at Boga illustrates how a group of communities changed their role from being health-care receivers to health promoters within a relatively short period (12 months). When communities change their role so radically there are inevitable implications for community life and public administration. New power structures emerge and existing authority figures need to be prepared to delegate and encourage decentralized decisions and action. In the evolution of this process, several groups played key roles.

Village Leaders and Committees

The greater the activity of the village development committees the wider and more profound were the implications. The implementation of the process brought a new incentive and authority for these committees to be involved in something more than supervising the hygiene and sanitation of the villages. It required that village leaders be dependable and have integrity and authority. Previously, these characteristics had seldom been put to the test. It was soon apparent which committees were going to work well. Traditional respect governed the extent to which committee relationships were productive or otherwise.

The Health Study Team

The health study team took the initiative of asking the community to define health. By doing so, the classical concept of health workers as 'Great Ones' or even 'Helpers' changed, and they became 'Collaborators' who did not assume that they knew more about the meaning of health than the community.

Once the definition of health had been composed and modified, the role of the health team was that of a resource, a facilitator and a collaborator. Sometimes it was called upon to be an arbitrator. It provided a link between the resource groups and the communities where this was appropriate. The team was later replaced by a facilitator, a health person who had also worked with the development resource team.

Subsequently, the health programme failed to follow-up and encourage the facilitator and to continue as an active party in the Collectivité Action Group. These weaknesses contributed to a general apathy which developed over the next two years. However, at the beginning of the following year (September 1990), the villagers, health programme leaders and the Chief, all recognized this deterioration and made a determined effort to improve the situation. Progress has been maintained since. From this experience it is clear that follow up and active participation by resource groups and personnel are essential to sustainability.

Technical Resource Groups

Not only were the resource groups from collaborating sectors available to the village development committees but they themselves formed a group through which intersectoral relationships could develop. This was for-

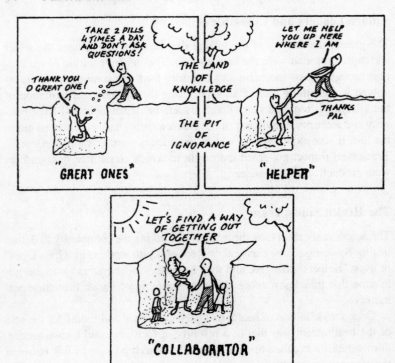

The change in the image of the health worker.

malized by the representation of each resource group at the weekly Collectivité Action Group meetings.

While priorities and strategies were being established, two seminars
were arranged for all members of village development committees (a total
of 120 people). The first of these, organized by the study team, discussed
how priorities could be and were being met. The second, promoted by the
Chief in collaboration with the study team and the development team, was
a forum where technical resource group leaders addressed specific development issues over two days. During the latter event the community-determined health development process was adopted by the Collectivité as a tool
for establishing priorities and devising a three-year health and development
plan.

The process of decentralized problem identification, community action
and problem-solving is a powerful means of addressing the wide variety of

health determinants in poor rural communities. It is the processes rather than the exact activities or outcomes which are most important. By their nature they empower the communities to mobilize their own resources as well as to call upon existing outside assistance to better meet their needs. The eventual impact on objective health parameters remains to be measured but the capacity of the community to identify and meet its own needs is unquestioned. It is this devolution of power to the people which underlies the processes of reaching health for all.

Reference

1. Zurbrigg, S. (1984). *Rakku's story*. George Joseph, Sidma Offset Press Ltd., Madras.

CHAPTER 4

Training Appropriate Health Workers in the Philippines

ROLANDO BORRINAGA AND ISABEL TANTUICO-KOH

*The authors describe how the rural Institute of Health Sciences (IHS) in Tacloban, Philippines, recruits and trains medical personnel. This innovative programme begins by training each recruit as a **barangay** health worker and assists them to become midwives, nurses, nurse practitioners or even full-fledged doctors if their communities so desire.*

***Rolando O. Borrinaga**, B.S.A., M.M.P.M., worked in the WHO-supported primary health care research project in the Philippines before joining the Faculty of the IHS, where he is presently Assistant Professor and Coordinator of Research.*

***Isabel Tantuico-Koh**, M.D., M.P.H., has held positions both in the Philippines government health department as well as in IHS since its establishment in 1976. Since 1988 she has been the full-time Director of IHS.*

INTRODUCTION

The Institute of Health Sciences of the University of the Philippines (UP) was established in 1976 in Tacloban, the capital city of Leyte Province in the Philippines. It was an experiment in medical education, aimed at developing a range of community-oriented health workers. The IHS represents a bold strategy to counteract the twin problems of the 'brain drain', and maldistribution of health manpower available in the Philippines. The exodus of Filipino medical professionals to affluent countries such as the United States had been alarming—about 50 per cent of medical graduates had left the country annually up to 1970. Within the country, the concentration of doctors in urban areas had left the 70 per cent of Filipinos who lived in rural areas without adequate health and medical services.

Many medical educators had dismissed these problems as being caused by economics and, therefore, insoluble. However, this was more a *post facto* rationalization than a true assessment of the situation. Crucial factors other than money contributed to doctors' desire to go abroad or practise only in urban areas. Foremost among them was the orientation of the curriculum towards the 'western system' of health care which was followed by all medical and allied educational institutions in the Philippines. Many features of this education were not relevant to health practice in rural areas. Consequently, most graduates developed skills, knowledge and attitudes which were not oriented towards the health needs or resources of rural Philippines.

An 'Extraordinary Curriculum Committee' was created by faculty members of the University of Philippines' College of Medicine (UPCM) in 1974 to prepare a medical curriculum geared towards health care delivery in under-served rural areas. These socially-concerned medical educators were joined by faculty members from other units of the University such as the Colleges of Arts and Sciences and of Engineering. They were headed by the late Dr Florentino B. Herrera, Jr, the Dean of UPCM at that time.

The Committee generated 'counter-culture' ideas for health manpower development that departed radically from traditional training programmes in curriculum design and admission policies. They followed educational principles that emphasized community relevance rather than academic excellence. With an invitation in 1975 from the Provincial Government of Leyte, the Committee proposed the Institute of Health Sciences to the Board of Regents of the University. The IHS formally opened its doors on 28 June 1976 in Tacloban.

Originally housed in a new two-classroom building constructed by UP behind the government regional hospital, the IHS also made extensive use of existing Department of Health (DOH) facilities and personnel for all academic training needs. The Regional Director of the DOH strongly supported the idea of IHS and was appointed concurrent Director of IHS. In 1981, the IHS transferred its campus to the town of Palo, 12 kilometres south of Tacloban.

Because of its location, a majority of the first group of 96 IHS students, who were chosen by their communities based on recruitment guidelines provided by IHS, came from the two major and two minor islands and numerous islets of the Leyte-Samar region.*

---

*The six provinces that comprise these islands in eastern-central Philippines make up a national administrative area called Region VIII, the Leyte-Samar or Eastern Visayas region.

EASTERN VISAYAS, HEALTH REGION VIII
PHILIPPINES

A PROFILE OF THE LEYTE-SAMAR REGION

The Leyte-Samar Region (Region VIII) is perhaps the most depressed and under-served among the Philippines' 14 administrative regions. It has 3845 *barangays* (villages) in 140 municipalities and three cities, with its regional capital at Tacloban City in Leyte. The region is home to some 3.1 million, mainly rural, Filipinos. Its low, 0.98 per cent, compound population growth rate during 1980–90 can be attributed largely to rapid out-migration from the region and not to a reduced birth rate. In an area covering more than 21431 square kilometres there were only 7259 kilometres of passable roads (in 1978), providing limited access between population centres. Such poor infrastructure has limited the social and economic growth of the population, which has been compelled to adhere to subsistence farming and fishing as a way of life.

The 1987–92 Medium Term Development Plan for Region VIII high-lighted the following realities and problems:

— Region VIII is among the most impoverished in the country, with 70 per cent of all families estimated to be below the poverty line.*
— A high rate of under-employment—25 per cent in 1985.
— Low labour productivity, estimated at only 37 per cent of the national figure, also among the lowest in the country.
— An active communist insurgency that had infiltrated about one-fifth (18 per cent) of the region's *barangays*, mostly in the island of Samar.
— Dependence on traditional export crops such as coconut, rice and sugar, which suffer from the adverse consequences of price fluctuations in the international commodity market.
— Imbalance in infrastructural development among provinces which had disadvantaged the island of Samar in terms of roads, irrigation systems, waterworks and rural electrification. For instance, the road density in Samar Island is only 0.28 kilometres per square kilometre while in Leyte the figure is 0.88.

Overlooked by the published official reports was the annual destruction caused by typhoons and such 'new' ecological concerns as the 'red tide' in Maqueda Bay in Western Samar. The latter first occurred in 1984 and randomly paralyses the area's shell-fish industry. The area also experiences frequent lowland flooding, a result of the decades-old commercial log-cutting, deforestation and swidden-farming activities in the region's uplands and public forests.

The major causes of mortality in the region are pneumonia, tuberculosis, heart disease, diarrhoeal diseases and cerebro-vascular accidents. Diarrhoeal diseases, bronchitis, pneumonia, influenza and tuberculosis account for major morbidity. Among infants the leading causes of death are pneumonia, diarrhoeal diseases, bronchitis, prematurity and malnutrition. *Schistosomiasis japonica* and malaria are also important public health problems. Neither the pattern nor the rate of these diseases has changed significantly in recent years, despite considerable government effort to control these conditions.

In 1990, the infant mortality rate was 52.8 per 1000 live births in the Philippines, one of the highest in the Asia-Pacific region. The figure for Region VIII was 56 per 1000 live births, in spite of the fact that the three Samar provinces are among the top 18 (out of 75) provinces with the highest IMR in the country. Region VIII has the second highest prevalence of

*In 1985, the World Bank estimated the Philippine poverty line at P 14 315 (about $770) family income per year. Forty-five per cent of Filipino families were below this line.

second and third degree child malnutrition in the country which affects 25 per cent of children aged 0–6 years.

Health facilities and manpower available in Region VIII are shown in Table 1. The hospital bed-to-population ratio is 1:1102. Rural Health Units are located in the towns, with one *Barangay* Health Station for every six or seven contiguous *barangays*. The physician-to-population ratio for the region improved from 1:9564 in 1970 to 1:5674 in 1987, but is still far below the national figure of 1:3135 in 1987. The nurse-to-population ratio is 1:2917, while the midwife-to-population ratio is 1:4117. The importance of the 16 000 active *Barangay* Health Workers can be readily seen from these professional staff ratios, especially considering that DOH manpower in the region is heavily hospital-based or curative-care oriented. Barely one-fourth of the DOH staff and resources are actually assigned or allocated to front-line primary health care activities.

THE INSTITUTE OF HEALTH SCIENCES

In the Institute of Health Sciences, we believe that health is a universal right. It should be made available even to the remotest rural communities. The IHS was an outcome of an increasingly resonant expression that the

Table 1. Region VIII—health facilities and manpower (1984)

Public hospitals	34 with:1925 beds	
Rural health units	160	
Barangay health stations	605	
Regional Health Training centre	1	
Private hospitals	34 with: 889 beds	
Hospital bed-to-patient ratio	1:1102	
Physicians	221	
Nurses	1039	
Midwives	736	
Dentists	83	
Pharmacists	27	
Health educators	7	
Nutritionists/dieticians	37	
Barangay health workers	16 657	(1988)
Physician-to-population ratio	1:9564	(1970)
	1:5674	(1987)
National physician-to-population ratio	1:3135	(1987)
Midwife-to-population ratio	1:4117	(1987)
Nurse-to-population ratio	1:2917	(1987)

delivery of health care in developing societies is a responsibility not solely of the physician but of a team of health development workers, a mutually supporting group of people with different levels of expertise, interests, needs and roles. Included in this team is the community itself which must play an active role in the promotion and protection of its own health.

We also believe in universal educability; that given the opportunity for appropriate education, rural communities can develop their own health manpower. To make this possible, the recruitment of students and the admission policies and procedures at IHS are not tied to the trappings of academic excellence but yield more to pragmatic imperatives of working within the human resources and constraints of the communities we serve.

The IHS emphasizes that the community, rather than the individual student it sponsors, is the primary consumer of IHS programmes. IHS students are thus viewed as extensions of their home communities. Linked to this view is the expectation that our students, as persons, have roots in rural areas and will be inclined to go back to serve their home communities after their training with us.

Finally, we believe that it is essential for our training to be relevant to community needs. In this regard, the IHS quite consciously veers away from the standard textbook-oriented courses and encourages its students to confront the grim realities present in their communities. Academic training is thus balanced with practical work, where abstract principles learned in the classroom are made concrete by field experience.

THE OBJECTIVES OF IHS

Thus, the objectives of the Institute are:

— to produce a broad range of health manpower that will serve the depressed and other under-served communities in Region VIII;
— to design and test programme models for health manpower development that are replicable in various parts of the country and, hopefully, in other countries.

To accomplish these objectives, the IHS operationalizes 'counter-culture' ideas for health manpower development that depart radically from traditional training programmes. These include highly democratized admission procedures that delegate most responsibilities for student recruitment to the community level, a step-ladder curriculum that offers a sequential yet integrated approach to health manpower education, and an educational principle that emphasizes community relevance rather than academic excellence. These principles are reinforced by a concept of 'service leave' between each stage of professional training, which serves to link students continually with their home communities. This generates an active partnership with communities in training and shaping the outlook of IHS students, a responsive entry–exit mechanism to and from the formal curriculum, linkages with other agencies for cooperation and support to IHS operations, and research and development activities that seek to root IHS academic pursuits within community realities.

PROGRAMME FEATURES

Democratized Admissions

Admission to the IHS is based on the assumption that a student recruited from a depressed and under-served area, when given relevant and appropriate training in health work, will return and become a committed worker in his/her place of origin.

Students nominated for studies at IHS must be between 17 and 25 years of age, high-school graduates with not more than one year of college experience, and financially unable to pursue their education. Their previous education can be described as 'handicapped'. Data show that the average IHS student has a literacy level of Grade Six based on the American Nelson Reading Test. This literacy level could still enable him/her to pursue college work, but only by using different 'success' criteria. Moreover, our experience has shown that a student with a literacy level of below Grade Four is already severely handicapped, and can only be taught relevant health knowledge and skills at considerable time and effort costs to the teachers.

Because IHS students come from rural communities and lack academic background it has been necessary to prepare teaching materials and pedagogic methods suitable for students whose life experience has been predominantly rural. Students are admitted on the basis of community need and target areas chosen on the basis of the availability of health workers, health statistics, population and economic status. The priority *barangays* screen and nominate their scholars based on recruitment guidelines provided by our Admissions Committee. Candidates are then reviewed and interviewed by faculty members, with a final choice among the candidates in a given community made by IHS.

The student evaluation system also avoids the traditional numerical grading system. Students are rated 'P' (Passed) or 'NT' (Needs Tutorial) at the end of each course. This system fosters team spirit and avoids the highly individualistic and competitive attitudes which generally prevail in traditional medical and health science schools. Students who received 'NT' ratings or were considered 'slow learners' were given informal one-to-one tutorials (one teacher per student) in the early years of IHS. Subsequently, group tutorials were conducted. More recently, students are grouped into classes of 'fast learners' and 'slow learners' based on their baseline literacy levels. The teachers are then expected to adopt more simplified teaching methods (e.g. group tutorials) to fit the learning capacities of the 'slow learners'. Admittedly this task is often a source of faculty anguish and frustration, especially when their best efforts fall short of imparting the minimum knowledge and skills to some students, who are still rated 'NT' and, therefore, have to be individually tutored.

The Step-Ladder Curriculum

The step-ladder curriculum is the main feature of the IHS academic programme (see figure on p. 70). The Philippines has a rather standard Western model of health manpower education, with separate schools for paramedical nurses, midwives and health technicians. The full medical degree requires four years of university with a B.A. or B.Sc. before entrance into a four-year medical course. An M.D. degree is granted, followed by one year of internship. The IHS curriculum is a reflection of our philosophy that all levels of the health team are equally important and must work closely together with mutual respect and understanding. Team members are best trained by receiving the same education to enable an appreciation of each other's skills and abilities, with those demonstrating the interest and capability advancing to the higher levels, eventually to become doctors of medicine.

All students admitted to the IHS initially go through the *Barangay* Health Worker (BHW) programme, or what is commonly known as paramedic training. After one quarter or 11 weeks of study, the student receives a certificate as a BHW, qualifying him/her to be a practising paramedic.

The BHW programme is not a terminal programme. Rather, it is intended to initiate the student to community work and enable him/her to determine his/her fitness and commitment for the community health profession. Fitness and commitment are further determined through the student's work as a BHW during the minimum three-month service leave after the BHW programme.

Following this leave, the *barangay* is asked to endorse further studies based on their satisfaction with the student's relationships and contribution

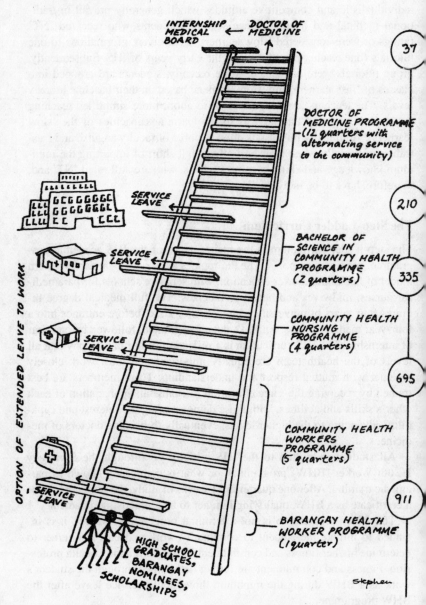

*The 'ladder' curriculum with service leave after each programme.
Numbers in circles are numbers of graduates through June 1992.*

to his own community. On a few occasions, the required '*Barangay* Resolution Document' has been denied to several BHW graduates. The student returns to school for an additional five quarters—some 15 months—to qualify as a community health worker. Completion of this programme entitles the student to the university-awarded Certificate in Community Health Work (CHW). This was originally termed, 'Certificate in Midwifery', but a change in title was necessitated by the fact that male students did not like to be called 'midwives'. Moreover, the CHW programme is broader than the standard midwifery programme. The courses prescribed for this programme are only partly determined by government regulations pertaining to the midwifery curriculum. The subjects covered include Logic and the Scientific Method, Ethics, Psychology, Sociology, Community Organization and Development, Basic Mathematics and English. After passing the National Licensure Examination for Midwives, the CHW graduate is employed as a licensed midwife for a variable period, depending on community need and the student's desire and ability to proceed further with studies.

After four additional quarters at IHS, the student receives a certificate as a Community Health Nurse (CHN). The CHN graduate is the equivalent of the graduate nurse from a hospital school of nursing and will become a registered nurse after passing the National Examination. Service leave again follows as graduates take jobs with increasing responsibilities in the health system serving their home area. Two more quarters of study qualifies the CHN graduate for the degree of Bachelor of Science in Community Health (BSCH). The BSCH graduate is the local counterpart of the Nurse Practitioner in other countries.

The final level of the IHS step-ladder curriculum is the Doctor of Medicine (M.D.) programme. It consists of an additional 12 quarters (three years) of studies, and a yearly interval of community experience capped by a full year's hospital internship, all spread over a period of five years. The M.D. graduate becomes a licensed physician after passing the National Licensure Examination for Physicians. Depending upon the length of time chosen for the various service leave options, a student may become a licensed physician in roughly the same time taken through the traditional nine-year course of university undergraduate degree, four-year medical college and internship.

Community-based health development work by IHS students is integral to the curriculum. In the *Barangay* Health Worker programme the students are immediately exposed to community work for three full weeks after eight weeks of classroom didactics. During these three weeks, groups of five to seven students conduct introductory meetings, a house-to-house survey, and feedback sessions in assigned laboratory villages, in the process of developing community profiles of these villages. The students replicate the same process individually in their home communities during the service leave that follows the BHW programme.

In the five-quarter Community Health Worker programme the students attend classes from Monday to Wednesday and undertake either hospital clinical duties or community practice from Thursday to Saturday. During their community practicum, spread over five weeks per quarter, groups of three to five students formulate, implement and evaluate community health development activities in their assigned laboratory communities jointly with these communities and with other agencies involved in primary health care. The students are expected to individually undertake a similar process in their home communities during their CHW service leave, which usually lasts for nine months.

The choice of laboratory communities has significantly changed through the years. In the early years of its existence, when IHS operated largely on extra-budgetary research funding, groups of students used to be simultaneously assigned to *barangays* in several municipalities as far as 70 kilometres north or south of Tacloban. Starting in 1981, when IHS started operating mainly on a government budget and with the costs of field supervision increasing, the laboratory communities were selected from towns closer to the new campus at Palo. At present, the laboratory communities belong to the central Leyte town of Alangalang, 20 kilometres northwest of Palo. The pattern has been to take one town at a time with each class having new communities in which to work. In recent years, however, it has become a pattern for a given laboratory community to have a BHW/CHW group, serially followed by a CHN group, then a BSCH group, and then an M.D. group, to match the growing expectation of communities for higher skill levels among the assigned students.

In the Community Health Nursing programme, the community practicum constitutes the last eight consecutive weeks of the fourth quarter of the programme. Groups of four students are assigned to a strategically-located *barangay*, preferably the location of the government *Barangay* Health Station (BHS) which covers several satellite villages. In their *barangay* assignments the students design and implement health care for a cluster of villages: a supervisory scheme for lower-level health workers, a family health care plan for 'risk' families, training for indigenous health workers, a community health research project, and an epidemiological investigation of a common disease occurrence (e.g. diarrhoea, measles, etc.) at the village level.

In the Bachelor of Science in Community Health programme the community practicum consists of six consecutive weeks in the second quarter of the programme. Groups of four students apply their clinical skills in minor surgery, basic medicine and therapeutics, preferably in the same communities in which they had been fielded as CHN students.

In the Doctor of Medicine programme, a three-quarter community clerkship in the second year and a full-year community internship in the fourth year constitute the community experience for the students. For these community practica, the students undergo alternate 'fielding' in the different levels of the district health system—the district hospital, a Rural Health Unit, a *Barangay* Health Station and a rural community. During these field placements, the medical students are expected to implement innovative approaches to community health development, rationalize the planning for health service resource allocation and utilization, and continue application of their clinical skills.

The IHS curriculum is innovative in the sense that the social laboratory for its courses is a real Filipino rural community and the student body is recruited from the community they will serve. IHS programmes have been designed with particular attention to community needs arising from the socio-cultural, economic and political conditions present in these rural areas. This system of designing programmes ensures that graduates of the IHS maintain continuity with the communities they are expected to serve. Their competence is tailored to fit the context within which it is applied.

Service Leave

Between each step of the curriculum ladder the students are required to undertake service leave. In practice this leave usually lasts for three months after the BHW programme, nine months after the CHW programme, six months after the CHN programme and six months after the BSCH programme. But a student may stay in service working in the government health system for an indefinite period without prejudice, remaining qualified and employable at the level of competence he or she has attained. He or she may return any time for the next level of training subject to favourable community endorsement and to IHS assessment of his/her capacity to pursue higher academic tasks when applying beyond the CHW programme.

The concept of service leave was derived from the need to integrate the instructional content and processes into a unified and understandable whole in the context of the realities and circumstances of the student's home *barangay*. During their service leaves the students are monitored and supervised mainly by the local DOH staff. For example, the rural health midwives servicing their home communities supervise CHW graduates, and public health nurses or municipal health officers supervise CHN and BSCH graduates. The graduates are expected to render voluntary health and related service in their communities. They receive a routine faculty visit while on service leave. During service leaves, the home communities are considered training venues where the students 'learn as they serve, and serve as they learn'.

Partnership with Communities

Students of the IHS are called '*barangay* scholars'. In addition to free tuition and other school fees, the government provides them a monthly stipend and board and lodging allowance for the entire duration of their stay at IHS, excluding service leaves. In 1990, this amounted to P1000 ($40) per month for each student.

Students are recruited primarily from communities which are badly in need of health workers. The recruitment of a student is the decision and responsibility of his/her sponsoring *barangay*. The endorsement of the *barangay* is a basic requirement for student admission and, later, for promotion to higher levels of the curriculum. This comes in the form of a public document called a *Barangay* Resolution which endorses the student for enrolment at IHS. It is signed by the local elected officials and at least 70 per cent of the household heads in the sponsoring *barangay*. Without this document, a student is refused admission at IHS.

The students are selected by their *barangays* at an open meeting of the community. Upon nomination, the student, with the consent of his/her parents, publicly pledges to return to the community to render services as a health worker. This pledge operates as a type of 'social contract' entered into by the student and his/her *barangay*, a service-oriented derivative of the Filipino cultural value of 'utang na loob', debt of gratitude. The *barangay* in turn pledges to provide a measure of support to the student while at the IHS. This support includes a transportation subsidy, the provision of medical kits, payment of a token 'local counterpart' fee, and community participation in the health programme that the student will implement upon his/her return to the *barangay*.

Mechanism for Entry and Exit

A student may exit from any level of the step-ladder curriculum and return to the community to serve with the knowledge and skills pertinent to the curriculum level he/she has completed. Thus, a student could exit as a *Barangay* Health Worker (paramedic), a Community Health Worker (midwife), a Community Health Nurse (registered nurse), with a B.Sc. in Community Health (nurse practitioner), or with a Doctor of Medicine (M.D.) degree.

If a student renders creditable service to the community beyond the minimum service leave time-frame, and thereby misses immediate (vertical) promotion, he/she may be re-admitted to a later session of the next level of the curriculum, subject to community need and endorsement. This is called the 'lateral entry' mechanism.

Similarly, deserving graduate midwives or nurses who have been working with the DOH, for instance, may seek admission later to the next level of the curriculum through the 'lateral entry' mechanism. DOH-employed IHS graduates were allowed to take study-leave without pay, and re-enter DOH on completion of the next step. At present, however, they have to resign from their midwifery or nursing jobs if their accumulated leave credits cannot tide them over the period of their absence from work. Of course, endorsement by their home *barangays* or by their present service communities is a basic requirement. Thus, if an IHS graduate who has left his/her home *barangay* is alienated from the community, he/she is deprived of the chance for further studies at IHS.

In this way the IHS has provided 'a progressive career structure' that offers different categories of health workers opportunities for lateral and vertical movement linked to a system of continuing education.

LINKAGES WITH OTHER AGENCIES

The IHS was established as a joint venture of the University of the Philippines, the Department of Health, the Department of Local Government and Community Development (DLGCD) and the Provincial Government of Leyte. The Provincial Government provided the political will that led to the commitment of generous support from various government agencies and enabled the establishment of IHS. This political support protected the IHS during its vulnerable years and 'kept the (political and academic) wolves at bay'.

The Department of Health agreed to make available to IHS the facilities and personnel of the government regional hospital, now renamed the Eastern Visayas Regional Medical Center, and of the various health units and district hospitals in Region VIII, which were necessary for training, teaching and supervision of IHS students. The University of the Philippines agreed to extend faculty appointments or provide honoraria or allowances to those DOH staff involved in teaching and supervising IHS students. The UP also cooperated in planning and implementing several continuing education programmes for DOH staff in the region. For a while, several DOH staff were sent on local or foreign fellowships on behalf of IHS.

For a period of ten years until 1986, the leadership structure also promoted integration of these systems by assigning the DOH Regional Director the additional role of Director of IHS. Since 1988, however, the IHS has been administered by a full-time Director. Attendant to this change in leadership was a weakening in the DOH-IHS relationship, manifest by the increase in bureaucratic procedures and arrangements.

The relationship with the Department of Local Government and Community Development has waxed and waned. It was hoped that in its community development function the DLGCD would be a source of funding for IHS operations and subsistence support for the *barangay* scholars. However, with the exception of a one-time contribution at the initiation of IHS, the DLGCD has not provided funds. In 1981 its community development function was removed and transferred to another agency, leaving the Department of Local Government to deal mainly with local officials in their efforts to obtain national funding for local projects and operations. The DLG staff remained involved in the recruitment of IHS scholars, a role they relished and even demanded in the hope of gaining political patronage. At this time, we remain hopeful that this agency will recognize the importance of IHS to the local communities and help to find the material support necessary for our programmes.

International agencies and organizations were also involved in the IHS. WHO and UNICEF provided technical and/or financial assistance to IHS during its fledgling years. The Nellie Kellogg van Schaick Charitable Trust provided 'seed money', including scholarship grants, during the first five years of IHS operations. WHO has kept the IHS on its mailing list for literature and publications, thus keeping IHS updated on the latest trends in the health field.

THE FACULTY

The nature of the IHS curriculum and students called for a special core of faculty members. Among the qualities required were flexibility, patience, compassion and, most of all, a sensitivity to the needs of depressed communities. Of equal importance was the need to have faculty in the behavioural and social sciences, in order to operationalize the 'holistic' approach to health care.

At present, there are 19 full-time faculty members at IHS. Two are physicians, 12 are nurses, and the five others represent various arts and sciences fields. This full-time faculty is supported by a pool of more than 60 part-time lecturers from different DOH facilities and from other schools in Leyte. The IHS recruits most of its part-time lecturers from the DOH on the assumption that IHS students can enhance their theoretical and academic perspectives with the first-hand experiences of their lecturers from the DOH. These lecturers are tapped on an 'as needed' basis, when their special expertise is required for courses offered in different curricular quarters. The Eastern Visayas Regional Medical Center (EVRMC), the government regional hospital, provides the largest number of lecturers—27 physicians and six nurses. The different facilities (district hospitals, RHUs) covered by the Leyte Integrated Provincial Health Office provide 13 physicians, a nurse and two nutritionists. The regional office of the DOH is represented by two physicians, a nurse and a regional sanitarian. Local private medical schools are also represented in the lecturer pool, along with the UP College at Tacloban.

There have never been more than 21 full-time faculty members at IHS at any one time. They teach a student population of approximately 150 students of all levels.

RESEARCH AND DEVELOPMENT ACTIVITIES

Initially, for want of more appropriate experience, the contents of IHS course offerings were derived from established midwifery and nursing curricula. Later it became necessary to develop a kind of 'educational compass' to guide future curriculum development so that IHS teaching could proceed in harmony with the evolving needs for development of rural areas. Thus, a Research and Development (R&D) arm became an essential and integral component of IHS. It was first necessary to validate or adjust IHS curricula which were new and still in the process of development. It was also important to ensure the continuous evolution of curricula to be relevant at all times to the dynamic and changing needs of the countryside.

In order to achieve these aims, the main thrust of R&D at the IHS was the development of an information system with 'internal' and 'external' components to generate data on which curriculum was to be based. The internal system dealt with methods, techniques and structures within the IHS, such as admissions procedures, teaching methods, course contents and alumni follow up, including their effectiveness in contributing towards IHS goals. The external system generated data regarding the perceptions, needs, expectations, programmes and structures of the communities to be served in the region.

The Carigara R&D Project

The R&D component of IHS initially operated almost independently of its academic training component. This autonomy was necessitated by the practical difficulty of simultaneously introducing innovations in both health manpower training and health care delivery in the late 1970s. With the general objective of developing an external monitoring system for both institutions, the IHS and the DOH in Region VIII jointly conducted the Carigara R&D Project in Primary Health Care from 1977 to 1982 with WHO support. Because its frontline implementors were DOH field personnel, the project had all the appearance of a DOH activity at the field level. However, official reports and documents cited the direct participation and collaboration of IHS personnel in the project. The first four batches of IHS students were assigned to over 20 laboratory communities in the Carigara area for their community practice during the project's lifetime.

The R&D project site, the Carigara Catchment Area (CCA) in north Leyte, is home to some 135 000 people living in 186 *barangays* of six towns covered by the 25-bed Carigara District Hospital, the main government health facility. The area is typical of socio-economically depressed rural Leyte with an economy based on agriculture (rice and coconuts) and fishing. Utilizing an 'action-research' approach, the project developed and tested various technologies by which the communities, the health services and other sectors (public and private) could jointly design, implement and evaluate health development programmes. These included methods and procedures for:

— re-orienting health workers from 'providing health services' to 'developing community health programmes' in the rural areas;
— training health workers to prepare and organize communities to participate in health development work;
— lay reporting of family health;
— planning and evaluating health development programmes with the community utilizing lay reports and official reports; and

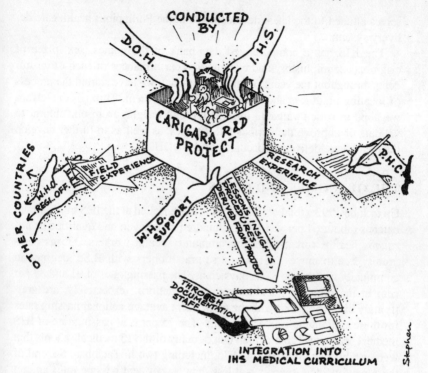

Research and development in the field guided the curriculum as well as new approaches to health care delivery.

— integrating hospital and public health services at the district level.

During its lifetime, the project provided the principal field experience for the formulation of 'Health for All' and Primary Health Care policy in the Philippines, and also for the Manila-based WHO Regional Office for the Western Pacific. From the IHS perspective, the research gave faculty and students a critical look at the needs and potential of our rural communities, at the shortcomings of existing health services, and opportunities to modify work patterns of health workers, their interface with communities and to measure the impact of these changes. The IHS curriculum grew out of this formative experience.

R&D activities are conducted continuously at the IHS. Because of them, we have maintained a leadership role in and developed practical experience for the goal of 'Health for All by the Year 2000'. We have also kept ourselves attuned to the latest developments in the Philippines health care delivery system.

The IHS has a computerized data-bank of the names, sex, place of origin, academic history and examination performances of each of its students throughout the years. With this data-bank we have started the process of locating graduates and communicating with them. Through this effort, we hope to solicit valuable information and insights from our alumni to validate or improve the various IHS courses, as well as to further develop the health care delivery procedures of the DOH.

THE OUTCOMES AND COSTS

Up to June 1992 a total of 963 students had enrolled at the IHS in 15 annual batches (about 64 per year). Nine hundred and eleven had qualified as *barangay* health workers, 695 as community health workers, 335 as community health nurses, 210 as nurse-practitioners with B.Sc. degrees in community health, and 37 as physicians. The passing rates of 91 and 87 per cent in the midwifery and nursing examinations, respectively, are gratifyingly high compared with the 60 per cent average national passing rates for these examinations over the years. The 75 per cent passing rate of IHS medical graduates is better than that of many of the 15 medical schools that were established after IHS in 1976, including two in Tacloban. Several of these new medical schools had less than 50 per cent passing rates among their initial batches of graduates. Thus, IHS graduates have not only overcome their pre-college educational handicaps, they have also outperformed their peers from traditional medical schools in nationally-administered academic tests.

However, these statistics reflect the academic capabilities of IHS graduates from the viewpoint of the 'traditional' professional regulatory boards of the Philippines. There is as yet no standard test to determine the community-related capabilities which comprise a significant part of the training of IHS graduates and in which they are unique in the country! It is estimated that about one-third of all government public health nurses and about 20 per cent of the rural health midwives in Region VIII at present are graduates of IHS.* In Western Samar province alone, 11 (44 per cent) of the 25 Rural Health Units are manned by public health nurses who are BSCH or CHN

---

*Region VIII is the home of 76 per cent of the IHS graduates; the remaining 24 per cent come from other regions of the country—more than half from the depressed Mindanao region in Southern Philippines. Females outnumber males in a 4:1 ratio.

graduates of IHS. Only eight (32 per cent) of the 25 RHUs have municipal health officers (MHO), two of whom are M.D. graduates of IHS. This MHO employment pattern applies also to the three Samar provinces, which have a combined population of 1.3 million in 72 municipalities and one city.

Of the 27 licensed M.D. graduates of IHS, 20 (74 per cent) have found jobs in Region VIII, mostly as MHOs or as resident physicians of different district hospitals. Almost all of these 27 physicians work in their region, province, hospital district or town of origin. Eleven (41 per cent) of the licensed M.D. graduates of IHS work on Samar Island, redressing the dearth of medical practitioners there.

A study done in 1984 found the cost of the IHS Medical Programme to be P10 000 ($714 at that year's exchange rate) per student per year, including room and board allowance for students, honoraria for part-time faculty members, and pro-rated salaries for the two physicians on the regular faculty. A 1978 study found the cost of the UP College of Medicine in Manila to be about P20 000 ($2500 at that year's exchange rate) per student per year without room and board allowance.

Field Performance Monitoring

Over the past few years, studies conducted by IHS faculty members have provided valuable insights to and lessons from the field performance of IHS graduates, many of whom are employed by the Department of Health. A general impression is that the existing, centrally-determined and vertical-programme-oriented health care system of the DOH has handicapped IHS graduates from delivering effective primary health care services at the community level.

A study conducted on the first 25 medical graduates of IHS, 21 of whom were already licensed physicians, showed that their performance as clinicians was satisfactory. A majority of them found work in rural areas, possessed high 'rural bias' (preference for rural work), and were moderately motivated and satisfied with their present jobs. However, they had not had the chance to perform their roles as community health developers because of the lack of expectation that they would implement this skill, and of consequent lack of opportunity. The people preferred their curative skills as physicians. The fact that they actually have been limited to performing administrative routines and clinical tasks is probably the reason for their 'moderate' motivation and satisfaction in their present jobs. In general, community residents have accepted IHS medical graduates as persons and as physicians, have availed of their clinical services and are satisfied with the outcomes of these interventions.

A majority of the IHS medical graduates have expressed the need for further training. This might provide a good entry-point for an enlightened continuing education programme that is separate from and beyond the step-ladder curriculum, relevant and appropriate to their work situations.

Another study of BSCH graduates from IHS showed that 78 per cent are based in rural and under-served communities. Many of them are connected with the DOH as public health nurses, with RHUs or with district hospitals as staff nurses. Unfortunately these BSCH graduates cannot fully utilize their skills as community nurse practitioners because some of their advanced skills (e.g. minor surgery) are not provided for in their job descriptions as PHNs, and they have no legal protection for utilizing these skills.*
Informal interviews conducted with several PHNs also showed that they have difficulty implementing the community organization and development skills that they learned at IHS, because they are hampered by having to spend a considerable portion of their time fulfilling official reporting and monitoring requirements. Although the DOH is keenly aware of this problem, most complaints from workers have been casually dismissed by statements such as: 'Orders are orders', or the more blunt, 'You can always resign; there are other job-seekers who can take your place'.

To its credit, however, the DOH has attempted to address the problem through projects to develop an information system, first in 1984 and again in 1989. Microcomputer technology was even introduced as part of the 1989 attempt which was called the Field Health Services Information System (FHSIS) project. However, instead of simplifying the field reporting tasks, the FHSIS project complicated the DOH field health information system even further, burdening frontline health staff—especially the public health nurses—more than ever.

A third study by IHS utilized disaggregated data from a UNFPA-funded community survey that monitored population, health and nutrition activities in six selected communities of Leyte in 1988. Included in this survey were the distant communities of two IHS graduates who were serving as government midwives. The study showed that the two IHS graduates were performing very well in their professional tasks, despite the constraints of distance and isolation imposed on them and the depressed socio-economic and educational status of their home communities.

---

*The nurse practitioner profession is not yet legalized in the Philippines.

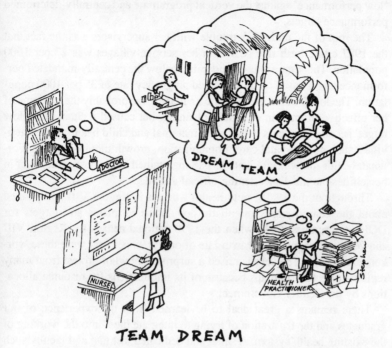

TEAM DREAM

IHS graduates, trained to work as a team in the community, often must accept jobs requiring more traditional work patterns.

The case of one of these midwives is very interesting. This midwife topped all other categories of health workers in covering her population with 11 out of 13 population, health and nutrition activities, including aspects as diverse as the motivation of mothers for family planning and consultations on diarrhoea and respiratory illnesses among young children. She was narrowly 'out-performed' in delivery attendance by traditional birth attendants, and she had fully delegated motivation of pregnant mothers for pre-natal consultation to the *Barangay* Health Workers that she had trained to assist in her work. The infant mortality rate in her nine villages (population of 4434) was only 8 per 1000 live births, the maternal mortality rate was zero, and the crude death rate was 6 per 1000 population. Yet despite these laudable achievements, the existing DOH monitoring and supervision criteria at the field level painted a negative picture of the midwife's performance. Indeed, she had been severely reprimanded by her superiors for 'low performance' against the vertical programme and centrally-determined performance targets.

The root of the midwife's trouble with her supervisors was the fact that the 1987 crude birth rate (CBR) in her service villages was 27 per 1000 population. This figure was considerably below the centrally-mandated performance target based on an estimated pregnancy rate of 35 per 1000 population. The low CBR in the midwife's villages was probably the outcome of her effective promotion of family planning, but caused a chain of 'below target' accomplishments in her other maternal and child health related activities, such as ante-natal care, immunization, growth monitoring, etc. Fortunately, this midwife-graduate of IHS maintained her honesty and belief in herself despite the disheartening official attitude.

Throughout the 1980s, field health workers in Region VIII complained about the centrally-set, unrealistic population estimates and targets for DOH programmes. Only when the 1990 national census for Region VIII showed a net population growth rate of only 0.98 per cent were these workers exonerated. The census raised a surprising howl of protest from many regional directors, perhaps because of its implications for resource allocations by the Central Government.

There remains a great deal to be learned from the experience of our graduates and the frustration of trying to integrate them into the working of the existing health system. A small and dedicated institute and faculty such as those at IHS can make immediate revisions in its curriculum, but to move a large health bureaucracy requires patience, time and extreme dedication.

THE FUTURE

During its 16 year existence, IHS narrowly survived three morale-shattering threats of closure instigated by influential, reactionary officials and vested interest groups. Nevertheless, the Institute has persistently addressed the problems it started out to solve and has achieved the objectives it sought to fulfil in Region VIII. Yet, it cannot rest on this success. It has unearthed new problems which it must help solve in the future.

One of the dilemmas of IHS is that its academic curriculum has remained an object of curiosity in the field of medical and health science education rather than serving as a model for health manpower development for under-served and unserved areas. The IHS approach has yet to be replicated in another region of the Philippines. In the past, several educational institutions have expressed their interest in replicating the IHS model, but have failed to pursue this actively. Their inaction may be due to the fact that replicating IHS would require a 'missionary' zeal and a very high level of commitment. Replication would directly challenge existing educational traditions in other schools and counteract the profit motive which underlies the establishment of most medical and health science schools, particularly private ones. Indeed, it may not be possible to replicate IHS where the profit motive exists.

Fortunately, various facets of the IHS concept are being replicated or adapted in some other countries such as Fiji and China (Heilongjiang Province). These include the step-ladder curriculum, the community-recruitment, training and service pattern for students, the integration of health personnel training and health service provision, community-based education, and several approaches and technologies developed by the Carigara R&D Project.

Only time will reveal the long-term impact of IHS. Meanwhile, we console ourselves with the thought that we have explored and continue to explore the limits of the possible in the fields of health manpower development and health care delivery. In order to reach 'health for all' we believe that it is necessary to press against these limits continually and that such effort will eventually prove rewarding.

A FINAL WORD

In October 1991, President Corazon Aquino signed into law the Philippine Local Government Code of 1991 (Republic Act No. 7160). The Code mandates the devolution of certain national government powers, including health, to local government units (i.e. provinces, cities, municipalities, and *barangays*). It increases the powers of these units to tax and their shares of national taxes. Under the Code, *barangays* now have the power to establish and maintain health and day-care centres. Municipalities now have power over the delivery of primary health care, maternal and child care, and communicable and non-communicable disease control. Provinces may establish and run hospitals and other tertiary health services. The purchase of medicines, medical equipment and supplies is also lodged with these local government units.

Ironically, the health-related provisions of the Code, which has legislated 'people's empowerment' features of the primary health care concept, are opposed vehemently by a majority of government health administrators and workers at all levels. Although their fears and apprehensions have some theoretical and factual ground, these health personnel appear to have forgotten that they once pledged to support and promote PHC as the approach to attain 'Health for All by the Year 2000'. Their effusive lip-service to PHC in the past is being put to a severe test.

In the IHS we keep a measure of optimism amidst the widespread despair in the Department of Health over the implementation of the Local Government Code, which is to start in 1993. In the past, not a few IHS graduates working with the DOH were handicapped or frustrated in their work by its centrally-oriented health care delivery system. A decentralized work situation would be more suitable for them. After all, they have been trained to be creative and to work effectively, despite the dearth of resources in distant and isolated rural settings. These areas will now have more resources available for health development.

References

1. Bonifacio, A. F. (1979). The Institute of Health Sciences: A strategy for health manpower development. In: *Development of Health Manpower for the Rural Areas* (A Report on the Philippines Experiment), Proceedings of the Scientific Session, 32nd World Medical Assembly, Manila, November 1978. Unladlahi Foundation, Manila, pp. 43–54.
2. Damian, A. C. Jr. (1978). The Institute of Health Sciences and the Future. In: *Development of Health Manpower for the Rural Areas*. Op. cit.
3. Estrada, H. R. (1978). The realities of Philippine medical education. In: *Development of Health Manpower for the Rural Areas*. Op. cit.
4. Lepreau, F. J., Koh, I. T. and Olds, R. (1990). Community-Based Medical Education in the Philippines, *Journal of the American Medical Association*, Vol. 263, pp. 1624–5.
5. Richards, R., Fulop, T., *et al.* (1987). *Innovative Schools for Health Personnel.* World Health Organization, Geneva. (The IHS is School B in this book.)
6. Siega-Sur, L. J. and Varona, Z. C. (1987). Elements in the institutionalization of the University of the Philippines Institute of Health Sciences at Palo, Leyte. In: *Innovative Tracks at Established Institutions for the Education of Health Personnel* (An Experimental Approach to Change Relevant to Health Needs), (eds. M. Kantrowitz, *et al.*), World Health Organization, Geneva, pp. 116–35.

CHAPTER 5

Enabling Primary Health Care through Disabled People

DAVID WERNER

The author shows the capacity of disabled people to meet their own needs for rehabilitation. At the same time, in Project PROJIMO in Mexico, disabled people provided a focal point for wider community-based activities in primary health care.

David Werner, M.D., is the founder of the Hesperian Foundation and is the motivating force behind innovative primary health care projects in Mexico and other countries. His first book Where There is No Doctor, which has been translated into many different languages and adapted for use in many countries, is widely considered the most consulted work in rural health care. It is additional testimony of the contribution that disabled persons can make to primary health care as David Werner himself has a progressive muscular disability. He has drawn most of the illustrations in this chapter.

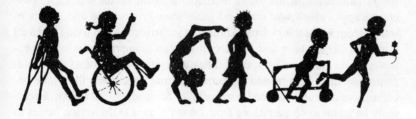

INTRODUCTION

It is now some 25 years since Project Piaxtla—an innovative villager-run health programme—began in the small town of Ajoya in the mountains of western Mexico. This community self-help programme has demonstrated the effectiveness of development efforts initiated and sustained by people themselves rather than with assistance and direction from the outside.

Early in the project, the different mountain communities chose their health workers. Since able-bodied adults were often hard at work in the fields and women had many responsibilities at home, physically-disabled persons were selected sometimes. As the years passed, some of these disabled health promoters proved to be—in many ways—the best workers of all. For the most part, disabled *promotors* came from communities in which they had not been appreciated. They had been pitied, secluded and marginalized. In Piaxtla their role changed completely. Once trained as health workers, they became central to the well-being of the community and, in turn, were valued and appreciated by their neighbours. Their new sense of self-worth, the satisfaction of serving others (not just being served) and the feeling of being appreciated drove these promoters to work harder than most, to stay longer with the project and to show the greatest commitment. In addition, because of their background, they were able to identify best with other disadvantaged people. In a way, their own weakness became their strength and they shared that strength with others.

STARTING WITH DISABLED PEOPLE

Some 15 years ago, Roberto Fajardo, a 15-year-old boy, was carried into the village on a stretcher. He appeared on the verge of death, his body emaciated and completely rigid with juvenile arthritis. The village health workers helped him as best they could with what amounted to basic physiotherapy exercises and simple pain-killers, such as aspirin, to reduce the inflammation in his joints. Perhaps most important was their 'psychotherapy', which was really no more than love, caring and efforts to interest him in the things around him, and in the prospect of living when all hope had already been lost. As Roberto began to improve, the health promoters gave him small responsibilities and jobs to do around the health centre. As time went by and he recovered from his chronic illness, he became more able and assumed responsibility for many different jobs. Eventually he learnt to do everything from taking X-rays to delivering babies to veterinary care. Gradually he moved into a leadership role in the health programme.

Because of his own very extreme disability and near-death as an adolescent, Roberto developed a real empathy for other disabled persons, especially children who were brought to the programme. Realizing he could help these children much more with the right knowledge, he traveled to a nearby city to learn brace-making. When he returned to the village he taught other disabled workers how to make and repair braces. Roberto was also the one to learn and then to teach others how to counsel children with mental disabilities and other problems.

By 1980, a number of disabled health workers came to be in leadership positions at Project Piaxtla. Although they recognized that they were meeting many health needs of the community, they were still very concerned that they knew so little about helping disabled people, especially children. Gradually they evolved the idea of forming a sister programme to Piaxtla. When they met with the community and discussed their needs they found a lot of interest and assistance. The men offered to help fix up an old building and turn it into a community centre. Women offered to take into their homes families from neighbouring villages who brought their disabled children to the new project for rehabilitation. The village children agreed to make a

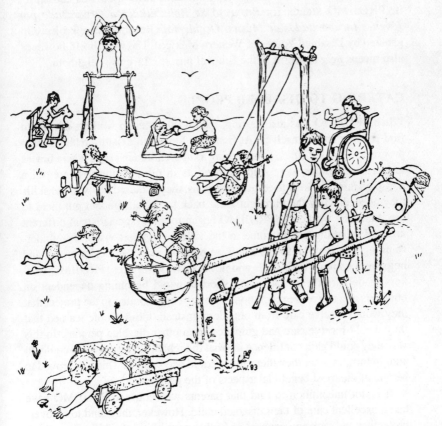

A playground made from local material became the first rehabilitation centre, bringing disabled and normal children together to play.

playground for all children—both able-bodied and disabled. In fact, the playground became the centre-piece of the new rehabilitation project. The children built it themselves with the help of their parents, using wooden poles, vines, ropes, old car tyres, and other locally-available materials. In the process they learnt how much they could accomplish by relying on themselves and the resources around them. For the visiting families, the playground provided an opportunity to try out different swings, parallel bars and other play-things to find those which best stimulated their own child's development. Once they were back at home they could replicate or adapt the equipment they had found most useful.

To reflect the spirit of the project, the name PROJIMO was chosen for it. PROJIMO stands for *Proyecto de Rehabilitación Organizado por Jóvenes Incapacitados de México Occidental* (Rehabilitation Project Organized by Disabled Youths of Western Mexico). The word itself, however, also means *neighbour*, as in the Biblical phrase, 'love thy neighbour'.

CATERING TO DISABLED PEOPLE

When PROJIMO was just starting, the disabled health workers needed to find training for themselves. At first they looked to existing rehabilitation programmes in the cities, volunteering as apprentices in shops where braces and artificial limbs were made as well as in other settings. There, on a non-pay, informal, hands-on learning basis, they acquired many of the skills they needed. They then brought these back to the village and put them to use. Later the workers at PROJIMO began to invite specialists in different areas of rehabilitation to come to the village for short visits. The understanding was that the specialists were there to train the local workers and help them upgrade their skills and not to provide services. PROJIMO workers made sure these visits were short to avoid becoming dependent on outsiders and to avoid expectations among people coming to the project that they would receive care from outsiders. Instead, these people learned that they would receive care and guidance from other disabled persons. In this way they could gain confidence in what the rehabilitation workers could do and, in turn, in what they themselves could accomplish. This has proved to be one of the most beneficial aspects of the programme.

It is not uncommon to find that parents who come to PROJIMO have taken excellent care of their disabled child. However, they tend to be over-protective and lack any concept of further possibilities for him. They think of the child as disabled, unable to do much of anything, and needing protection. They will not send the child to school, afraid that he would be teased, or would be unable to learn quickly. They often do not allow the child go out on the streets to play with other children, afraid that he will get hurt. They expect that the child will need to be taken care of for life. When they arrive at PROJIMO they see, to their amazement, that the people providing care for their child—as consultants, as therapists, or as producers of braces or wheelchairs—are all disabled themselves, many of them more so than the child being brought for consultation. Some workers are in wheelchairs or even on wheel-gurneys.*

For the family with a disabled child seeing severely disabled persons working and providing services, living together and obviously enjoying life, contributing to other people's needs, even more than the average able-bodied person does, is a revelation. Sometimes children who arrive at the project one day, withdrawn, timid and unsure of themselves, leave within two or three days with a whole new sense of self-esteem. Their family has a new feeling of pride in them and their progress, and higher expectations for their future. This rarely happens in the standard rehabilitation centre with professional workers, high-tech equipment and a caring but often condescending staff. PROJIMO's disabled counsellors really appreciate the problems of the child and can look through the child's eyes, often because they have seen life from a similar perspective. They have a much greater sense of equality, of empathy and pride. Disabled people are the best leaders in the provision of care for other disabled people, just as village health work is best done by village health workers and not privileged members of the community or outsiders.

BUILDING FROM THE BOTTOM UP

Some of the children who come to PROJIMO have conditions and deformities that the PROJIMO team cannot correct—usually conditions that require plastic or orthopaedic surgery. In order to save these children, several plastic surgeons from Stanford University in California, U.S.A., have visited the project. At one point Dr Donald Laub brought to the programme a team of plastic surgeons to carry out some important and basic plastic and reconstructive procedures. Their visit turned out to be the beginning of Project Interplast, now a $40 million-a-year programme with centres in Thailand and several areas of the United States, and branches in several countries of South America and Africa. Today Interplast actually involves

*A wheel-gurney is a narrow bed on large wheels that a person can drive while lying down.

Third World plastic surgeons in outreach programmes to poor communities. The surgeons work as volunteers, levying no charge for their services.

Our own organization, the Hesperian Foundation, started in a village when Project Piaxtla, the first village programme, needed the support of more specialized services. Hesperian is now well-known around the world, yet it remains responsive to the needs and demands of the village in which it was founded. The real meaning of 'building from the bottom up' lies in projects like these, in which a village initiative seeks help from outside and those who are skilled and capable recognize and participate as colleagues and helpers in the village-directed effort. In contrast, standard programmes are built 'from the top down'. We feel this process should be reversed. Programmes should grow from the ground up, the 'grassroots', from the concerns of people who have analysed their own problems and are taking action with some encouragement (not 'directives') and resources supplied from outside.

DEVELOPING RELATIONSHIPS

Through the years, the disabled workers of PROJIMO have developed a heightened social consciousness, self-awareness and pride in their lives and work. They have also contributed to an explosion of understanding and appreciation of disabled persons. When the programme began, the village still looked at disabled people as poor unfortunates, useless people who needed help and had no future. It was thought that disabled people had no right to a love-life, to marriage or to a family. Many disabled persons had a similar image of themselves. In spite of all this, a few of the disabled workers at PROJIMO began to develop close relationships, some of which became real romances and eventually led to marriages. At first these relationships developed among disabled people only, but later they came to include non-disabled men and women of the village as well. In the beginning, the community looked upon this with disfavour. For example, a few years ago the mother of an able-bodied girl would have been terrified at the idea of having her daughter marry—or even date—a disabled man. Now such relationships are more acceptable and the community and families discuss them openly. Disabled children and young people have come to play such an integral and natural part of village life that today nobody looks down on them, takes pity on them, or looks the other way because they feel embarrassed to see them.

An interesting aspect of the programme which was unplanned and occurred of its own has been the development of women's rights and their

A DISABLED CHILD GROWING UP HAS THE SAME NEEDS AS OTHER CHILDREN, FOR . . .

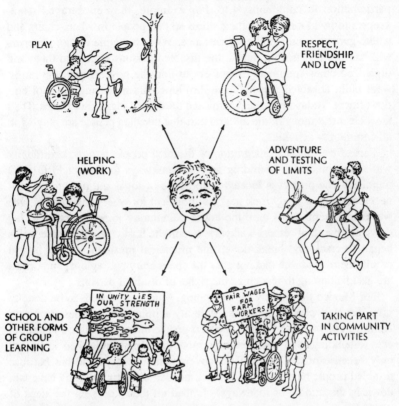

PLAY

RESPECT, FRIENDSHIP, AND LOVE

HELPING (WORK)

ADVENTURE AND TESTING OF LIMITS

SCHOOL AND OTHER FORMS OF GROUP LEARNING

IN UNITY LIES OUR STRENGTH

FAIR WAGES FOR FARM WORKERS!

TAKING PART IN COMMUNITY ACTIVITIES

increasing freedom from sexual exploitation. But the process was not easy. When the disabled people recognized their need for and the possibility of love relationships and a sexual life, there was a flurry of sexual activity, which created a scandal in the community. The disabled people went through a process of liberation, in the course of which some disabled girls were taken advantage of. Several of the older women and girls became very concerned, as did some of the more conscientious young men. They held meetings in search of a solution; and gradually established a relatively liberal set of rules, along with measures that protected young girls, at the same time ensuring an environment where positive and beneficial relationships could blossom. Young girls were able to get counselling and guidance from older girls and women.

FULL PARTICIPATION AND EQUALITY

Disabled people have wrought many changes in Ajoya through their full participation in community life. For example, they encouraged store-keepers to build ramps into their stores so that people in wheel-chairs and wheel-gurneys could gain easy entrance. When a couple of store-keepers still had not constructed ramps, the disabled persons boycotted them and organized other community members to join the boycott until the ramps were built. Disabled persons have developed an increasing sense of empowerment. Today, even the cinema and the central plaza have ramps. They are a clear testimony of the integral part that disabled people are playing in all community activities.

Part of the physical integration of disabled people into the community was accomplished by building smooth walkways to Project PROJIMO premises. The project is located at the edge of town and used to be connected only by a sandy rock trail, not practical for wheel-chair riders. One weekend several years ago, the entire community joined together to lay down a network of cement walkways overnight. Last year when these walks began to crack and break down, the municipal presidency came in and rebuilt them, evidence that not only the community but regional authorities are also beginning to recognize the rights of disabled persons.

For Mexico this is only the beginning. Much more needs to be done to give disabled people rights and equality within communities. In North America and much of Europe disabled people have more rights, better access to buildings and transportation, more job opportunities and so on, not only because of the goodwill of governments or of people but because disabled people have organized and demanded these rights. They have lain down in the middle of roadways, climbed on their knees up the steps of post-offices, and actively protested in other ways until the public responded. Similar organized action is necessary in every community where disabled people and their families are denied their rights. Interestingly, when these rights are finally won, the whole community takes great pride and pleasure in the accomplishments of their disabled citizens, as well as in their assimilation into community activities.

PROVIDING CARE FOR ALL DISABILITIES

The disease spectrum causing disability in western Mexico is typical of many developing countries. For instance, polio is still the most common disability in western Mexico. However, in the population of about 15 000

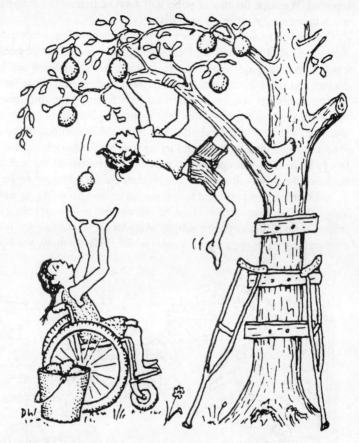

As much as possible, disabled children should get their exercise in ways that are useful and enjoyable.

covered by the Piaxtla primary health care programme, there have been only two cases of paralytic polio in the last 20 years. In contrast, children disabled by polio have been brought to PROJIMO in great numbers from surrounding areas and now total 240. Ironically, as the word has spread about the programme, we have seen more and more city children (mainly from slums) coming to the village with their families. The records of PRO-JIMO and other community rehabilitation programmes in western Mexico indicate that the incidence of paralytic polio is still far higher than officially reported. We hope the day of polio will soon be behind us, eliminating so much unnecessary suffering and disability.

Cerebral palsy follows closely behind polio and is often accompanied by multiple disabilities—hearing, visual and mental as well as physical. Epilepsy is another major problem. Many children with epilepsy are taken to doctors and receive standard treatment prescriptions with little follow-up. Their convulsions continue. Placed on high doses of the drug phenytoin, they often develop hypertrophy of the gums until their teeth cannot even be seen, and yet they still have fits. The PROJIMO team has become quite expert in evaluating epilepsy and trying alternative medicines, helping the family to decide—through an experimental approach—on the best medications and the proper doses to deal with their child's recurring seizures.

Another common problem is spinal cord injury (including *spina bifida*). Tragically, the commonest cause of spinal cord injury is bullet wounds among teenagers and young adults. Many of these injuries are related to drug-trafficking in the mountain areas which, unfortunately, has been pro-

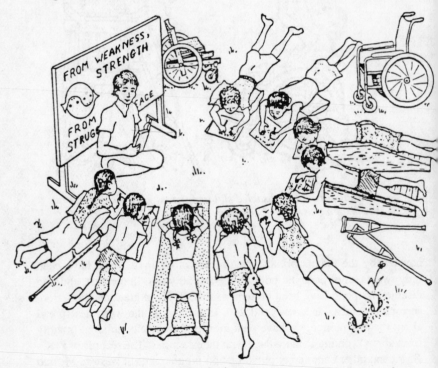

Disabled people are often the best and most understanding teachers.

moted in part by the very soldiers who are waging the so-called 'war on drugs'. The soldiers often supply the seed, take a cut of the profits from drug harvests, and sometimes beat up those who refuse to grow drugs. Not a few of the bullet wounds causing spinal cord injuries are inflicted by the soldiers or police.

Typically, in under-developed countries persons with spinal cord injury do not live more than a year or two. They die either from pressure sores or urinary tract infections. Usually pressure sores develop in hospital and patients are sent home with no instructions on how to treat or prevent them. Many have no place else to go for help and their sores and infections worsen steadily until they die.

As the word got out that PROJIMO was not only providing treatment for pressure sores and urinary infections but also helping people to develop bowel control and urinary care, and providing overall rehabilitation, including skills-training and work opportunities, people with spinal cord injuries began to arrive from all over the country. Almost 200 paraplegic and quadriplegic young people have been treated.

Some stay for months or years with the programme, learning skills such as wheel-chair making, brace-making and counselling other disabled people. Some have entered the programme on the edge of death; often they have learned skills while lying on their wheel-gurneys, remaining active while their pressure sores heal slowly over many months. For the most part they go about their work exuding good spirit and encouragement to others. Some have assumed a leadership role in the programme.

The PROJIMO team sees children with a very wide range of disabilities, including less common problems such as muscular dystrophy. In quite a few cases their families have gone from doctor to doctor, as the child's health worsens continually. One family came to PROJIMO after reading the chapter on muscular dystrophy in our book, *Disabled Village Children*. They explained that up to that point they had used half their family income on doctors and a wide range of prescription medicines. Nothing was working.

The village team discouraged all medication as it is useless for muscular dystrophy. This saved the family an enormous amount of money which they used instead to provide their child with education and other opportunities. The PROJIMO team encouraged the family to help the child draw and use his hands and to get him into a school. They also adapted a wheel-chair to the child's needs so that he could use his hands more effectively and interact more positively with other children as well as his family.

We have found that, no matter how severe the problem, there is always

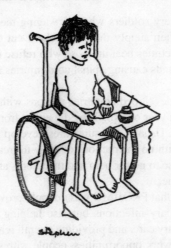

something that can be done. In the process of doing something, not only the disabled person but his family and community feel better and in greater control over their situation.

From the beginning, the programme has been a rural one. It has focused largely on physical disability in response to the felt need within a physically-oriented, farming community. In a rural setting a mentally slow child or one with Down's syndrome is not really that out of place. He can learn to do physical, repetitive jobs like carrying water or working in a field, getting along quite well and contributing to his family's needs. In this setting it is the physically-handicapped child—who cannot walk on steep mountain paths or help with physically-demanding farm work—who is often isolated and perhaps left in a corner for his brief life. In the cities the opposite is true: the mentally-disabled child is at a greater disadvantage. An urban setting may place very few physical demands on the child, but if he is unable to read, write and do other tasks that require thought, he will suffer a great deal.

Whatever the situation, the role of other disabled persons as care-takers can be critical to success. Sometimes nothing more is required than helping the whole family learn how to cope with a disabled child. At times it may be enough to work with neighbours to set up a support system in which people from the community take turns at watching the child, allowing the family (usually the mother) to take care of their other needs. Families and their friends, when they understand the problem, can do much to solve it.

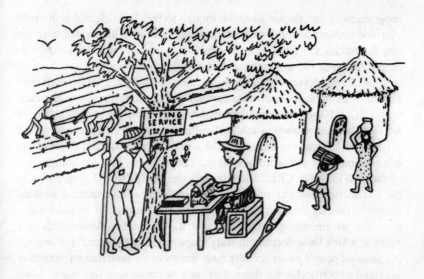

In a village, skills learned through schooling can be important for the disabled person.

RELATING TO THE STATE

People often ask us about the relationship between the villager-run programme and government health and rehabilitation services. When PROJIMO began a decade ago there were no rehabilitation facilities in our state (Sinaloa). Two or three years later, however, a new national programme called 'The Centre for Rehabilitation and Special Education' (CREE) was opened in the capital city. Fortunately the young director of this programme did not view PROJIMO as a threat because it was run by non-professionals, but came to visit the programme and was impressed by it. He began to bring his own trainees and therapists to visit PROJIMO and to exchange ideas with the disabled workers. He said this helped his workers understand the importance of listening to the ideas of disabled people on how to solve their own problems. After these visits the PROJIMO village workers were invited in turn to visit the government centre, 150 miles away. Later the director of CREE contracted the PROJIMO team to make prostheses, orthopaedic appliances, braces, calipers, wheel-chairs and other aids for the government programme.

The Mexican government is faced with very limited resources as the country has been going through a severe economic crisis. Rehabilitation programmes often do not have the money to buy the aids and equipment disabled children and others need, although facilities are available in the city for making this equipment. The private brace and limb shops charge so much that even the government and middle-class families cannot afford their products. Moreover, the quality is often not good despite the high cost. For this reason the government programme has continued making contracts with PROJIMO to produce the necessary equipment. These contracts have boosted the programme towards self-sufficiency, and they have represented a vote of confidence in the team. The workers have gained a sense of accomplishment, of self-worth and of the value of what they are doing.

Not too long ago CREE tried to replicate the PROJIMO programme in the 13 counties (districts) of the state. It went as far as encouraging disabled people to take on local leadership. Unfortunately in spite of its good intentions the government programme found it very hard to decentralize to a point at which local people felt truly empowered and 'owned' the project. As disabled people never actually took charge of the government centres or accepted responsibility for them, they have not been very successful. None the less something is happening, and the government has not abandoned its efforts. At one point the director of CREE very much wanted to incorporate PROJIMO as one of his district programmes. He met with our team members to encourage them to come under government auspices. He offered salaries three times as high as those they were earning. In a group meeting, the team decided by consensus to forego this offer, preferring their independence and autonomy. However, they did agree happily to continue close collaboration with the government programme in other ways.

HEALTH FOR *ALL*

Today in various parts of Mexico several programmes are emerging and growing, inspired by PROJIMO's example. Each has its own distinct approach to meeting local needs and dealing with local situations. In the city of Mazatlán a programme has developed which places much greater emphasis on special education for mentally disabled children. This group has set up special classes at a local prep school after normal working hours. It also makes a trip to PROJIMO every few weeks, partly as an exchange with the village programme but also to learn more about making braces and other aids, counselling and developing other skills. The name '*Los Pargos*' was chosen by the children in the programme. *Pargo* is the name of a colourful fish—much of the funding for the programme comes from the sale of artificial flower arrangements made from fish scales! The children in the project make the arrangements with help from their parents and sell them in the tourist city of Mazatlán. So far, they have done quite well.

In the city of Culiacán, the capital of Sinaloa, a different programme arose after two disabled men from that city went to PROJIMO for their own rehabilitation. The two were so impressed that they decided to start their own programme upon returnung home. Their first step was to organize a group of people and take them to PROJIMO. They stayed there for about three months, learning skills in wheel-chair and brace-making as well as other aspects of rehabilitation. Today the Más Válidos project is able to provide counselling, simple physical therapy and a wide range of aids, including braces, standing frames, special seats and wheel-chairs for those with disabilities. Recently they held a meeting with a group of speech therapists from the US to evaluate the needs of children with speech and hearing disability and learn how to serve them. The majority of the workers at Más (more) Válidos are themselves disabled, lending appropriateness to the group's name. 'Más válidos' was chosen in response to the term *minus válidos*, which is often used to describe disabled people. *Minus válidos* means 'less valuable'. The workers at Más Válidos ('more valid') are proving in many ways that disabled people can do more for other human beings than the majority of able-bodied people.

Programmes modelled after PROJIMO have also started in the states of Oaxaca, Michoacán, and Jalisco. The basic idea of people helping themselves has also produced spin-off programmes focusing on other needs. For example *Campamentos Unidos* is a programme in Mexico run by young architects. Their purpose is to help people who were left homeless after the 1985 earthquake to rebuild their houses. Over time they have expanded their focus to include primary health care, and now also disability. A young doctor, himself paralysed by polio, is a leader in that programme.

PROJIMO has even influenced people and programmes beyond Mexico: in Nepal, Philippines, Mozambique, South Africa, Angola, Nicaragua, Colombia, India and Pakistan. Projects all over the world use our books and adapt our methods and ideas, though we have no way of listing them or knowing who they are. In Central America UNICEF has helped to organize study visits to PROJIMO by people involved in community health programmes and rehabilitation efforts. This has provided important interchange. We have frequent exchanges with Nicaragua where there are new programmes and some of our trainees are helping the many people disabled by war in that unfortunate country.

A new income-generating programme provides work for extensively disabled persons, at the same time promoting lively interchange between disabled people and activists in community health from other countries. This is an intensive, Spanish-language training programme which invites disabled persons, rehabilitation activists and those concerned with progressive people-centred health care from English-speaking (or other language) cultures to spend time learning Spanish. The instructors are disabled people from PROJIMO, mainly young persons who are quadriplegic. Although they have difficulty doing physical work, they earn incomes through this programme—and contribute meaningfully to health for others.

Around the world, at least in part as a result of our booklets, drawings and the book *Disabled Village Children*, there are many projects starting to incorporate disability programmes into primary health care activities. Up to now, disability has been kept separate like dentistry or an unusual specialty, but it is important that there should be full integration so that primary health care workers can understand disability and the role that disabled people can play. Few people have realized the extensive contribution that can be made to broad-based PHC programmes by incorporating disabled persons as part of the health team and as full members of the community.

PROJIMO has taught us that disabled people are indeed an enabling part of community health, an integral part of the human family in any community, who often can participate more fully than those without disability. To include them in village programmes not only heightens their dignity, self-respect and quality of life, but also completes the concept of Health for All.

Reference

1. Werner, D. (1987). *Disabled village children—A guide for community health workers, rehabilitation workers, and families.* The Hesperian Foundation, Palo Alto, California.

CHAPTER 6

Participation, Poverty and Violence: Health and Survival in Latin America

FRITS MULLER

The author chronicles the difficult choices faced by five Latin American communities in which participation and action have often resulted in political backlashes and repression. In the three countries in which these 'cases' are situated—Peru, Colombia and Guatemala—community struggle for equitable development is occurring amidst growing poverty and violence.*

Frits Muller, Ph.D., M.D., worked in Peruvian villages from 1972 until 1977. He returned ten years later to study the progress of primary health care in Peru, Colombia and Guatemala. He now works as a primary health care consultant based in Holland.

POVERTY AND DEVELOPMENT, 1977–87

Peru, Colombia and Guatemala suffer from deep economic, social and cultural disparities. These social divisions grew even deeper between 1977 and 1987. The extreme inequality in chance for work, land, housing, income and health is the basic reason for increasing violence and guerrilla warfare in these three countries. Disparity also discredits governments, leading to a power vacuum which is being filled by national armies, drug mafias and other anti-democratic forces.

In addition to the existing inequalities, these countries suffered an economic crisis in the 1980s. All three experienced moderate economic growth initially but suffered severe setbacks between 1982 and 1985. Per capita output in Latin America as a whole, with the possible exception of Colombia, fell by 6.5 per cent between 1980 and 1988.[1] This economic crisis increased inequalities even further (Table 1).

*This chapter presents a summary of case studies made in 1977 (described in Practising Health for All) and again, in the same communities, in 1987, which are described in a new book: Poverty, Participation and Health: Latin American Case Studies, by Frits Muller, Antioguia University Press, Medellin, Colombia, 1991.

Table 1. Income distribution in Peru, Colombia and Guatemala[2-4]

	1975	1985
Peru: Per cent of national income taken by the richest 10 per cent	58	62
Guatemala: Per cent of national income taken by richest 20 per cent	47	57
Colombia: Per cent living in absolute poverty	45	43

It is clear that the past decade has seen not only the persistence of poverty but also a worsening in several countries, e.g. Peru and Guatemala, where more than half of the population lives in poverty. Also, averages are obscuring the important pockets within countries where both economics and health have deteriorated.

DEVELOPMENTS IN HEALTH

According to official national statistics health improved between 1977 and 1987. The overall infant mortality rate in Peru decreased from 110 to 99 per 1000 live births, in Colombia from 65 to 50 and in Guatemala from 95 to 70.[5] However, gross inequalities remained in mortality, morbidity, fertility and the use of health services. For example, the IMR in Peru in 1988 was said to be 88, while it was 134 in the poor area of Huancavelica.[6] In Colombia the IMR of children born to mothers with six years of education was 34 in 1981, while it was 92 for illiterate mothers.[7] In Guatemala the children of the poor had twice as many bouts of diarrhoea (667 per 1000 in the 14 days preceding the interview) as middle class children (365/1000).[8] In these 'pockets of health poverty', statistics indicate deterioration during recent years, especially in the cases of slum areas and high-risk groups. In the department of Narino, Colombia, the IMR went up from 114 in 1976 to 125 in 1983.[9] In the poor Andean province of Canas, Peru, the IMR went up from 166 to 199 in the same period.[10]

Not all changed for the worse. Some preventive health programmes that were supported over the years in Latin America were successful in increasing coverage and thus probably in reducing disease. For example, coverage of under-ones with DPT, polio and measles vaccination increased dramatically between 1975 and 1990 (Table 2).

Table 2. Per cent coverage of children under one year with
DPT immunization, 1975–90[8,11]

Country	1975	1980	1989	1990
Peru	19	28	57	72
Colombia	9	54	75	87
Guatemala	?	49	51	66

To better understand the significance of these economic and health changes in Latin America, I studied six projects in rural and urban areas, two in each of the three countries of Peru, Colombia and Guatemala, during the year 1977 and again a decade later in 1987. Following a brief description of the programmes in five of these six areas, this chapter analyses the changing health profiles of the poor in Latin America, paying specific attention to progress in primary health care and its implications for 'reaching health for all' in these countries.

RURAL PERU: QUISPICANCHIS

Quispicanchis is a rural Andean province of Peru with altitudes between 3500 metres (valleys) and over 6000 metres (*nevada* peaks). Of the 80 000 inhabitants, about 80 per cent are Quechua-speaking Indians, the rest *mestizo* (of mixed Indian and Spanish blood). The *mestizo* group lives in villages, dominating bureaucracy, trade and transport; the Indians live in scattered communities.

Daily life in the countryside is characterized by a struggle to survive. Small plots of land, one or two acres per family, are worked intensively to produce mostly potatoes, some wheat and corn. All families keep some animals: llamas and sheep being their capital. As the land does not produce enough to feed a family and provide for their needs, most men (50 to 70 per cent) leave temporarily in search of paid jobs. They find work either in the Amazonian jungle (gold-washing) or in the cities (carrying loads).

Social and health conditions are poor. Less than 30 per cent of adult men and 10 per cent of adult women can read and write. Infant mortality is around 200 per 1000 births. Common health problems are respiratory infections, diarrhoea, tuberculosis, obstetric difficulties and accidents.

The survival strategies of these communities include their traditional system of health care. There is a network of traditional healers who specialize in reconciling patients with their ancestors and the gods. Other healers, largely 'empirical', specialize in herbal treatments, bone-setting and deliveries (traditional birth attendants). Another important survival strategy is an elaborate system of barter trade and mutual aid. The whole community meets frequently to discuss common problems. However, there is also a lot of strife between families, and old disputes flare up on nights of heavy drinking and special festive occasions.

Western health care was introduced into the region in the 1960s through the sale of drugs in shops and markets and through the governmental health centre and health posts (eventually nine in number). The major service provided by these health facilities was to issue official documents registering births, marriages and deaths. In general, the health services were distrusted. Only when an especially-dedicated and sensitive health worker was assigned to one of these facilities did the traditional population begin to use these modern health services.

In 1974 a health centre team comprising a doctor, a nurse and two auxiliaries tried to improve the official health services and their responsiveness to community need. Linking their activities with the work of a team of Jesuit priests who practised the 'Theology of Liberation',* they trained rural school-teachers as village health workers (VHWs) and later some additional 40 chosen community members as VHWs. The initial VHW training lasted for two weeks. Emphasis was given to supervision: once every six weeks personally on the spot and once every three months in inter-village meetings of two to three days. All VHWs were volunteers. The community received health equipment worth US $100, and each VHW an initial stock of 12 drugs (worth $50). Prices were discussed by the community and established in order to allow repurchase of necessary items through a revolving fund. Curative activities formed the basis of initial work, as it is not possible to preach prevention when infant mortality is 200 per 1000 births and no other sources of medical care are available. Preventive work followed later with protection of wells, introduction of vegetable gardens and health education. By 1977 some 9000 people had been added to the 18 000 already having access to some health services including first aid, essential drugs, health education and sanitation. The costs were low, with an initial

*In the Theology of Liberation, liberation is not supposed to wait until heaven. Liberation is first of all, here and now, liberation from misery and oppression. Therefore, priests will not only preach Christianity, but also work with their people towards a better economic and social fate.

investment of $0.70 per capita per year and running costs of $0.60 per capita per year. The success of the programme was dependent on the presence of caring and charismatic health workers in the health centre.

By 1987 the health infrastructure had increased. An additional health centre was built and the number of health personnel had doubled. The output of services, however, varied. On the one hand, curative care diminished from 6500 to only 2600 consultations per year at one health centre. On the other, preventive programmes extended their coverage, including immunization (from 15 to 40 per cent coverage of under-threes), school lunches (from zero to almost all rural schools) and well-baby clinics (zero to 815 clinical examinations per year).

About 20 of the 40 originally-trained VHWs were still serving as volunteers; in some cases, sons of former VHWs had taken their place. The VHWs had maintained their work in spite of periods in which the health services showed no interest in them. To survive they had 'commercialized' the sale of drugs. This enabled them to repurchase drugs which they used and serve the major felt needs of the community. The attitude of the health service staff in 1987 was rather critical. They had meetings with VHWs every month and they provided them with drugs, but they engaged more in control as supervisors than in support as medical colleagues. VHWs were seen as particularly useful in organizing the yearly immunization campaigns.

While this case study illustrates how local health services can flourish under a caring staff, it also shows that 'improvement' in health service quality by the addition of professional staff may easily lead to the alienation of communities and a fall in health services. When it was ensured that village health workers could respond to local demand, in this case for curative services, they continued their work despite years of neglect or outright abandonment by health service personnel. They remained active in helping services such as immunization, achieve important results. A continued, close working relationship between the health services and VHWs might have advanced health and social development even further.

URBAN PERU: VILLA EL SALVADOR

Villa el Salvador is an outstanding case of urban primary health care. Its development was strongly participatory and amply demonstrates the ups and downs of this approach.

Villa was born of an illegal invasion of Church-owned land in 1971. After a week of conflict, negotiations and an outright fight between the people and the authorities, the police and the army transported some 5000 people to a piece of desert, some ten miles out of the centre of Lima, and settled them there. From the very beginning there was tension between the organizations representing the local people and the state. The government had a strong populist appeal and wanted to support Villa el Salvador, partly out of solidarity with the needs of its population and partly to make Villa a showcase of slum development. On the other hand, they also wanted to control the politically-active population living there.

Government officials had laid out a plan for eventually harbouring 125 000 people in the desert. The planning started with carving out individual plots, 6×15 metres in dimension. Twenty-four plots made up an 'apple', 16 apples one 'group', and a varied number of groups one 'sector'. In December 1971, eight months after the original resettlement, there were 70 000 inhabitants; in 1976 there were 123 000; and in 1984 there were 186 000 inhabitants in Villa.

There were many urgent needs to be attended to by the people themselves. For security they organized watch groups. Meals were prepared collectively by groups of women ('common pots'). Water had to be bought from tankers and carried a mile or more through the deep desert sand. Schools were built from reed-mats (as were the houses) and volunteers started teaching. In health, unused drugs were collected house-to-house by a person chosen to be responsible for health. Special collections were organized to raise money for a clinic and a doctor. In this way, spontaneous and popular organizations were born around the issues of security, food, education and health, the basic needs. Committees were formed in every 'apple' and people were chosen to be responsible for each of the tasks described.

In the first General Assembly, a meeting of community leaders in November 1973, two competing models of social organization were proposed. The state officials promoted the idea of cooperative groups based on membership and contributions. The popular organizations, however, promoted the idea of neighbourhood organizations aimed at the complete self-sufficiency of Villa el Salvador. The latter concept won and thus, CUAVES, the Urban Community of Self-sufficiency, Villa el Salvador, was formed. This organization, with representatives from the smallest neighbourhoods called 'apple-groups', proved to be the real force of change. By 1976 a community bank, managed by CUAVES, was financing public works, including water, electricity and small community-owned enterprises. Community hardware shops provided cheap building materials.

The original health committees had reached an understanding with volunteer doctors and nurses from San Marcos University to start a health project to train and provide a network of Village Health Workers rather than of clinics and doctors. Approved by the People's Assembly in 1973, the first task of the VHWs was to monitor health through monthly home-visits and to provide first-aid. Furthermore, they cooperated with health staff in immunization efforts and organized the burning of waste. With around US $20 000 of community money, a community health centre-cum-pharmacy was built. Volunteer professionals held their clinics here—totalling some 12 000 consultations in 1976. In 1977 there were 60 VHWs actively collaborating with the community health centre. Nine TBAs were trained but were later lost to the programme. Some 60 school-teachers were also trained in primary health care. Still, with such a large population to serve, only 10 000 people received curative services in 1977, a mere 7 per cent of the community. The whole project relied exclusively on volunteers and the money needed (about $1000 per month for running costs) was raised locally. The community-based health survey implemented in 1974 showed that only 15 per cent of adults had a stable job, 5 per cent of the houses were decently constructed and one public tap served 75 houses. The infant mortality rate was estimated at 60 per 1000. The most frequent diseases were diarrhoea and dehydration, skin diseases and fever. Between 1978 and 1983 the community organization fell apart and the health project all but stopped. The reasons were not specific to the health sector. Indeed, one could even say that the health sector kept the community organization alive for a time. Initial basic needs: water, roads, transport, markets, shops had been satisfied. As private doctors began to settle in the area people took less interest in community activities and tended to look after their own personal and family needs. The need for social organization diminished. Moreover, small left-wing political parties were by now dominating local politics, each claiming certain sections of the population and thus setting one group against the other. A similar effect was caused by the 'invasion' of Villa by non-governmental organizations. While they provided badly-needed services, each also practised its own ideas in health and claimed its own followers and loyalties, thus undermining community solidarity. Lastly, the political climate had changed: the new government did not support the slum community.

Technically, the management of a variety of community services faltered for a lack of management experience and support. The community bank and other services eventually had to close. The community health centre was also closed between 1979 and 1982, although some VHWs continued their work at home, still being supervised and supported by professional staff from the community, acting as volunteers. The decline of community participation and services between 1978 and 1983 was eventually reversed by a new participatory surge. This revitalized spirit was kindled by the original settlers who, feeling that they had lost control over Villa's destiny to political parties and competing NGOs, led a resurgence of self-help. This was further catalysed by the declining levels of living of the poor, caused by liberal governmental economic policies and decreased social budgets. Liberal price policies after 1978 had caused prices of basic food commodities and transport to rise. These changes were felt earlier and more intensely by the urban poor than by the rural poor. Their effects were shown in a second health survey carried out by CUAVES in 1984, ten years after the first one. People were poorer than in 1974. Prices of primary products had gone up 1542 per cent while salaries had risen only 881 per cent. More important, about 20 per cent of the families interviewed said they had to live on $20 per month, and the average family income was only $70. This clearly showed the extent of pockets of poverty within the urban slum.

The crude birth rate was 41 per 1000, and the IMR 63 per 1000, about the same as ten years earlier. Thirteen per cent of children under-five were malnourished (under 75 per cent of the standard), while in 1974 malnutrition was virtually unknown. Accidents at work caused 13 per cent of the mortality in Villa in 1984, and tuberculosis 6 per cent.

The reconstruction of the CUAVES health project was based firstly on the revitalization of CUAVES itself. Door-to-door campaigning led to a newly-elected CUAVES board which picked up many themes of struggle. The most important one was creating an 'industrial park' for small-scale industries. The community clinic was reopened and a new health plan was drawn with the main purpose of unifying official health services and the many (more than ten) NGO health projects under CUAVES leadership. By 1987 more than 100 VHWs were again active in Villa. Health made an important contribution to the rebirth of community organization in Villa.

In 1982 the municipal government of Lima started a programme called 'a glass of milk a day'. Hundreds of women's committees were formed to implement the programme. In Villa alone there were 160 committees in 1984. They soon dealt with issues other than the daily glass of milk: education, health and local elections. 'Glass of milk' and a parallel programme of soup kitchens run for 20 to 100 women comprised the urban slum nutrition programme. Thus the medium of food aid created and supported strong population-based organizations which eventually became a political power in themselves. This led to the birth of a series of feminist NGOs from

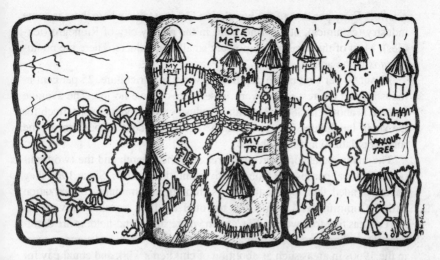

Initially united by adversity, people participated less as basic needs were met and politicized. Economic crisis brought a new sense of solidarity and mutual assistance.

among the popular organizations running nutrition programmes within the urban slum—a feminization of social participation.

The experience of participation in Villa provides an important example of the forces which underlie participatory development in primary health care. The original threat to survival was the main force in creating participation which extended beyond the health sector. The decline resulted from the satisfaction of individual basic needs, politicization and the invasion of well-meaning but nonetheless competing NGOs. The rebirth of participation was provoked by the economic crisis and fuelled by the sense of identity as a community which the people gained during their original success in overcoming substantial adversity. The importance of continued dialogue, ownership and of a shared purpose in this experience is a reminder that participatory primary health care requires constant leadership, vision and nurturing.

COLOMBIA: EL CARMEN DE VIBORAL

El Carmen is a rural municipality of 25 000 inhabitants in the eastern part of the Department of Antioquia, Colombia. The population is *mestizo* or

criollo.* Forty per cent of the population live in a town where there is some
industry (ceramics); others find work in the nearby city of Rionegro (tex-
tiles). Most of the rural population are small-landholders. There are no *ha-
ciendas* in the area.

About 50 per cent of the population works in agriculture, 25 per cent in
industry, and the rest either work in services or have no job. The average
income is about US $80 per month in industry and about twice as much for
the small-landholder. The poor are the landless (about 10 per cent of the
rural population) and the jobless.

The main social forces in rural areas are the Church and the two traditional political parties, the Conservatives and the Liberals. Since 1962 they
have extended their political favours through a community organization
called Community Action. The national landless peasant movement,
ANUC, has few followers in El Carmen where small land-holders are dominant. The urban workers are organized into unions which had some success
in the 1960s in areas such as abolition of children's work and equal pay for
women. The unions have been weakened by the system increasingly used
by industry of contracting workers for only one year. At present 80 per cent
of workers are contracted in this manner which does not allow for unioni-
zation.

Health conditions are relatively good, with an IMR of about 60 per 1000.
Cardiovascular disease is the first cause of death. By 1986 homicide had
reached second place, responsible for 9 per cent of overall mortality, though
it did not appear among the first ten causes of death in 1977.

A health project was started in 1975, supported by the Medellin School
of Public Health. It was originally an attempt to integrate the services of the
Ministry of Health with those of the Social Security agency which served
about 10 per cent of the population—the regularly employed. The health
needs of the population and their active participation in shaping the health
services were considered the basic forces for this integration. The School of
Public Health which had many teachers interested in promoting and practising primary health care was in charge of coordinating and stimulating the
project. No external funds have been involved at any time.

The project contributed to the local health services by training Village
Health Workers. Twenty-two young women were given six weeks of initial
training in 1975. The better ones surveyed their communities and drew a
map, performed periodic home visits (about 30 per month), provided first-
aid and attended patients with acute and chronic diseases (about 75 per

*Of mixed Spanish and Indian origin or of purely Spanish origin.

month). They participated in selective programmes, especially EPI and diarrhoea control. Although they started as volunteers, they quickly pressured the health services to pay them and, not long after a strike, they began to receive the minimum wage. They soon became employees representing the local health services rather than representatives of their own communities as had been envisaged originally. Not only did the VHWs wish to join the formal health system, but the system also pressed for professionalization. As the system demanded that VHWs perform a broad range of functions, they wished to improve their skills. In 1987 the Regional Health Director said that he wanted only women with two or three years of secondary schooling, and that they would be trained initially for six months! Thus, the institutionalization of the VHW as the lowest rank in the health services has deprived communities of their own responsive spokesperson. This has also happened in the rest of Colombia where, by 1987, some 5000 VHWs were contracted under similar conditions.

However, the community has participated in the project in a broader way. Locally-chosen *Responsables de Salud* met with local health authorities for a dialogue on local needs and on utilization of health institutions. This participatory board formed an effective bridge between the communities and the health services, resulting in more effective utilization of existing facilities and more responsive policies in the health services. The board discussed issues such as having more convenient hours for clinics, home visiting, complaints about staff and the lack of drugs, and solved several problems. The improved contact between the communities and health services led to a substantial increase in consultations, which doubled in only three years, and to rapid improvement in preventive programmes. The health team itself became democratized and responded not only to decisions from the Director and the Ministry of Health but also to their own perceptions of community needs which emerged from dialogue with the community on the means to improve health care.

However, political changes in Colombia led the Social Security authorities to withdraw from the project after two years. The local health services and now-active communities were both interested in pursuing the main lines of action: participation in health care services through the *Responsables de Salud* and a Health Committee working to respond to the felt needs of the community. After only three years, these participatory aspects of the programme gradually disappeared, although collaboration continued until 1980 when key project persons left and the School of Public Health lost interest.

Previously permanent health-care staff were now changed on an annual basis, with doctors performing only their required 'rural year' of social service before leaving to practise. In this way they had little contact or commitment to the community. One day in 1980, a newly-named director literally put a lock on the door to keep community representatives outside the hospital. Thus the *Responsables* disappeared as they had no formal role. Their participation and influence depended only on the good-will of health-care staff. In that same year, the participatory board was dismissed. Long afterwards in 1987, the board was replaced by a committee representing different social institutions (Church, schools, etc.) but not the community themselves.

The experience of El Carmen shows how primary health care can be generated within existing health services by an inspiring outside influence, in this case the Medellin School of Public Health. The approach led to a doubling of health services in three years. However, the extent of community participation depended on the goodwill of the present staff, and once this changed, participation became an empty phrase.

GUATEMALA: CHICHICASTENANGO

Guatemala is a beautiful country of eight million, mainly rural, inhabitants. Sixty per cent of them are Indian and most of them live in the mountains, the *altiplano*. The distribution of income, power and land is very skewed. A study by USAID mentions that 16 per cent of cultivable land in the country is owned by 90 per cent of the rural population. Sixty-five per cent of the best soil is owned by only 3 per cent. The mortality rate is 169 for infants born to illiterate mothers and 26 for infants born to mothers who have more than ten years of formal schooling.

Chichicastenango is an Indian rural *altiplano* municipality. Of its 1987 population of 64 000 only 6 per cent live in the capital, the rest in 65 rural communities. Eighty-five per cent of adults are illiterate and only 28 per cent of children go to school. Ninety-five per cent of the population work in agriculture as small-landholders or as day-labourers. Their incomes are not sufficient to feed most families. Therefore, the men generally go down to the coastal *fincas* (plantations) where coffee, rice and bananas periodically need labourers. There they earn about $1 a day. The people are deeply religious. Traditional beliefs and Catholicism are the major influences, although Protestant sects, mainly fundamentalist, are rapidly gaining ground in rural Guatemala. Some 60 denominations are estimated to have a membership of about 40 per cent of the Guatemalan population.

Social organization, originally strongly traditional, has weakened considerably during the last 25 years. A civil war raged across the countryside between 1978 and 1985, killing some 40 000 peasants country-wide. The militarization of the countryside resulted in new forms of local power, with armed self-defence patrols exercising nearly complete control over the communities. In 1983 about 300 000 armed men participated in these army-created and controlled patrols.

In Chichicastenango health conditions are poor. The infant mortality rate in 1977 was officially 81 per 1000 births, but might actually have been twice as high. Childhood malnutrition was widespread—between 60 and 80 per cent—and diarrhoea and acute respiratory infections took a heavy toll. Violence accounted for 17 per cent of deaths nationwide in 1981.

The one private 20-bed hospital in Chichi provides exclusively curative services for a fee. It operates outside the formal health services. The national primary health care project, started in 1974, had three main elements: introduction of Rural Health Technicians (RHT), training of Village Health Workers and Traditional Birth Attendants in rural areas, and promotion of preventive health.

The RHT received two years of training geared towards promoting rural health at the community level. Using motorbikes, RHTs visited all the communities in their charge regularly. They improved the availability of potable water and trained local volunteer promoters who collaborated with the immunization campaigns. They were the main outreach from Health Centres into communities, and represented community interests to the health services. In addition, some 80 VHWs were trained between 1974 and 1978 to provide simple curative services on demand. They organized health meetings in their villages, gave health education talks, and were supposed to refer patients to the Health Centre, though they generally treated them themselves.

Indians were not treated well in the Health Centre and they preferred to care for their health problems at home. Traditional Birth Attendants were also given training for ten days and received a UNICEF delivery kit for their work. After their course, the relation between TBAs and the Health Centre quickly deteriorated as the latter showed contempt for these 'uncultured women'. With each side literally speaking a different language, the initial training remained an isolated phenomenon.

By my return in 1987, much had changed in Chichicastenango. The civil war had devastated complete communities. Community leaders had fled the area or had been killed, and most communities were now controlled by army civil-defence patrols. The Rural Health Technicians ceased work between 1978 and 1985 except in the health centre itself. In 1986 they restarted their work, concentrating on concrete activities such as building rural water systems and rebuilding schools and roads.

By 1988 there was one health centre with a doctor, a nurse, ten auxiliaries and three Rural Health Technicians. There were seven rural dispensaries built in the 1970s as part of the PHC approach, all of which have been ransacked and some burned. None is functional today. Instead, five Health Posts were built with a loan from the Inter-American Development Bank, and each of them is staffed by an auxiliary nurse. Over the ten-year period, consultations with the doctor fell from 7000 to 1600 per year, but the ten auxiliaries undertook about 10 000 consultations in 1987, against only 400 in 1977. Thus, there seems to have been a deprofessionalization of medical consultation. In preventive programmes, coverage remained low, reflecting the deep breach in relations between the health services and communities, as a result of the civil war. In 1987 only 20 per cent of under-fours received

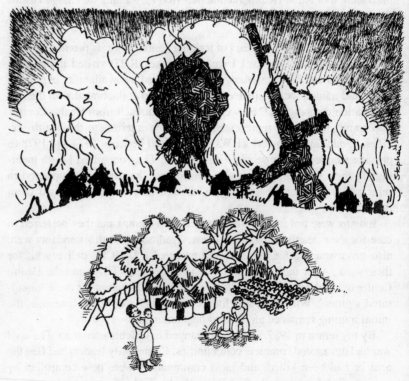

In the midst of violence health is a most elusive state.

DPT and polio whereas in 1977 immunization coverage had reached 70 per cent for the same vaccines. During the decade, distrust of the government led to substantial alienation and avoidance of all government institutions, including health services.

Only 12 of the 50 VHWs who were functioning in 1977 have remained. The rest either fled the area or were killed. The remaining VHWs gradually restarted their work, mainly along curative lines, and charged heavily for drugs, thus becoming self-sufficient. Now they do not feel they need the Health Centre any more. Meanwhile, 48 new VHWs have been trained by the Health Centre, most of them young men who play no leadership role in their communities. They are taught preventive health care rather than curative—immunization, oral rehydration, promotion of the use of latrines—and how to refer patients. They are mainly involved in these 'selective' programmes which make up most of the primary health care in Guatemala today. The TBAs, who had lost their contact with the Health Centre before the civil war broke out, continued their traditional work delivering babies, but some of them reached the extreme point of burying their UNICEF equipment for fear of being recognized as community leaders! Though training of TBAs restarted in Chichi in 1986, there is still no supervision and support for their work.

Chichicastenango provides an example of a nationwide, donor-supported primary health care effort that achieved little or no support at the local level. While minimal programme activities were carried out, certainly to some benefit, contact between VHWs, TBAs and the local health centre staff remained superficial. The civil war brought death and destruction, increasing the importance of VHWs and TBAs in the communities. As staffing of the government health centre increased, their service output actually decreased. The restructured programme of the last few years has placed major emphasis on preventive and selective programme interventions, much in line with international trends. This may be the best compromise for a system attempting to provide a minimum basic level of care without true community involvement and participation. The activities of VHWs and TBAs are certainly relevant and well appreciated.

GUATEMALA: CHIMALTENANGO

The Chimaltenango Health and Development Project (the Behrhorst project) is one of the oldest and best known Latin American primary health care projects. It started in 1962 and had a pioneering trajectory in which new approaches were discovered and tried with variable success. Since 1979 developments have been dramatic.

The province of Chimaltenango (with 285 000 inhabitants in 1988) is only marginally different from the Municipality of Chichicastenango, described earlier. The civil war of 1978–85 raged in Chimaltenango as in Chichi. As a result, in many communities there are between 50 and 100 widows and orphans today, a group at high risk in health.

Health conditions in Chimaltenango in the 1970s were very bad with an estimated infant mortality rate of 200 per 1000. By 1986 the IMR was estimated as 81 per 1000, on the basis of inaccurate official data. The main causes of death in children are said to be: acute respiratory infections (28 per cent), diarrhoea and dehydration (35 per cent), malnutrition (9 per cent) and other causes (29 per cent).

In 1977 health services consisted of one maternity clinic, eight government-run Health Centres, one Social Security Clinic and the Behrhorst clinic. There were six MDs in the province, four private practitioners and four private pharmacies. By 1986 these services had expanded considerably. At present the Government runs a 50-bed hospital and 12 health centres. The Social Security clinic is integrated with the hospital, as is the former Maternity Ward. The Behrhorst Clinic still exists and is functioning, but at a very low level. There are now 25 MDs in the city of Chimaltenango. On the main street I counted 21 private practitioners, eight private pharmacies, four private dentists and one private undertaker in 1988! Privatization is apparently taking hold quickly in Guatemalan health services.

The project of health and development was started by a young missionary doctor, Carroll Behrhorst, in 1962. Because the founder had a pervasive influence in the first 15 years of the project, it is usually called the 'Behrhorst project'. It started as a clinic providing curative health services to the poor in the central market of Chimaltenango. As there were few health services at the time, demand was great, and the possibility of one doctor being effective was limited. Thus in 1964, Behrhorst started training Village Health Workers. 'I wanted to multiply myself to be able to reach more people', he told me later. The VHWs, all men and not chosen by the community, worked along with Dr Behrhorst one day a week. They soon started practising medicine in their communities but continued to learn. In 1977 Behrhorst trained another group chosen by their communities as the community perspective was better appreciated by then.

By 1978 the project had expanded and developed a broad range of activities. There was a flourishing clinic with 20 000 out-patient consultations and 6000 hospitalizations a year. The 40 active VHWs, still being trained weekly and now supervised by the most experienced VHW, were treating between 25 and 35 thousand patients per year. The main focus of their work was curative and many had built their own community clinics. All of them had a relatively good income from their work, about $300 per month, eight times the minimum wage of that time. They were handling about 60 different drugs which they bought from a cooperative pharmacy functioning on a rotating fund. In addition they had initiated various community development projects which were of considerable value to the rural poor. For example, there was a land purchase project, a rural extension project, a water and sanitation project, and a Health Education and Nutrition project aimed mainly at women.

Since 1978 dramatic developments have overtaken the project. Increasing social polarization and the civil war forced the project to 'take sides'. The project's board was practically taken over by the national elite, and the project itself started working with both the *finqueros* (large landholders) and the army. It proved impossible to protect the community work at this time. All community-based programmes ceased to exist. Massive killings occurred in communities, forcing the VHWs to flee the area. In 1987 I found that ten VHWs had either been killed or had 'disappeared', one had died from natural causes, four had fled the country, 17 had dropped work and only eight VHWs were still active. Seven new VHWs had been trained, bringing the active total to 15. Such a disaster needs little further comment. After this devastating experience the project started its activities again only in 1983. Since Dr Behrhorst left in 1985, it has been under Guatemalan leadership. Productivity has remained low: only 6000 out-patient consultations by two doctors and 1400 hospitalizations in 1988. The work of the VHWs remains curative and the social and economic development activities in the community have been curtailed.

The Behrhorst Project demonstrates some important stages in the evolution of primary health care. Curative work came first as high rates of illness and death required care. Then, curative care was extended into communities, preventive care was included and, finally, community development with a health perspective was begun. However, the project could not withstand the external pressures which had led to the civil war and to army control. It broke down, leaving some VHWs to act commercially to maintain curative care, which they managed effectively. Sadly the project is now directed by the Guatemalan elite and has lost its social and liberating characteristics.

The 'one-man charismatic leadership' aspect imposed technical limitations on the project: no systematic MCH care was developed, and coordination with national authorities was always minimal. This led to rejection from the official side. Thus, the project illuminates both the potential and the serious limitation of charismatic leadership: the same power which opened so many perspectives for health care development limited its social impact and caused its dissolution under social and political stress. Today there is no social basis for the project, which has been left to the whims of the Guatemalan rich. No technical cadre was created that could take over from Dr Behrhorst when he left.

This project also raises the question of the vulnerability of VHWs and others trained in projects run by outsiders. We foreigners do not usually bear the risk, though we may be responsible for the vulnerability of these workers in difficult times. Perhaps the role of the foreigner is not so much to create institutions as to allow things to happen. There was and still is an obvious need for care, cure and prevention in the Guatemalan highlands. The project provided an effective solution, accepted by the people, and widely appreciated. Today some of the children of the original VHWs are carrying on the work. It is their choice and that of the communities they serve despite the blinding violence disrupting their society.

THE HEALTH PROFILE OF THE POOR

Overall, during the past decade, health indicators have improved in the countries studied. However, improvement seems to be concentrated among the better-off. Among the poor, health status has stabilized or even deteriorated. Socially-differentiated health statistics supported by data from my field studies in six communities show striking changes in the health profile of the poor in Latin America.

— Violence became a major cause of death. In El Carmen 9 per cent of deaths were caused by violence, the second cause of death for all ages in 1987. In Guatemala, violence alone accounted for 17 per cent of all deaths in 1981 although it had not been among the top ten causes in 1977. In Colombia, violence was not among the top ten causes of mortality in 1975. It rose to fifth place in 1981 and to third in 1988, with 18 000 victims (9 per cent of all deaths). Accidents at work caused 13 per cent of all adult deaths in Villa El Salvador in 1984.
— Poverty and poverty-related diseases increased. In Villa el Salvador clear-cut malnutrition did not exist in children under-five in 1974, while in 1984 13 per cent were malnourished.
— 'Development-related' diseases, such as acute intoxication with insecticides, increased. In the Andean province of Quispicanchis no insec-

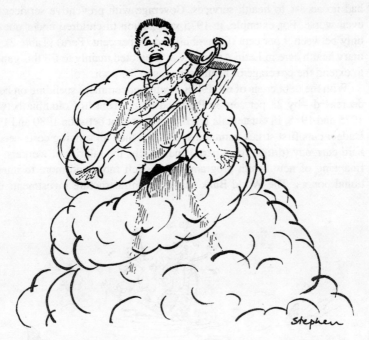

Aerial spraying and other uses of pesticides have become major threats to the lives of the poor.

ticides were used in 1977. In 1985, in only two villages, 21 children died of acute intoxication with insecticides. In rural Colombia crops are now 'cured' with pesticides ten times as frequently as in 1977. In one community of 40 families (La Chapa, Rionegro, Antioquia, Colombia), eight non-fatal cases of insecticide poisoning presented in adults in 1987, whereas there were none in 1977.

Although these data have a local character, they are supported by national statistics wherever these are socially-disaggregated, demonstrating the existence of 'pockets of health poverty' in health care development.

CHANGES IN HEALTH SERVICES

Health services in Peru, Colombia and Guatemala, already weak in the 1970s, suffered from the economic and political crises of the 1980s. In 1977 the three countries admitted that 30 per cent or more of their populations had no access to health services. Coverage with preventive services was even worse. For example, in 1975 vaccination of children under one was only between 9 per cent (Colombia) and 19 per cent (Peru) (Table 2). Primary health care in Latin America was promoted mainly to fill this gap and to extend the coverage of health services to the poor.

With the debt crisis of the 1980s, central government spending on health decreased—by 28 per cent in Peru and 58 per cent in Colombia between 1975 and 1985. In Guatemala it fell by 58 per cent between 1980 and 1985. Budget cuts first struck capital investments, then all running costs needing hard currency (drugs, spare parts) and, finally, the salaries of workers. The financing of new health programmes was left more and more to international donors. The World Bank supported infrastructure investments on a

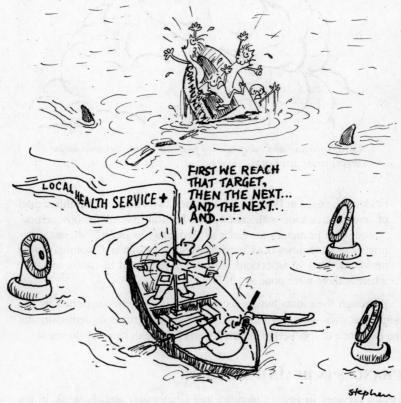

Encouraged by donors, health services have pursued performance targets, often to the exclusion of community concerns and participation.

large scale in Colombia and Peru, but withdrew when Peru's financial policy became unacceptable to the Bank in 1985. The Inter-American Development Bank financed new hospitals in Guatemala. In spite of decreased budgets, all governments employed more personnel between 1977 and 1987, increasing the percentage of spending on doctors and nurses.

During this time USAID, the World Bank, UNICEF and other donors became the main sources of finance for primary health care. Promoting the 'selective' approach, UNICEF and USAID financed child survival programmes mainly, including immunization and family planning. These efforts clearly did improve specific services in many communities in the countries under study. The best results were obtained in immunization (Table 2). All three countries studied changed their approach from the integrated, continuous immunization which was practised in the 1970s to vertical immunization campaigns in the 1980s. Though these were a medical success in terms of increasing coverage of children under one year, they did little, if anything, to promote a comprehensive development of local health services or participation. The same was true of efforts to control diarrhoea and acute respiratory infections. Thus, donor-financed PHC left little space for social mobilization or community participation.

The interests of the governments of these countries also did not promote participation. Dealing with popular unrest and increasing guerrilla warfare, the governments avoided community-oriented approaches. Meetings were seen as dangerous. In Guatemala, community meetings were completely forbidden between 1979 and 1985. In Colombia, the original Government Decree which demanded popular participation in local health boards was changed. Now an intersectoral representation in the board is sought which substitutes institutions such as scouts or Church for fully-responsive and elected community representation.

NGOs had to manoeuvre carefully in the field of primary health care. Where the concentration of NGOs was high, as in Villa el Salvador, Lima, Peru, there was a time when each NGO could develop its own programme independently. Participation thus was 'patronage', which bound entire populations to specific NGOs, rather than submitting the NGOs' work to the felt needs of their communities. Interestingly, in Villa the original popular organization, CUAVES, regained a degree of control, forcing the NGOs to cooperate in a local planning exercise in 1985. Among other things, this resulted in a distribution of tasks among the 'participating' NGOs. However, such an approach was not possible in rural Guatemala where the existing NGOs in health (some 150 of them) were forced either to make a deal with the military government (and stick to institutional health care as community work was ruled out), or to go underground.

Health promoters, a pioneering category in the 1970s, were either institutionalized, i.e. made government employees on a minimum wage, as in Colombia, or left entirely on their own to become 'privatized', as in Peru and Guatemala. In the latter country, a few of them were actually killed by the army (10 of the 40 in the Behrhorst project). The others disappeared and gradually reappeared to resume their curative work. With no support forthcoming, they commercialized their activities so as to become independent and self-supporting. This is an interesting phenomenon in itself: when properly trained and after years of supervision (as was the case in the Behrhorst project), VHWs apparently can make a living out of their curative work even in areas as poor as the Altiplano of Guatemala. The task is seen as so important that in various projects (Quispicanchis, Chichicastenango) one now meets a second generation of VHWs: the children of VHWs who have also become VHWs.

PARTICIPATION IN HEALTH

The acute economic crisis of the 1980s brought about a change in the pattern of participation in the projects studied throughout Latin America.

First of all, survival became a more urgent matter every year, in terms of income and food. Especially in the urban slums (e.g. Villa el Salvador), where people depend on a cash economy (in contrast with rural areas where people at least have access to their own harvest), development strategies moved away from collective goals and struggle to individual survival efforts. Thus, the informal economy blossomed at the expense of community participation.

On the other hand, food aid had different effects in different communities. The 'one glass of milk a day' programme in Villa el Salvador and the soup kitchens promoted social organization, especially among women, and reinforced their potential to solve their own problems. In rural areas of Peru the social effect of food aid was just the opposite. Women organized themselves into women's clubs with the exclusive aim of gaining access to food aid. Women were 'mobilized' to do the cooking and to distribute school lunches based completely on outside aid. Dependency was the rule. Participation was negatively affected.

The verticalization of primary health care was another factor influencing participation negatively. The two worlds of the community on the one hand and local health services on the other continued to grow apart. While communities were increasingly involved in daily survival, local health services were more and more occupied with meeting preset targets. Special training, conditional financing, separated registration and supervision decreased the 'community sensitiveness' of the health services. At one extreme in 1985, the health services in Ocongate (Quispicanchis, Peru) continued their concentration on food aid, diarrhoea control and immunization in the face of a devastating epidemic of acute insecticide poisoning about which they did nothing. At least 100 children died that year (nine in Pinchimuru and 13 in Pachhanta, two communities with a total of about 100 families). No preventive campaign was undertaken and Village Health Workers were questioned on whether they were doing their work in EPI and diarrhoeal disease control, rather than in supporting communities which were facing an epidemic of poisoning among children.

While there is no recipe for involvement, some of the lessons of these cases provide insights to effective and sustained community participation. Chances of participation are higher when a project provides services which are needed and wanted. An intersectoral team, like the ones in Quispicanchis and Villa el Salvador, Peru, increases the likelihood of people's involvement. The El Carmen case shows how important it is to inspire workers continuously and to train local health staff to allow people to be represented in the services. If this is not done, community interest can be lost and participation killed. True participation has a way of resurging despite adversity. For example, even when severe repression occurred in Guatemala, the young community health volunteers stood up again at the first chance and resumed work.

CHALLENGES TO PRIMARY HEALTH CARE

Health care developments are dynamic. Thus, existing trends are the result of various forces and counter-forces. During the 1980s the winners clearly were: cuts in social spending, the medicalization of health services, and the verticalization of primary health care. The 1990s offer new opportunities for health care development.

Governments, political parties and the international community admit the need for more resources for health and a more equitable use of these resources. Health care financing is much more open in Latin America at present than it was in the 1970s and 1980s. All three countries in this study are attempting to extend health insurance through social security, focusing on workers and creating openings for volunteer insurance schemes. A de-

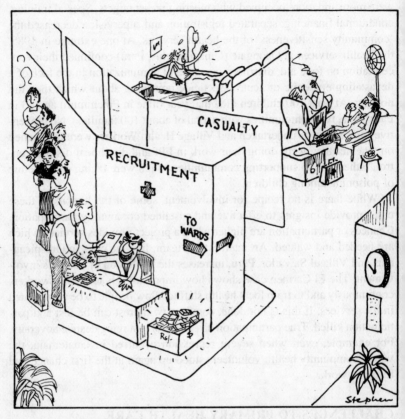

Cost recovery all-too-often releases the worst elements of the market economy into social services.

gree of cost recovery has been introduced or this has been strengthened, for example, through payment for drugs at cost.

More emphasis is being laid on prevention even in the Social Security health services. While vertical primary health care programmes have weakened community participation they have clearly shown the possibility of rapid increase in coverage.

The private sector is no longer excluded from health care planning. In Colombia 'packages' of health services defined by the Ministry of Health are to be contracted out to groups of private physicians or NGOs.

Even with an increasing share of government budgets going to health, the need for external financial support will remain strong in the 1990s. However, the main challenge to health financing will not be garnering resources as much as improving their distribution. With so many hospitals neglected for so long a time, and so many doctors wanting to practice the skills they have learned, there will be strong pressure on governments to invest in medical jobs, medical technology and maintenance.

On the other hand, the needs of an impoverished population (at least 30 per cent of whom have no access to health services) will not be served only by improved investments in medical services. They will require community-based health care. Elements of primary health care have been developed and implemented on a large scale. Many lessons have been learned and should be used.

Primary health care is not cheap and so requires a greater share of health care resources. These resources do not need to be exclusively national government funds; they can be increased by cost recovery schemes, NGO and donor contributions. In the 1990s structural adjustment programmes carried out explicitly in Peru and implicitly in Colombia and Guatemala should be expected to have a 'human face'.[2] Funds made available for poverty reduction, employment and basic needs must be used to strengthen district level health services. As these funds are multisectoral by nature, they offer a chance for integrated local development. The health sector can provide the stimulus for local leadership in planning, community commitment to development, and the design of services which are responsive to the articulated needs of the people. An important lesson is that progress can only be made through people's involvement.

Primary health care cannot be implemented by governments alone. It should include coalitions of implementors, like local governments, NGOs and private providers. Communities have to be seen as partners in planning and control of local health services. As the cases in this study demonstrate, these groups are capable of and willing to assist in health care provision if given a chance. Given a share in planning and control they are willing to raise money for local investments. The undying enthusiasm of communities to participate and of Village Health Workers to continue their work, even in the face of neglect or severe repression, is well demonstrated by these studies. The difficulty in participation is not so much that communities are not interested but rather that local health services are unable to open their doors, or unwilling to accept community influence through partnership in their work.

Planning, implementation and control of health services can best be implemented at district level. Here, intersectoral coordination is also best achieved. The chances for district development are greatly enhanced by the wind of decentralization of government that is blowing over Latin America today. National governments now realize that centralized government has not been effective in all aspects and that their control does not include the district level. Local government is seen as more effective, especially in the field of social services, and it is hoped this will increase the democratic content of the political process. Decentralization is being promoted by major donors like the World Bank.

Selective disease control, especially immunization, has been effective but remains largely isolated within the health services. Moreover, it is vulnerable as a donor-dependent phenomenon. Integration of these activities in district services and, especially, integration of the many important lessons learned in training, supply logistics, supervision and reporting may help to develop primary health care further and strengthen local health services.

The existence of 'pockets of health poverty' demands a redefinition of the risk focus in health. If a social definition of risk is included in health care planning and primary health care is geared more specifically towards the needs of the poorest, a rapid improvement is likely to occur in overall levels of health.

References

1. United Nations Economic Commission for Latin America and the Caribbean, Preliminary overview of the Latin American Economy, Official Document LC/G 1536, 1989.
2. Figueroa, L. (1988). 'Economic adjustment and development in Peru: towards an alternative policy'. In: Cornia *et al. Adjustment with a human face*. Clarendon Press, Oxford. Volume 2, pp. 156–83.
3. DANE (Departemento Administrativo Nacional de Estadisticas). (1987). 'La pobreza en Colombia, resultados preliminares' cited in Negocios, Julio, pp. 20–2.
4. Inforpress 'Guatemala 1984–1986' Inforpress Centroamericana, Guatemala. 1984.
5. Pan American Health Organization. (1981). *Malaria in the Americas*. Scientific Publication no. 405, Washington.
6. Ministry of Health. (1989). Triannual, Multisectoral Plan to Protect Children's Health, PAHO, Lima.
7. Gomez Serrano, L. C. (1984). 'La situacion actual de salud en Colombia' in Foro Salud siglo XXI ('The present health situation in Colombia' in Health Forum in the XXI century). University of Antioquia Press, Medellin, Colombia, 2 Volumes: 1–279 and 1–402.
8. Pan American Health Organization. (1986). 'Health conditions in the Americas 1981–1984, Scientific Publication no. 500, PAHO, Washington, USA, 2 Volumes: 1–416 and II: 1–250.
9. Servicio Seccional de Salud de Narino, Analisis seccional de salud. (1983). (Regional situational health analysis), Mimeo, Pasto.

10. Convenio Peru-alemania Proyecto de atencion primaria y desarrollo de los servicios de salud. (1985). (Primary health care and health services development project), Mimeo, Ministry of Health, Cusco, Peru.
11. UNICEF. (1992). *The study of the World's children.* Oxford University Press, New York.

II

Reaching out to Larger Communities

SUSTAINING COMMUNITY INVOLVEMENT

Beyond the experiences of specific communities which have designed and implemented their own approaches to health, there are examples of community-level action in larger-scale programmes. By and large, these efforts are aimed at tackling a critical, widespread health problem and, thus, are catalysed from 'outside' individual communities. But community involvement is ensured from the inception of the programme through careful design and introduction of programme elements. It is sustained by continuous assessment and feedback. Accountability is the cornerstone of these larger-scale community-based programmes.

Many of these programmes have recognized that 'Health for All' cannot be achieved without the provision of basic needs such as nutrition. Thus, some have focused on improving nutrition as a means to better health, integrating other health activities with a range of nutrition-improvement measures. Changes in household behaviour have been viewed as the key to success, and a variety of interventions have addressed this need. Important among these has been growth monitoring—a recurring activity which not only facilitates interaction between the health system and needy children and their mothers but is also an instrument which helps workers target their efforts and measure their achievements, thus enabling accountability. Regular growth monitoring is a communication strategy to improve child-rearing behaviour, addressing nutrition as well as overall health care. It calls upon households to utilize their own resources, thus potentially reducing dependence on outside technologies and resources. It calls for continuous attention to the needs of each child, thus introducing 'care' as the critical factor in nutrition rather than health or even food itself.

The four chapters in this section describe different approaches to improving the health of large populations by community-level activities. In three programmes, the Indonesian *Posyandu* Programme described by Jon Rohde, the Tamil Nadu Integrated Nutrition Project in India discussed by Jayshree Balachander, and the Iringa Nutrition Programme in Tanzania described by Urban Jonsson, Björn Ljungqvist and Olivia Yambi, growth monitoring and promotion were the prime activities, although participatory decision-making and action varied tremendously among the programmes. In the fourth chapter on the Bangladesh Rural Advancement Committee (BRAC), Catherine Lovell and F. H. Abed show how a comprehensive, community health and development programme evolved step-by-step from an effort initially based on a single health intervention. The process of adding activities to the initial house-to-house training of mothers in oral rehydration has engaged both non-governmental and governmental resources and workers, always responsive to the needs and involvement of communities.

NUTRITION AT THE FOUNDATION OF HEALTH

It is not mere coincidence that the larger-scale community programmes described in this section have focused largely on nutrition. Communities easily recognize nutrition needs and can be prepared to accept outside help in fulfilling these, whether this help is in the form of food supplements, education or organization. Conversely, actions to promote nutrition are most effective at the community level, in households and in the hands of mothers. Growth monitoring itself is inherently a community-based activity, with the involvement of health workers facilitating the analysis of growth problems, leading to the identification of practical remedial actions to promote growth.

The *Posyandu* Programme in Indonesia is a large-scale, standardized, low-cost, community-based education and participatory primary health care effort. At the outset a decision was made not to provide food supplements so that the programme is affordable and expandable. The regular monitoring of growth at village-level *posyandus* provided a forum for discussion and promotion of proper nutrition. Later, regular supplies of family planning commodities and a few primary health care services became available at the *posyandus*. Recognizing the potential of these monthly village gatherings to achieve high coverage with immunization, the Expanded Programme of Immunization assigned a professional health worker to the *posyandus* to provide immunization and, eventually, curative medical care. In the process, the community-based activities became increasingly medicalized, the communities more passive, and the effectiveness of communication and behavioural change strategies declined. Today, Indonesia is once again seeking the community roots of the *posyandu* system to ensure attention to self-help and self-reliance in meeting overall nutritional goals and to restore the primacy of control by community women's groups. Medical care, family planning and other service inputs will then again become supporting elements rather than the primary functions of the community self-help programme.

The Tamil Nadu Integrated Nutrition Project (TINP) uses many of the same technologies as the *posyandu* programme but has a far greater investment in actively addressing growth faltering or malnutrition with more than just nutrition education. The selective feeding component of TINP, absorbing over half the cost, is an important contribution and appears to have been a major nutrition education strategy. TINP has measured its success predominantly on the basis of nutritional improvement, which has been impressive in the midst of a poor environment. Although its health care delivery component and community participation have been weak, these elements are being strengthened in the second phase of the programme through better integration and management structures. Together with the community-based nutrition activities, these improvements promise to be the foundation for a sound primary health care effort.

The Iringa Nutrition Programme used malnutrition as the starting point for a broader community self-analysis and undertook a wide range of actions to address the causative factors underlying malnutrition. Using regular community-based growth monitoring, communities were called upon to analyse the causes of poor growth. They then took action, utilizing government extension resources to improve the situations of families with malnourished children. This required development efforts as widely different as food production, credit, creches and latrine-building to improve the care of children. At the household-, community- and district-levels, the success of the programme was measured by the reduction of malnutrition. As the section on community health and development emphasizes, communities must spend the time and effort to analyse their own situation, develop alternative actions, and actually see the effects of their actions in order to be truly involved. At Iringa, they plan for and recognize improved growth among their children. Heavy initial costs have led some observers to question the applicability of this approach on a wide scale. The cost per child of the

Iringa programme was comparable to that of TINP, but was five to ten times that of the Indonesian *posyandu* system. The expansion of the Iringa approach throughout Tanzania has built more on existing resources with far lower unit costs. The impact of such large-scale expansion is yet to be measured.

FROM HEALTH TO DEVELOPMENT

In the BRAC programme, teaching mothers to make and use oral rehydration solution was the central health intervention. Starting with this nationwide activity, the programme expanded to include other health services such as immunization and vitamin A prophylaxis. With help from BRAC, government services successfully provided immunization to more than 80 per cent of infants in a quarter of Bangladesh. The programme later evolved into a more comprehensive primary health care system based on community volunteers dealing successfully with such difficult problems as the treatment of tuberculosis and family planning. However, nutritional improvement remains a major challenge because of the persistence of widespread poverty. Today, with the recognition of the factors underlying ill-health and malnutrition, BRAC's new women's development programme will incorporate the education of young girls, adult literacy, credit and income-generation with the array of primary health care activities. This should make for truly healthy and self-reliant families.

These studies raise a number of important questions:

— How is scaling-up of community-level activities achieved? What is gained or lost in the process? Can flexible, community-based programmes such as Iringa go to scale, or are more rigid standards necessary, like those of TINP or the *posyandu* programme?
— What interventions work for nutrition? What is the role of growth monitoring? Of health care? Are food supplements necessary? What costs are acceptable? Unnecessary?
— Can nutrition and health be improved amidst poverty?
— BRAC and Iringa focus more on the very poor than TINP or Indonesia's *posyandus* which involve entire communities. Should programmes focus on the poorest or cater to all groups?
— These experiences show that health, nutrition, agriculture, education, employment, are all important. How can different development sectors be integrated to achieve synergy and increased impact?

CHAPTER 7

Indonesia's *Posyandus*: Accomplishments and Future Challenges

JON ROHDE

The author chronicles the expansion of the Indonesian village-based nutrition and primary health care programme that has spread throughout the country's 68 000 villages. Indonesia's posyandu programme has evolved over the decade into the basic implementing strategy for comprehensive primary health care in that country.

Jon E. Rohde, M.D., *a paediatrician, taught community health in the medical faculty at Yogjakarta, Indonesia, in the 1970s. He lives in New Delhi, India, where he serves as Special Adviser on health and nutrition to the Executive Director of UNICEF, dealing with programmes for children throughout the world.*

INTRODUCTION

The 1973 National Nutrition Survey of Indonesia, an evaluation of the small but comprehensive intersectoral Applied Nutrition Programme of the previous decade, exposed the extent and severity of malnutrition. With half its children undernourished, the nation embarked on a multisectoral effort to improve child growth, exploring numerous approaches through the 1970s. By 1979, an affordable village model, organized by the local women's organization (*PKK*) with technical help and guidance from the health, agriculture, and religious affairs ministries had evolved and was operating in nearly 1000 villages (Village Family Nutrition Improvement Programme—*UPGK*). In the early 1980s, with the considerable organizational abilities of the National Family Planning Board (*BKKBN*), the programme increased services to include contraceptive supply, as well as growth promotion; and expanded into nearly half of the nation's 68 000 villages, covering almost all villages in the densely populated islands of Java and Bali. With the acceptance in 1984 of the goal of universal immunization by 1990, programme services enlarged still further. A massive increase in *posyandus* (integrated health service posts) resulted in nearly a quarter million posts by 1990. The expansion process, while achieving the target of 80 per cent infants fully immunized, saw a modification of post activities. Less attention was paid to child nutrition and growth, and ownership and participation by village women declined. Today, steps are being taken to decentralize control, to reduce dependency on technical medical personnel, and to return primary responsibility to the community. With improvement in quality, the *posyandu* system offers a highly equitable, affordable, and practical approach to reaching health for all in Indonesia.

THE EARLY YEARS: RECOGNIZING MALNUTRITION

The earlier chapter in PHFA[1] chronicled the development of awareness of the nutritional problem in Indonesia, the processes leading to a policy, and the political will to undertake a nation-wide programme to improve nutrition in 68 000 villages, covering over 20 million children under the age of five. The National Nutrition Survey found half of Indonesian children to be undernourished. Existing efforts in nutrition only treated established malnutrition, and had placed a major emphasis on protein, rather than overall food intake. In 1974, President Suharto established a coordinating board for nutrition comprising ten ministries, to explore ways to address this massive problem.

ESTABLISHING A VILLAGE APPROACH

The village family nutrition improvement programme (*UPGK*), an intersectoral activity, grew in the 1970s out of the increasing interest in mobilizing village volunteers to improve health and nutrition using simple, affordable and effective interventions. In Java, the most populous and poorest part of the country, the women's Family Welfare Programme, *PKK*, was already reaching into most villages, organizing women around practical, useful and socially-attractive activities to improve family and community welfare. Their monthly meeting, the *arisan*, primarily a social gathering, became an opportunity for health and nutrition education, often guided by staff from the nearby health centre. In many villages, the opportunity was used by women to weigh children, plot weights on growth cards, and discuss nutrition and child growth as they prepared a common meal for their children from locally available foods using a wide range of local recipes. As the activities were conducted entirely by volunteers or cadres, the education and communication was based predominantly on local knowledge and experience with successful mothers counselling and guiding others. The importance of weight gain was popularized in a national slogan, 'A Healthy Child, As He Gains in Age, Gains in Weight'.

EXPANDING THE VILLAGE MODEL

The Department of Health adapted this village model, providing standardized activities and training, and eventually reaching 800 villages throughout Java and Bali by 1979. However, the *UPGK* became excessively expensive because of the provision of daily food supplements to identified undernourished children. Not only was it costly, but the feeding also diverted attention from nutrition education and the importance of growth. Earlier in the village women's clubs, small groups of mothers or neighbourhoods had taken responsibility for remedial action for children not gaining weight. However, this self-reliance was substantially eroded in the expanded programme. Dependency on Health Department funds and workers limited expansion and, unfortunately, reduced village participation.

From this experience, several principles became evident:

— a programme must be village-based and affordable with local resources;
— communities need to take responsibility for both identifying the nutrition problem and its solution, and to be held accountable for measuring the outcome of intervention; this requires clear, unambiguous and locally understandable goals;
— emphasis must rest on prevention rather than treatment of malnutrition; only in this way can malnutrition be effectively and affordably dealt with.

LINKING NUTRITION TO FAMILY WELFARE

During the 1970s, the National Family Planning Programme expanded rapidly, with 7000 village based lay workers (*PKKB*) responsible for identifying new contraceptive acceptors, and arranging for the monthly resupply of commodities, particularly the popular and widely used oral pill. Family planning acceptor groups were formed in every village in Java and Bali (see chapter by Suyono *et al.* in this book). These became the primary motivators of other acceptors. Membership as a family planner became a widely recognized social attribute. Villages openly discussed and advertised their success. As more and more villages reached current user rates of 60 or even

80 per cent of eligible couples, interest shifted from family planning to overall family welfare. The attractiveness of a monthly health and nutrition activity within the context of these acceptor groups became obvious, and the Family Planning Coordinating Board (*BKKBN*) adopted village-based growth monitoring and promotion as a central theme. This fitted well within the Third Five Year Plan which emphasized 'equity and sharing the fruits of development'. This focus on nutrition transformed the view of malnutrition from that of an unfortunate and inevitable concomitant of poverty to that of a developmental challenge. Healthy growth and good nutrition for all became a national goal.

During the Third Five Year Plan (1979–84), monthly weighing and nutrition education activities expanded to 80 000 weighing posts located in 41 000 villages. The *BKKBN* and the Health Department played the major role. Their field workers were trained to organize, establish and supervise the village posts. Agricultural extension workers were trained in the basics of nutrition, and particularly of growth. They attended the monthly weighing sessions, offering guidance in home gardening, small animal raising, and improved home food preservation. The Religious Affairs Ministry took major responsibility for interpreting health and nutrition goals through religious documents, particularly the scriptures of Islam, the religion of more than 80 per cent of the population. A major publication provided to all mosques cited holy works in their support for health, nutrition and responsible parenthood, providing a useful reference work from which religious leaders could develop sermons and talks in direct support of participation in the village weighing posts.

Policies and procedures became highly standardized and uniform in order to facilitate rapid expansion, while preserving quality. The 7000 family planning field workers (*PLKB*), who would organize and oversee the posts, were trained for five days using a set curriculum. The training featured slide-sound instructional materials which illustrated and explained each task they would perform. Each worker demonstrated competence in the basic steps of growth monitoring, and the 'nutritional first-aid package'—iron-folic acid tablets for anaemia prophylaxis in pregnancy, high dose vitamin A, and oral rehydration salts for diarrhoea.

At the village level, the programme was run by village volunteers, who received a five-day standard training (later reduced to three days to facilitate larger numbers) on the process of weighing, plotting, interpreting and counselling. Each post was provided with '*dachin*', a locally made, robust and standardized beam balance familiar to virtually every mother throughout Indonesia. Locally made cloth pants with long 'suspenders', or woven

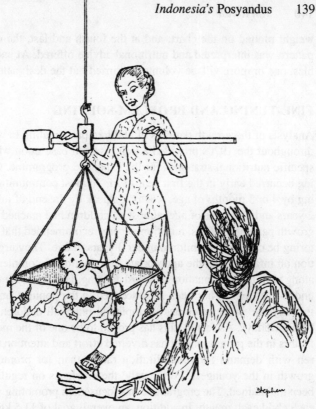

Each mother weighs her own child suspended in a gaily painted box or basket using the familiar 'dachin' beam scale. This scale is widely used in the markets and villages of Indonesia.

baskets, wood chairs, or gaily painted boxes suspended the child. The amusement provided to children through this colourful swing has been an important element in the acceptability of weighing to mothers and children alike! The standard growth card was redesigned, removing nutritional status indicators and emphasizing growth through a series of narrow, coloured channels. Printed on indestructible plastic paper in gay colours, the card substantially enhanced mothers' desire to participate regularly in the weighing programme.

The weighing sessions were structured to be uniform from village to village to ensure that the critical aspects of growth monitoring and promotion were carried out. At each post, four tables were organized. At the first, the child was registered; at the second, she was weighed; at the third, the weight plotted on the chart; and at the fourth and last, the child's growth pattern was interpreted and nutritional advice offered. At each of these tables, one or more village volunteers carried out the designated procedures.

FINE-TUNING AND PROBLEM-SOLVING

Analysis of the growth patterns of children participating in weighing posts throughout the 1970s provided a rich research base upon which to design specific nutritional strategies for the expanded programme. Growth faltering occurred early in the first year of life in most communities, often starting by 4 or 5 months of age, reaching a peak by the end of infancy. By 2 or 2 years and 6 months of age, almost all children had reached their eventual growth percentile. Thus, nutrition experts recommended that growth monitoring be confined to children under 3 years of age. They urged concentration on infancy, with the appropriate introduction of complementary foods along with the continuation of breast-feeding. However, the concept of the under-five (*balita*) has been so ensconced in the popular language that, to this day, the programme has attempted to reach all children through their fifth birthdays. As feared, this has proved to be one of the most weakening factors in the programme. It has diverted effort and attention to older children with demand for rehabilitation rather than for promotion of good growth in the youngest. Fortunately, the emphasis on regular growth has been maintained. The programme has focused on promoting weight gain in each child each month. In addition, an overall goal of 11.5 kg at 36 months (80 per cent of standard) for every child was established. This enabled the dynamics of growth, and also the nutritional status of each child to be tracked.

In an effort to standardize nutritional education, a behavioural change strategy was adopted. Twelve basic action messages were embraced. These prescriptive instructions were illustrated on a flip-chart. If followed, they would ensure regular growth. More often than not, the flip-chart was used hastily at 'table four' as the weight chart was returned to the mother. While attempting to ensure a minimum standard of behaviour, the standardized format of these messages diminished the spontaneity and relevance of earlier efforts to let successful mothers counsel others using local wisdom.

The nutrition intervention strategy was based entirely on behavioural change and local self-reliance. The 60 000 family planning-nutrition posts (*KB-Gizi*) provided only a small amount for a demonstration meal once a month, an extension of the village meal prepared in the original *PKK* nutrition *arisan* posts. The Health Department programme, expanding to over

13 000 posts, continued provision of daily supplementary feeding for the undernourished for several years. However, high costs and lack of evidence of impact led to its phasing out in all except the two poorest provinces. While most children grew well, 10–15 per cent eventually became significantly undernourished and 2–3 per cent severely malnourished (II and III degree). Referral to health centres or hospitals helped little in the absence of rehabilitation programmes at these facilities.

In order to facilitate local measurement of outcomes and accountability, a standardized and simplified monitoring system was established for all villages. The *SKDN* score was recorded each month in each village. This identified the total number of children, S; those enrolled in the programme, K; those participating in the monthly activity in a given month, D; and those gaining weight, N, the ultimate objective. A graphic display of these parameters became a means to stimulate inter-village competition to achieve higher *SKDN* levels. A single-page report form recorded these data, as well as information on the supply of critical materials such as ORS packets, vitamin A and iron tablets. An identical monitoring system was used at the sub-district, district, province and national levels, to oversee and measure progress.

COMPREHENSIVE VILLAGE SERVICES: THE *POSYANDU*

By late 1984, more than 80 000 posts in 34 000 villages provided basic nutrition and growth monitoring services to ten million children, one-half of Indonesia's total. Extensive and in-depth evaluation of these village programmes late in the Third Five Year Plan demonstrated conclusively the power of village-based activities to reach a previously unexpected and large proportion of the population with essential services.

In preparation for the Fourth Five Year Plan (1984–89), meetings and workshops hammered out an expanded array of activities which would come to be known as Village-based Integrated Service Posts, *Pos Pelayanan Terpadu*, the *Posyandu*. To the basic *UPGK* activities of monthly weighing, nutrition information, food demonstration, provision of vitamin A capsules, iron tablets, oral rehydration salts, and advice on home gardening had already been added a reliable supply of contraceptives and family planning advice. As Indonesia embraced the goal of Universal Childhood Immunization (UCI) by 1990, which would require complete primary immunization of 80 per cent of all infants each year, monthly immunization services were added to the package. This would require, for the first time, the presence of a trained health worker at each post. Thus, the Department of Health assumed full responsibility for the technical guidance and operational supervision of all *posyandus*.

The *BKKBN* would transform its involvement. Its workers who previously oversaw the entire activity would now confine their attention to communication and behavioural change strategies and monitoring. The Agriculture Department was to continue to intensify its efforts to reach families in need with improved food production; and the Religious Affairs Department would intensify motivation of the community to increase acceptance of and participation in the programme. The Home Affairs Ministry, responsible for all development activities at the village level, was assigned the role of intersectoral coordination, with particular attention to greater involvement of village decision-makers, and increasingly of the *PKK* women's family welfare groups.

Not only was a wider range of services to be provided in all existing posts but, more importantly and ambitiously, the programme was to be expanded to all villages in all provinces. The ratio of target children per post was decreased from 250 to 100, requiring a proliferation of service posts even within existing village programmes. The management challenge of this vast expansion was staggering.

MICROPLANNING

An intersectoral body, the Area Nutrition Improvement Council (*BPGD*) which had been functioning at sub-district, district and provincial level for some ten years was expected to oversee the district microplanning process. Clear guidelines were established which included:

— introduction of the integrated post approach to community leaders by the health centre staff;
— a community self-survey to identify nutrition and health problems and increase awareness among all citizens;
— a community-wide meeting to discuss the survey results and the role of the community in seeking solutions by developing the *posyandu*; and
— identification and training of volunteers to take responsibility for activities at the post, as well as for problem-solving in the various sectors outside normal post activities.

In a nation-wide evaluation in late 1986, it was found that some three-quarters of health centres were undertaking all these steps in their effort to expand the number of *posyandus*. During this 12-province (out of 27) sample survey of 35 000 households, programme activities were as shown

Table 1. Selected integrated family health package indicators by programme
(Sample: 35 000 households, 12 provinces)[2]

Programme	Indicator	Sample average	Highest province	Lowest province
		Per cent coverage		
Maternal and child health (MCH)	Ante-natal care	64	82	36
Family planning	Current users	49	56	31
Nutrition	Children weighed last month	52	65	39
Immunization	DPT1, 1–2 yrs	49	62	33
	Polio3, 1–2 yrs	34	48	14
	TT2, last pregnancy	46	56	20
Diarrhoea	Children with diarrhoea treated with ORS	34	51	20

in Table 1. By 1988, 200 000 posts in 49 734 villages were serving 18.2 million target children under the age of 5, estimated to be over 80 per cent of the target group in the entire country. In 1991, over 20 million children were enrolled in 250 000 posts. Some 60 per cent of these posts submit reports each month which record the services given and the results of weighing 6–7 million children.

INCREASED INVOLVEMENT OF HEALTH WORKERS

While the Health Department had taken only a facilitating role in *KB-Gizi* until the mid 1980s, the formal responsibility for expansion and service delivery resulted in health workers becoming the key operational personnel in the programme in each of the 3500 sub-districts. A fifth table was added to the village monthly activities, at which medical services were provided. Initially, immunization was the main service; later, in response to widespread demand, medical care was provided for common symptoms. As a result, demand and participation in post activities increased and the credibility of the *posyandu* as a health delivery point was enhanced. Previously, referral to the health centre, perhaps miles away, was rarely acted upon and consequently was not considered an effective health response to felt needs.

An unfortunate consequence of this new approach was the medicalization of the programme, due to the presence of a health worker at each monthly weighing session. Each health centre had 60 or more posts and five to ten health workers served a population of 30 to 40 000. Lay cadres continued to conduct the weighing programme, but many became reluctant to provide specific advice to mothers on child care, nutrition, and feeding issues in the presence of a health professional. They referred any child from the fourth table to the new fifth table for medical intervention, regardless of the problem. As the health worker was often a sanitarian or other paramedical, untrained in nutrition, nutritional advice and guidance was frequently missing. Vaccines were offered and, too often, a further injection or medicine provided for a fee. There was a visible decline in the quantity and quality of educational interaction between cadres and participating mothers.

Ultimately, the quality of community participation changed, as mothers increasingly came to *posyandus* to receive services provided by health professionals, rather than to conduct an information-sharing and motivational session between themselves. The strong role played by the *PKK*, in which village women determined the site, timings and activities, particularly in nutrition education, of the weighing posts, receded in importance as medical workers scheduled and ran the *posyandu* sessions. Health workers determined timings to fit their own convenience. While posts had earlier conducted activities in the evenings or on weekends to suit the busy work schedules of village women, weighing sessions were now held mid-morning to suit the work schedule and travel patterns of the health centre staff. Whereas earlier the health post had often been a social gathering in the village, marked by the preparation of a common nutritious meal and extensive interaction of village women with their young children, it now became a formalized health delivery activity, a mini-clinic conducted in the village. Nutrition advice previously offered and shared among mothers became medical advice dispensed with tablets or even an injection from an overworked health worker. The rising emphasis on reaching EPI targets and the technical demands of immunization contrasted with previous emphasis on self-reliance and communication, with a resulting loss in community ownership and participation.

RECORD-KEEPING

With the addition of major services at the *posyandu*, the burden of record-keeping burgeoned. The original simple record containing weight gain information (*SKDN*) was replaced by numerous registers recording family planning acceptors, ante-natal care assessment, immunization, distribution of vitamin A, ORS and iron tablets, and sometimes details of medical treatment, vital events, supply inventories, and even names of visitors! Because of demand for reports from the health centre, individual weights, previously recorded only on the mother-held child weight card, were now kept in a master register to ensure their availability during supervisory visits. Targets were set and monitored for the provision of each service. Emphasis on qualitative elements of communication, education and behavioural change shifted perceptively to the quantitative accomplishment of targets, numbers of posts, participation percentages, family planning acceptors, injections, cases treated, and so on.

TRAINING

With continued expansion in the number of posts, reaching nearly one-quarter million by the end of 1990, the need to train new cadres exceeded the capacity of training resources. It had always been expected that *volunteer* nutrition cadres would serve for several years, but eventually be replaced. With up to five cadres per post, there were now nearly a million of these field-trained workers, with an estimated average turnover time of two years. The training course was abbreviated from five to three days, and participatory learning activities were reduced accordingly. While the evaluation of cadres in 1989 showed an overall appreciation of how to weigh children, mark weight cards, and assess the health of children, a far smaller percentage were found to be capable of giving meaningful nutritional advice or interacting in a collegial or productive way with mothers.

PARTICIPATION AND COVERAGE

A 1989 UNICEF-sponsored study in four provinces showed 80–98 per cent enrolment in the programme, 35–70 per cent monthly participation, and 46–52 per cent of those participating gaining weight each month. This latter percentage has been rather constant since the programme began. Coverage figures of target children (under five) have hovered just over 40 per cent for the past five to seven years. More careful analysis, however, shows 80–90 per cent participation in the first year of life, and 75–80 per cent in the second year, the most critical and important age groups (Fig. 1). Low overall attendance is accounted for largely by the striking fall of participation in 3-, 4-, and 5-year-old children, dipping to 20 per cent or less. There has been a consistent tendency for mothers with higher education, higher socioeconomic status, and overall higher participation in government pro-

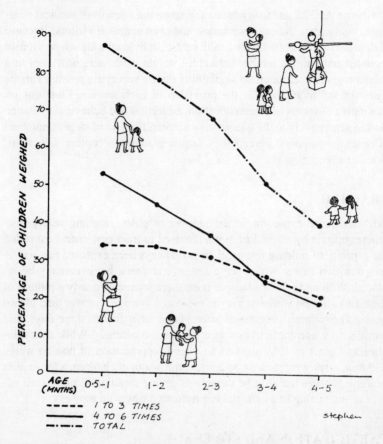

Fig. 1. Participation in monthly weighing by age of
child—attendance, initially high, falls with age.

grammes, to participate more regularly in *posyandu* activities. Nonetheless *posyandus* reach a higher proportion of poor, illiterate and marginalized village persons than any other government health effort in Indonesia.[3,4]

A recent study of mothers' attendance has shown a high positive attitude towards the post, with improved nutritional knowledge correlating well with frequency of attendance. Mothers believe that weighing is an integral part of the monthly activity. But they are often unable to cite any benefit or, indeed, demonstrate understanding of the weighing process. Mothers still express greatest appreciation for the fifth medical table. Unfortunately, there is evidence of large use of unnecessary drugs provided for virtually

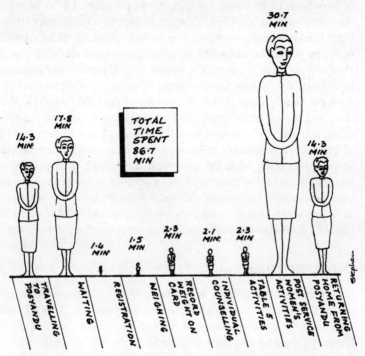

Time spent by an average mother attending monthly 'Posyandu' activities.[3]

all conditions and complaints. This increases costs and, most likely, iatrogenic problems. Mothers spend an average of 90 minutes per month at the weighing post with half an hour related directly to health activities: 18 minutes of waiting time followed by registration, weighing, recording on the card, individual counselling and Table 5 activities.

COSTS

Numerous cost studies have been conducted, showing that start-up costs for new posts are between $2 and 4 per child beneficiary. Recurring annual costs range from US $0.33 to 0.75 per child per year. Eighty-two per cent of costs are expended at the post in the village, 17 per cent at the level of the sub-district health centre, and 1 per cent at the district or regency (of which there are 265 in Indonesia). Government sources provide an average of two-thirds of this money (range 39–88 per cent). Up to 70 per cent of these costs are for supplies, although in certain settings, especially in the outer islands, transport can take a larger proportion. Medicines, particularly in recent years, have claimed an increasingly large share of expenditure. However, as these are generally sold at a small profit, their value need not be calculated as a programme expense. The cost of staff, particularly those from the health centre, is 14–40 per cent of the total; supplies, 35–40 per cent; and capital investments, such as weighing scales and pants, growth cards, and other simple paraphernalia, between 5 and 25 per cent. The cost of cadre time is difficult to evaluate, yet increasingly more mothers are serving, becoming educated, and eventually giving their place to others. Becoming a nutrition cadre is clearly a form of active health education for young mothers in Indonesian villages. Some villages openly state their goal as the training of each mother to serve as a nutrition cadre, thereby increasing her knowledge and skills, as well as her stature in the community.

INTERSECTORAL ACTIVITIES

Recent evaluations suggest diminished activity in other sectors participating in the programmes. With the heavy emphasis on Health Department activities, agricultural extension workers became a rarity at *posyandus*. However, the new emphasis on community control gives hope of a resurgence of earlier home-garden activities. Religious leaders have given strong support to the EPI effort which also became the indicator programme by which the Department of Home Affairs monitored community participation. *Posyandus* are the source of contraceptive resupply for more than 25 per cent of current family planning users. Thus, while predominantly a rural health activity, multisectoral participation remains an important element of the *posyandu* programme.

THE CURRENT SITUATION

Today, in Indonesia, a quarter million health posts function each month providing an integrated array of primary health care services within easy access to almost 90 per cent of families, spread throughout the archipelago. Nearly a million village volunteers sustain the work of the programme in close conjunction with, and under direct supervision of, 15 to 20 000 health workers from nearly 5000 health centres. Previously confined largely to their institutions, health workers, doctors and paramedicals alike, now each take full responsibility for the integrated services in several villages, bringing about a new level of accountability of the health system to the community.

HEALTH ACHIEVEMENTS

Through this system, Indonesia has achieved remarkable improvement in its immunization coverage of children under one year of age, reaching over 80 per cent immunization by the end of 1990. Family planning participation has continued to rise, with 50 per cent current users throughout the country. In East Java and Bali as many as 80 per cent of couples use contraception (see chapter by Suyono *et al.*). Knowledge of ORT is universal, with high ORS use rates and a sharp decline in dehydration as a cause of hospitalization or death. From an estimated 600 000 deaths per year in 1974, two-thirds from dehydration, diarrhoea is estimated to have claimed 175 000 lives in 1989, only one-third of which were due to dehydration. Recent estimates (1987) show that infant mortality fell from 125 to 58 per thousand over a 15-year period. In those areas where *posyandus* have functioned longest, infant mortality fell below 50, with under-five mortality approaching the 1990s goal of 70 per 1000. In the province of Yogjakarta, the IMR is less than 20, and malnutrition is unknown—a dramatic change from the situation in 1974 when the programme was piloted there. Knowledge of the importance of growth in children is now almost universal. Indeed, one reason women give for not participating in the monthly weighing programme is that they feel embarrassed if their child has lost weight due to illness in the past month. They feel this is an adverse reflection on their own mothering.

NUTRITIONAL IMPACT

In spite of an increased appreciation and knowledge of common nutritional messages by almost all women, the impact of the programme on the nutritional status of the nation is still debated. As the programme expanded rapidly, baseline data were not carefully collected, and substantial intra-province variations were obscured by averages. Studies consistently show levels of severe PEM (<60 per cent weight for age) to have declined to 1 per cent or so (range 0.5 to 1.8 per cent) from 3–5 per cent 15 years ago. Moderate degrees of PEM vary by definition (Gomez II 60–75 per cent; or Indonesia 'undernutrition' 60–80 per cent of standard weight for age), averaging 12 per cent (range 8–20 per cent), only marginally lower than the mid-1970s.

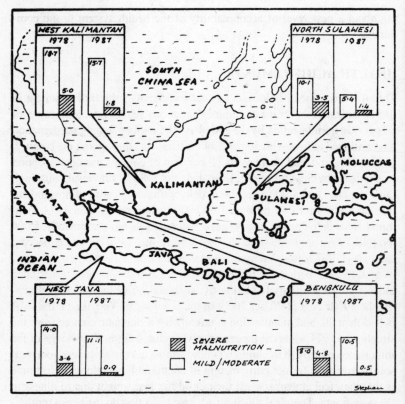

Change in nutritional status in various parts of Indonesia over ten years of programme expansion.

While at first glance these figures may suggest the programme's nutritional impact to be rather modest, one must take into consideration the dramatic decline in mortality and the consequent likely rise in undernutrition attendant upon such improved survival. Those who would most likely have died in the 1970s under prevailing mortality levels were disproportionately the undernourished, who are surviving today. With a halving in infant and child mortality (from 180 to 75 per 1000 children under 5), one would have expected as much as a 5 per cent rise in malnutrition. The deaths of 80 out of 1000 children would have occurred predominantly among the moderately and severely malnourished. Their survival would have been expected to augment the numbers of malnourished by 50 or more per 1000 children. Instead, severe malnutrition has been almost eliminated and moderate malnutrition remains at very modest levels, 10–15 per cent or less.

OTHER DEVELOPMENT BENEFITS

Associated with many *posyandus*, particularly in Java and Bali, has been the development of an array of ancillary activities. Health insurance, or *danasehat*, schemes have proliferated, underwriting the costs of referral curative services and providing simple medical care in the village by trained cadres available every day of the month, even when the *posyandu* is not functioning.[5] With the recent concern for cost recovery and self-reliant services, community-based insurance schemes for health, for family planning supplies, and for small credit for agriculture and women's development have proliferated through the *posyandu* system. Both governmental and non-governmental organizations (NGOs) use the system as a convenient community forum in which to initiate new activities and through which to encourage broad participation in development.

CHALLENGES OF THE 1990s

During the past decade there have been more than a hundred research projects conducted in and about the *UPGK-posyandu* programme. Major evaluations involving numbers of provinces and thousands of households have been conducted at intervals of two to three years. These have been supported by international agencies including UNICEF, USAID, the World Bank, UNFPA, and a variety of NGOs. The government and, particularly, the Directorate of Community Health Services, Ministry of Health, *BKKBN*, and a variety of national institutions have conducted intensive evaluations and prepared recommendations and reports. These provide a wealth of information upon which policies can be reformulated and activities redesigned to optimize *posyandu* performance.

The evaluations have highlighted major problems and proposed practical solutions, many of which have already been acted upon:

— Coordination of the many ministries operating at the village level has been hampered by the lack of a common budget and sectoral lines of authority. A national level coordinating committee has at last been established under the Ministry of Home Affairs, with the authority to set norms and ensure adequate resource allocations from all participating ministries.

— At the same time, the decision has been made to decentralize, allowing greater flexibility, depending on the level of development of existing posts. Provincial levels will similarly be encouraged to decentralize management functions to the regency or district (*Kabupaten*) level (roughly 200 to 400 000 population). Here, careful microplanning will enable evolution of the most appropriate systems for training, supply, logistics, monitoring, supervision, and information. Responsibility for monitoring programme activities and accomplishments has now been formally given to the top civil authority at each level, with each participating ministry accountable to the local administrative chief. Health and nutrition goals will be locally determined and monitored by the highest authority at each level of government.

— Quantifiable goals within a set time-frame for the reduction of malnutrition, as well as for sustaining healthy growth will be established at the national and provincial levels. Similarly, locally-set targets will strengthen the degree of participation, the sense of accomplishment, and the effort to achieve tangible goals of reducing malnutrition in each village. Action to achieve these goals will need to extend beyond the health-nutritional-medical sphere to involve the community in a dialogue, analysis and action to address underlying causes of malnutrition in their own setting. The range of activities addressing problems at the village level must be expanded and deepened to include areas such as water supply, food production, environmental sanitation, and other health promotion activities. This will depend on innovative action from the departments of Agriculture, Home Affairs, Religion, etc.

— Cadre selection will be more firmly based in the community with the understanding that the community must choose and supervise their own members to ensure that they gain maximally from the resources allocated.

— There will be greater intersectoral cooperation between cadres and outreach workers in sectors other than health to ensure a broader approach to identified village problems.

— A social marketing effort in support of the village-based nutrition programme, building up the role of the cadre and of self-help activities, would make the entire programme more credible.

— Attention will be given to improving the quality of training of cadres and the nature of their interaction with health workers to ensure a continuing flow of information and improvement of their skills.

— Some experimentation with cadre training will be necessary with the possibility of increasing the duration from the present three days to as long as eight days of initial training for at least one super cadre per post.

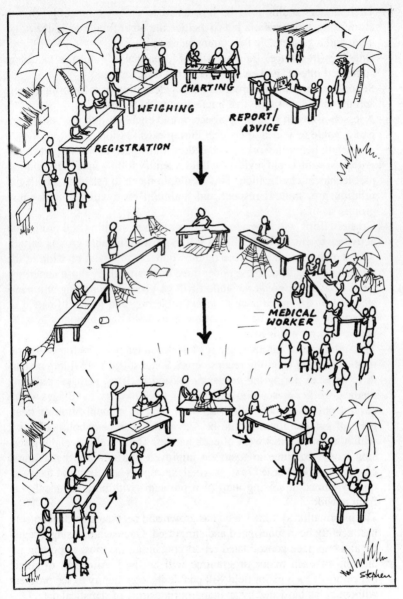

The original four-table focus on growth promotion atrophied as mothers flocked to the 'fifth' table for curative care. A new emphasis on participation and child growth is restoring the balance.

— Their understanding will be broadened to embrace not only growth monitoring and nutrition, but to include the other functions of the *posyandu* and a greater role for communication.

— Ongoing (in-service) training will need particular emphasis to ensure continued interest and enhance the skills of volunteers.

— Supervision must move from its narrow definition of monitoring targets and numbers to a supportive interaction with cadres.

— A lesson-a-month type of approach would enable health workers to impart a single new idea or concept during each session.

— A meeting between workers and cadres immediately following each *posyandu* session could review findings, identify follow-up action, and impart technical clarification. This would do much to establish a collegial relationship, mutual respect and maintain motivation among these groups.

— Greater efforts will be made to target growth monitoring and promotion activities to ensure that children in the most vulnerable groups participate. Emphasis will be placed on the younger child with revision of the target age to focus on those under three and particularly those under two years of age. Far greater attention will be given to imparting an understanding of the importance of growth faltering and to identification of affordable actions to be taken at the household or community level to ensure that growth is resumed.

— The shift towards curative services and dependency on doctors and paramedics is being carefully reconsidered. Some suggest providing no curative services during the *posyandu* session itself or, perhaps, reducing medical worker presence to only once in three months. In villages where several posts are functioning, services such as immunization or treatment of genuine illness could be provided at one neighbourhood post, within a few minutes walk of each hamlet. The monthly weighing session would continue to focus on improved nutrition and behavioural change, and be returned to its original concept as an activity of the community, aimed at solving their own problems with only technical help from outside.

— The information system, which has grown and become a burden in itself, has recently been redesigned and simplified. Once again, a single register and one-page consolidated report containing the most important indicators of each major programme will be used. Attention to single indicators in each major field will enable the community to see progress without being burdened by an inappropriate array of statistical data. Display of the indicators on village boards, a technique already widely used for many socio-economic parameters (e.g. population, electricity, roads, livestock, farm-land) will enable the entire village to view the changing pattern of the most important parameter—the health and nutrition of children. Were the village evaluation system of the Home Affairs Ministry to incorporate indicators such as an *SKDN* score, EPI coverage, and reduction in malnutrition (as they have done already for family planning), this would provide a nation-wide incentive for greater local resource allocation to this important element of village development. It would give real meaning to the claim that good nutrition and good health are legitimate national goals, reflected in the priority activities of each village. Then, not only would *posyandus* and services be universalized, but the outcome of healthy growth would also become a locally-salient national objective.

— Most important, major efforts are already being undertaken to return *posyandus* to the control and responsibility of the community. A recent instruction of the Home Affairs Ministry clearly charges each local authority with overseeing and facilitating the technical services to support basic community ownership and decision-making regarding *posyandus*. This will not be an easy task for there is always the tendency to bureaucratize when government workers are involved, to standardize, and to create dependency on technological solutions. Women's groups (*PKK*) will be asked to take a greater role in determining when and how the posts should function.

CONCLUSIONS

The dynamic nature and evolution of the *posyandu* system is its greatest guarantee of increasing relevance and effectiveness in the decade ahead. This programme evolved from a small village pilot project in the early 1970s in which women's groups initiated community-based growth monitoring and nutrition promotion. It received a major boost from the family planning network when tens of thousands of village contraceptive resupply posts adopted the monthly child growth promotion activity, run by village volunteers under the guidance of *BKKBN* field motivators. In the early 1980s, the opportunity to include immunization, health care, family planning and ante-natal care services resulted in a vast expansion of the system, to bring these benefits to virtually all families in urban and rural areas of Indonesia. The expansion process resulted in remarkably high coverage, especially of immunization, but took its toll in terms of reduced quality of services, particularly those relating to nutrition and behavioural change. Worst of all, the level of community participation and ownership of the programme declined as the *posyandus* shifted to a more medical and health focus.

The challenge today is to shift ownership back to the community while retaining the desired health services and convenience of health and nutrition at the doorstep. Additionally, the community must take a greater role in identifying the underlying causes of persistent nutritional problems. They must be facilitated in drawing on other sectors to join in addressing these underlying developmental issues. Through greater participation and control at the community level will come broadened appreciation of the determinants of ill-health and undernutrition, and an intersectoral development process which will provide more definitive and long-range solutions to these underlying problems.

It is interesting and important that the monthly weighing has continued to provide the recurring opportunity for a universal programme capable not only of delivering primary health care services but, more importantly, encouraging a high level of involvement in health care of all families, and particularly of women. The attention to monitoring child growth and well-being has been a major factor in making this programme viable at the village level. As each mother has recognized the importance of assessing her child's growth and development monthly, she has benefited from the regular contact with the health services, and with agriculture and other government outreach services. This will continue to be the cutting edge of community nutrition and health improvement in Indonesia in the decade ahead.

References

1. Rohde, J. E. and Hendrata, L. H. (1983). Development from below: transformation from village-based nutrition projects to a national family nutrition programme in Indonesia. In: *Practising Health for All,* (eds. D. Morley., J. Rohde and G. Williams), Oxford University Press, Oxford, pp. 251–71.
2. Directorate General of Community Health (1987). *Assessment of Integrated Family Health Package—Part I: Summary of findings and recommendations and Part II: Basic data tabulations by province.* Ministry of Health, Jakarta.
3. The Community Health and Development Unit, Dipongoro University School of Public Health, University of Indonesia, and The Centre for Research and Development of Nutrition, Bogor in collaboration with the Government of Indonesia and UNICEF. (1990). *Rapid Assessment of Growth Monitoring and Promotion Activities in Indonesia.*
4. Berman, P. A. (1992). Community-based health programs in Indonesia: The challenge of supporting a national expansion. In: *The Community Health Worker,* (ed. S. Frankel), Oxford University Press, Oxford, pp. 62–87.
5. Johnston, M. (1983). The ant and the elephant: Voluntary agencies and government

health programmes in Indonesia. In: *Practising Health for All*, (eds. D. Morley., J. Rohde and G. Williams), Oxford University Press, Oxford, pp. 168–89.

6. Ministry of Home Affairs, Indonesia. Improving the quality of *Posyandu*. Instruction No. 9, 5 April 1990.

CHAPTER 8

Tamil Nadu's Successful Nutrition Effort

JAYSHREE BALACHANDER

The author describes the community-based integrated nutrition project
undertaken by India's southern state of Tamil Nadu with assistance from the
World Bank. The Tamil Nadu Integrated Nutrition Project (TINP) has been
considered by many to be the most successful large-scale public health
nutrition effort of the 1980s.

Jayshree Balachander, a member of the Indian Administrative Service, was
Project Coordinator of TINP and Director of Social Welfare in the
Government of Tamil Nadu for three years. She became administrator of the
district of Madras in 1991 and joined the World Bank in 1992.

INTRODUCTION

The Tamil Nadu Integrated Nutrition Project (TINP), implemented in the
South Indian State of Tamil Nadu by the government has generated considerable interest in the international nutrition community for a number of
reasons. First, independent evaluation has shown that the project has had
substantial success in reducing levels of severe malnutrition. Second, the
project has demonstrated how a large-scale nutrition programme with a
complex design including growth monitoring, supplementary feeding, nutrition education and health interventions can be implemented successfully
with the help of community-based nutrition workers. Third, the project has
proved cost-effective in tackling the problem of malnutrition within a context of low economic levels. Fourth, the project's design and implementation offer a number of do's and dont's for efforts in the nutrition and health
sectors of developing countries.[1] This chapter describes the project's objectives, content and impact and highlights key features of design and implementation which contain lessons for programmes elsewhere.

Tamil Nadu's poor nutritional profile is not commensurate with its relatively better position among Indian states in respect of many other indicators of development. Although the state has comparatively lower birth and
infant mortality rates and a higher literacy rate, it is among the worst-off

Table 1. Indicators for selected states[2,3]

	Birth rate: Births/1000 population (1989)	IMR: Infant deaths/1000 live births (1990)	Female literacy rate (1991) (per cent)	Annual per capita income (1987) (Rs)	Daily per capita calorie intake (1988) (kcal)
Tamil Nadu	23	67	52	2980	1910
Kerala	20	17	87	2371	2203
Andhra Pradesh	26	70	34	2333	2401
Karnataka	29	71	44	2802	2592
Gujarat	29	72	48	3636	2608
Orissa	30	123	34	1983	2700

states in terms of average calorie consumption (Table 1). In the 1970s, levels of undernutrition among children under five years old were among the highest in the country. About 85 per cent of children were estimated to be less than 90 per cent of the recommended weight for their age. Malnutrition was identified as a leading or associated cause of more than 75 per cent of deaths among children under three. The very young child (6 months to 3 years), pregnant and nursing women (PNW) and adolescents (particularly females), in that order, were the most deprived groups in terms of the gap between recommended and actual calorie consumption.[3] In the late 1970s about 25 different nutrition programmes were operating in Tamil Nadu at an annual cost of Rs 162 million (approx. US $15 million). However, less than ten per cent of the groups identified as most vulnerable were actually receiving benefits under these programmes. These programmes had very limited success because:

— They did not reach intended beneficiaries as feeding was on a 'drop-in' basis rather than aimed at those who were identified as being at risk.
— Most programmes did not cater adequately to the nutritionally most-needy group, those under three years of age.
— The food distributed tended to *substitute* rather than supplement food normally consumed at home.
— Take-home rations were usually shared among members of the family, thus diluting the impact on the intended beneficiary.
— Most programmes placed little emphasis on nutrition education although food habits were a major determinant of nutritional status in Tamil Nadu,

particularly of weanlings whose growth faltered dramatically across all income groups.
— Existing maternal and child health services were inadequate to support the healthy growth of mother and child.

Therefore, the government's main concern was to design a programme that would avoid these common pitfalls of nutrition programmes. Because of the large numbers to be covered and potentially high costs associated with feeding, it was decided to provide food to only the most vulnerable. In view of the relationship between nutritional status and factors such as health, household food security, water supply and sanitation, it was believed that the project should integrate all these components. However, the potential difficulties of such broad intersectoral collaboration in a large project were daunting. Project activities were confined finally to those components which were thought likely to have the greatest impact on nutritional status: health services and nutrition education with a core of nutrition services including growth monitoring and selective nutritional supplementation.

OBJECTIVES AND ORGANIZATION

TINP's overall goal was to improve the nutrition and health status of pre-school children, especially those under-three, and of pregnant and nursing women. It aimed at a 50 per cent reduction in the prevalence of severe and moderate protein–energy malnutrition, estimated at about 60 per cent among preschool children. In addition the project aimed to contribute to a 25 per cent reduction in the infant mortality rate (then 125 per 1000 live births); a reduction in the proportion of children below five years showing signs of vitamin A deficiency from about 27 to 5 per cent; a reduction in the prevalence of nutritional anaemia among pregnant and nursing women from about 55 to 20 per cent; and increases in the provision of antenatal services and trained attendance at deliveries from about 50 to 80 per cent.

TINP covered about 40 per cent of the state's rural population, 17 million people living in ten of the state's 22 districts. After an initial year-long trial in one block* the project expanded at the rate of 35 blocks per year to cover a total of 173 blocks at the end of five years.

A Community Nutrition Centre (CNC) housed in a rented dwelling was opened in every village of approximately 1500 persons. Nine thousand such centres were opened, each staffed by a Community Nutrition Worker (CNW) and a helper. They were responsible for growth monitoring, select-

---

*A block is an administrative unit with a population of about 100 000.

ing children for feeding, distributing the nutrition supplements, organizing people to participate in health activities, and nutrition education through demonstrations, house visits and organization of women's groups.

The CNW was a local village woman, herself the mother of a healthy child. Special emphasis was given to her leadership potential, communication skills and acceptability in the community. She was expected to have a high-school certificate but this qualification was less important than the others and was often waived. The CNW received a monthly honorarium of Rs 90 (US $6) and the helper was paid Rs 30 per month.

The CNWs were given an initial two-month practical training course in groups of not more than 25 at the block headquarters. The training curriculum included segments on nutrition, health and communication skills, as well as on record-keeping and administration of the CNC. CNWs also received at least two days of in-service training each month at the block headquarters on specific project activities, and one at a selected CNC. At these sessions, project progress and problems were discussed.

The CNW's immediate supervisor was the Community Nutrition Supervisor (CNS), usually a college graduate. There was one CNS for every ten CNCs. This low ratio of field workers to supervisors was designed to permit maximum support, direction and encouragement to the CNWs. The supervisor was expected to visit each CNC at least twice a month, and 'weak' CNCs more often.

In each project block a full-time Community Nutrition Instructress (CNI) conducted the initial training course and continued the bimonthly in-service training sessions for CNWs. The CNI was required to have a postgraduate degree in Home Science, Nutrition or a related field. She was the second-line supervisor of project implementation and used monitoring data to review work performance in the block. She also had to help organize the extensive communication activities.

A Taluk* Nutrition Officer was the lowest level administrator in the project, responsible for disbursing salaries, distributing supplies, liaising with the Health Department and monitoring project activities. She was expected to tour extensively and to check CNCs randomly. A District Nutrition Officer was appointed to oversee the project's nutrition component at the district level. A Project Coordination Office (PCO) was created at the state level, headed by an officer of the Indian Administrative Service. The PCO managed the project, also overseeing training, communication, information processing and evaluation.

---

*A *taluk* usually consists of three blocks.

COMPONENTS AND STRATEGIES

Growth Monitoring and Supplementary Nutrition

Nutrition services, the core of the project, centred around monthly growth monitoring of children. Short-term supplementary feeding was provided for those found to be malnourished, those showing signs of growth faltering, and selected pregnant and nursing women. All children under three were to receive deworming medicines and a mega-dose (200 000 IU) of vitamin A twice a year. Daily iron-folate tablets were provided for three months to pregnant women. Intensive counselling was given to mothers to improve home care and feeding of children. Education on the home-based management of diarrhoea with fluids and feeding was an important component of the nutrition strategy.

Growth monitoring was the basis of the nutrition programme. The female Multipurpose Health Worker (MPWF), a health department auxiliary serving four or five villages, was expected to record all births and birth weights and to monitor the growth of infants up to 6 months of age, after which the task was taken over by the Community Nutrition Worker.*

Monthly weighing of children aged 6–36 months by CNWs was scheduled from the twenty-fifth to the twenty-eighth of each month. This facilitated supervision, orderly collection of data and the monthly indent for supplementary food required. Weighing took place at the CNC on the first day. On the remaining days those who did not come to the CNC were weighed in or near their homes. A light-weight bar scale that could be suspended from any hook or hung in a doorway was used for weighing. The child's weight was entered in a growth chart retained by the mother, and in the CNW's register.

Children were enrolled in the supplementary feeding programme only if they were 'at risk', i.e. if they were identified as severely malnourished** or if their growth pattern faltered, indicating incipient malnutrition. While children in Grades III and IV were admitted to feeding immediately on the

---

*The first step for the CNW was the registration of all children under three in the area covered by her Community Nutrition Centre. She spent her first month surveying families in her area. Records were prepared listing under-threes, and pregnant and nursing women. These were updated continuously, with all subsequent pregnancies, births and deaths listed.

**Severe malnourishment corresponds to Grades III and IV in the classification of the Indian Academy of Paediatrics which utilizes the Harvard weight-for-age standard, i.e. 80% and above median – Normal; 70–80% – Grade I; 60–70% – Grade II; 50–60% – Grade III; under 50% – Grade IV.

detection of their malnourishment, those losing weight or failing to gain weight (in Grades II, I and normal) were admitted to feeding only after two successive weighings (30 days) in the 6–12 month age-group, and four successive weighings (90 days) in the 12–35 month age-group. Enrolment in feeding was accompanied by intensive nutrition education of the mothers of these children.

The project provided feeding for a limited duration (90 days) only.* Those who had gained at least 500 grams over three months exited from the feeding programme. Children who did not gain adequate weight during this period were referred for medical evaluation and treated for any illness detected. After treatment these children continued in feeding for 30-day periods with monthly checks to determine if growth had resumed. It was found on average that 20 per cent of children who had graduated would again be eligible for supplementation or 'relapse' within six months of their exit from feeding. Thereafter, children who had received feeding experienced the same probability as others of becoming malnourished. Children also exited from the feeding programme on reaching 36 months of age or, if they were being fed at that time, by 39 months of age at the latest.

Pregnant and nursing women were also selected for feeding on the basis of objective criteria :

— having a child enrolled for supplementary feeding,
— lactating simultaneously with pregnancy,
— being of fourth or higher parity,
— having oedema,
— being 'single' mothers, or
— carrying twins.

These women received food supplements daily during the last trimester of pregnancy and the first four months after child-birth. At the beginning of the project female health workers were required to certify a mother's eligibility for feeding. However, since MPWs lived in only a few villages and were often absent from their health posts, this task was re-assigned to CNWs. Initially, the food was given in fortnightly 'take-home' rations. This was modified to on-site feeding to ensure that the mothers consumed the food themselves.

Three-quarters of the project's food requirement was met by a govern-

---

*Children below 24 months received a food ration containing approximately 140 calories and 6 grams of protein a day. Those between 24–36 months, severely malnourished children and mothers received double this amount daily.

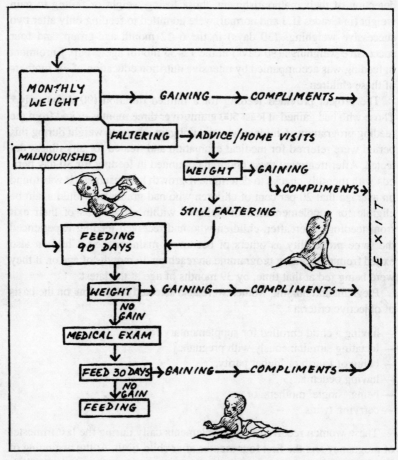

Children, weighed monthly, receive individual advice during home visits and supplementary feeding until gain in weight resumes.

ment-owned factory in neighbouring Karnataka state. The rest was produced by 322 village women's groups set up under the project. There were no breaks in supply from either source. Local food production had the advantages of contributing to the incomes of local women and of educating women to produce a low-cost weaning food. However, there were problems of quality control and supervision with such an extensive production network. Towards the end of the project, women were organized into larger production groups under the auspices of cooperative societies and these were stabilizing as well as viable and profitable ventures.

The nutrition component also paid attention to home-management of diarrhoea, the most common illness of young children. Frequently the traditional home treatment was to discontinue all feeding. The CNW was responsible for teaching mothers the importance of continuing feeding and instructing them in the preparation and use of sugar–salt solution and in the use of oral rehydration glucose–electrolyte solution (ORS packets).

Health Care

Health care was intended to back-up the nutrition effort. It included antenatal registration and care, tetanus toxoid immunization, deliveries by trained persons, child immunization, and examination and medical care of children found sick or not gaining adequate weight. Coordination between health and nutrition workers was considered particularly important for malnourished children who failed to respond to therapeutic feeding.

In the project the existing rural health system was strengthened to provide improved maternal and child health services and preventive care. The supply of drugs and medicines to the block level Primary Health Centre was also augmented.

The project constructed some 1300 Sub Health Centres in the villages, each with an outpatient clinic and residence for the MPHW. Training facilities were created or improved for MPHWs. As the Government of Tamil Nadu had rejected the Central Government's Community Health Guides' scheme there was great potential for using CNWs to improve the spread of primary care services, which were estimated to be reaching only 30 per cent of villagers.

Communications

Communications were designed to familiarize families with and involve them in project goals, encourage them to accept services and influence them to perform activities at home to improve the health and nutrition of mothers and young children. The interpersonal communication skills of nutrition and health staff were strengthened by training. They were provided communication materials for use in the field and encouraged to produce materials of their own. A staff newsletter informed and motivated them. Mass media campaigns reinforced interpersonal communications. Films, radio spots, wall posters, advertisements and folk theatre were used.

Villages were 'prepared' to receive the project by its objectives and design being explained to village elders and opinion leaders. Communication materials were used to describe the activities. In the last week of the CNWs training, joint training with the MPHW was aimed at informing the community of and involving it in initiating the CNC.

The CNW was the prime communicator. Her ability to communicate effectively was a criterion for her selection. This skill was enhanced further by training and the supply of a wide range of communication materials to assist her in her role as educator. The Community Nutrition Instructress played an important part in enhancing the CNWs skills, and the supervisor provided back-up support to the CNW as communicator. Unfortunately the communications effort did not involve the health worker to any extent, although the project originally intended to provide such support to the health system.

A key to winning community support was the Women's Working Group (WWG): 15 to 20 women identified by the CNW as progressive, capable of working together and interested in the activities of the CNC. The groups met once a month at a cooking demonstration where nutritious and easy-to-make weaning food recipes were demonstrated by the CNW. They were given health and nutrition training and some members became quite proficient in using flip-books and flannel-graphs to spread messages to their neighbours. To sustain the interest of WWG members, the project recently experimented with a community self-survey and with 'adoption' of several families by each WWG member.

Another recent innovation in the communications effort was the formation of Children's Working Groups. The facility with which children communicate and the enthusiasm with which they learn and relay project messages through poems, songs and skits has made this a highly successful activity.

A crucial communication strategy was the monthly growth monitoring session. Children's growth patterns were discussed and mothers complimented for good growth. The causes of and remedial actions for faltering were suggested. At follow-up home visits CNWs continued mothers' education. 'Graduation' from feeding provided ample demonstration of the effect of extra feeding on growth which could actually be *seen* on the growth card. Selective feeding was, therefore, a key communication strategy.

The Project Coordination Office had a Joint Coordinator for communications and some technical staff including an Assistant Communication Officer, a Communication Research Officer, a Training Support Officer, an Editor and a Research Assistant. A District Communication Officer or ganized the communication programme in each district, assisted by a Teacher Educator and Community Nutrition Educators in each taluk. The component had no separate grass root level workers. The CNW was the prime communicator and special attention was given to her communication skills and ways of supporting and improving them. The health personnel were simply too busy or uninterested.

MANAGEMENT SYSTEMS AND EVALUATION

The project design included a monitoring system, planned evaluation and the conduct of special studies.[4] The main purpose of the monitoring system was to assist project managers to monitor project inputs and implementation, assess project outcomes and to validate or provide a basis for changing project design. The management information system was designed to measure project benefits in terms of improved maternal and child health and nutrition and to document the process by which these gains occurred (or did not occur). Evaluation was intended to assess project impact by comparing changes from baseline, measuring the achievement of targets and objectives and contrasting changes in control areas. Together the monitoring and evaluation activities were intended to help determine whether the project was progressing according to plans, targets and implementation schedules and to ascertain the impact of the project on nutritional status, morbidity and mortality among beneficiaries. The provision for special studies allowed inquiry into issues of operational relevance allowing midproject redesign where necessary.

The monitoring system was based on three important principles:

— collect only what information is needed, not what is possible;
— devolve responsibility for data interpretation and remedial action to the lowest possible level; and
— manage by exception.

Since each of the three major project components were managed by different persons—nutrition by the Director of Social Welfare, health by the Director of Health and communication by the Project Coordinator, each person also had responsibility for monitoring the specific component. However, a Monitoring Division attached to the Project Coordination Office was responsible for overall monitoring. This division relied first on data generated by the component managers, but also had its own personnel in the districts to verify the quality of the data through surprise checks and frequent visits to villages. Project management received and consolidated certain 'key indicators' of project performance—ratios intended to capture coverage and effectiveness at each level, starting at the CNC. Initially three key indicators were thought sufficient to capture the essence of the project:

— the percentage of children in the project area weighed each month;
— the percentage of those weighed who were not gaining weight; and
— the percentage of those who were being fed and not gaining weight.

The first was an indicator of participation, the second of children at risk and the third indicated levels of 'treatment' under the project. The high quality of TINP data has been widely recognized. CNWs received careful training in data collection and in its use for self-evaluation and village action. CNIs were involved in data collection at the block level. Data were verified both by the supervisory line functionaries and by an independent person from the monitoring wing.

There were many feedback loops in the Management Information System (MIS). An information blackboard was maintained by the CNW at the village centre. This displayed up-to-date information on the village health and nutrition profile using the standard indicators. On the twenty-fifth of each month, each supervisor met with her group of ten CNWs to collate monthly figures and discuss their implications. Around the twenty-eighth the supervisors met the CNIs to consolidate the block report. A monthly performance review was conducted by each District Nutrition Officer on the third of every month. Instructions following from these reviews then flowed back at a meeting of each CNI with all the CNWs in her block on the fifth or sixth of each month.

At the state level, data reviews by the Project Coordination Office deteriorated into routine monthly exercises because of the absence of contact with front-line health and nutrition functionaries. The duplication of monitoring systems in each Directorate (sometimes yielding different results) was a problem. Data processing became progressively more cumbersome as the number of key indicators was increased from the initial 3 to 17. Consequently, monthly feedback also began to receive less attention in the field.

While the difficulties and uncertainties of nutrition project impact evaluation were well-recognized, the Project did plan for an elaborate evaluation and hoped to advance the state of the art in this regard. The purpose of the evaluation was to assess levels of malnutrition, morbidity and mortality in the pre- and post-project period, compare these with levels in non-project areas, and relate any changes observed to the interventions and their costs. The evaluation was also intended to assess in depth the target group's acceptance and adoption of recommended practices as well as their actual effectiveness. It was hoped that results of such an evaluation would help to fine-tune project strategies as well as provide lessons for interventions in all sectors affecting health and nutritional status.

Evaluation surveys were to be conducted at the beginning, middle and end of the project period. The phased implementation of the project made it possible to establish control groups who would receive project benefits only toward the end of the project. A district in which the project was not implemented at all was to provide 'control' data. Particular attention was paid to questionnaire development, the conduct of the survey and the choice and application of statistical procedures and analytical tools.

However, the control area was abandoned after a year due to operational difficulties. Moreover, the Expert Committee formed to guide the evaluation effort failed to provide the necessary support, especially in the final analysis of the evaluation data. While World Bank Supervision Mission reports provided a comprehensive, timely critique of the evaluation, they could not empower the PCO to implement most of the suggestions.

Nutritional Surveillance

The Project also proposed to generate and analyse nutritional information that would provide early warning of nutritional deterioration in a specific village, block or district. It was hoped that this would enable the government to initiate suitable action, beyond planned project interventions, to deal with the cause of the problem or at least to mitigate it. The surveillance system was to make use of the Project's growth monitoring data and the three key indicators. This information was to be made available to the District Collector each month. District officials were to monitor changes in the nutritional status of their populations closely and continuously. Unfortunately, although the data were available they were never used for this purpose, and no response mechanisms were ever instituted.

During the project, more than 60 special studies were conducted in order to resolve problems, understand processes or outcomes and develop new approaches (Table 2). These studies were done by project staff or independent institutions on contract with the PCO. Most relied on independent data collection. Some were based on detailed analysis of monitoring data. The findings of several studies were used in mid-project revisions and in the major redesigning which was undertaken for the Second TINP project (TINP-II).

Table 2. List of study titles drawn from 63 special studies conducted during TINP-I

1. Reports on nutritional dimensions of pilot blocks and control blocks.
2. Efficiency of various nutrition interventions and changes in nutritional status.
3. Diet survey and intra-family food intake.
4. Mid-term impact review in trial block.
5. Efficiency of health service delivery in pilot block.
6. Choice of beneficiaries by weight gain vs. nutritional grade methods in pilot block.
7. Evaluation of CNW and health worker performance.
8. Study of absenteeism in CNCs.
9. Changes in nutritional status of expectant women and nursing mothers.
10. Special study on home management of diarrhoea.
11. Nutritional surveillance—approach and methodologies.
12. The efficiency of communication approaches in pilot block.
13. Supplementary feeding—why results are not very impressive?
14. Field worker job satisfaction and worker interaction.
15. A note on critical areas of project implementation as revealed by process evaluation in extended blocks of Madurai district.
16. Women's working group in Madurai district.
17. Study on community responsiveness under TINP.
18. Revision and rationalization of CNW recording and reporting systems.
19. A special study on delivery assistance.
20. Report on weight gain versus nutritional grade methods for selecting beneficiaries.
21. Evaluation of children showing no or late response to project feeding.
22. Special study of health worker performance in the TINP.
23. Evaluation of behavioural changes associated with TINP activities.
24. A note on neonatal mortality in Madurai district.
25. Evaluation of training programmes of CNWs.
26. Results of nutritional surveillance in study blocks.

TINP'S ACHIEVEMENTS

Independent mid-term and end-line evaluations of the project found an impressive improvement in the nutritional status of children. Severe malnutrition was reduced by 25 to 55 per cent in different blocks depending upon the duration of the project.

There was a corresponding shift in the proportion of children in the 'better' nutritional grades indicating improvement in the entire child (0–3) population. The proportion of children in feeding at any time (children fed/children registered) declined from 40 per cent to 25 per cent. On an average, 80 to 85 per cent of children entered feeding for at least one 90-day period. Fully one-half of these required only a single period of intervention to maintain healthy growth. Some 40 per cent required two or more periods of supplementary feeding and a group ranging from 5 to 10 per cent required almost constant feeding, never emerging from the lower grades of undernutrition.

Thus, each child in the community received personalized attention and supplementary feeding when required at a cost equivalent to feeding only 25 per cent of children at any one time. Some 2.4 million children participated in the TINP project. The total cost of the project (covering food, salaries, construction and administration) was $26 per beneficiary or roughly $9 per child per year. If total costs are attributed exclusively to the reduction of third and fourth degree malnutrition, the cost per malnourished child was about $90 per year or $270 per child saved from third and fourth degree malnutrition. Of course, this notional calculation does not consider the extensive benefits provided by the programme to other children in the community.

Evaluation also found the nutritional benefits of the project to be long lasting. Children in the age-group 37–60 months who had been in the project enjoyed better nutritional status than their counterparts in other communities who had not. The terminal evaluation estimated that 77 per cent of children were reached by the project. The shortfall in coverage was due to the fact that CNWs had not covered outlying hamlets in less accessible

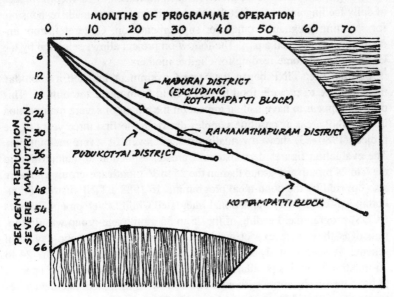

Fig. 1. *Percentage decline in III and IV grade malnutrition (age 6–60 months).*[5]

areas of their villages adequately. This error has been corrected in the follow-on project (TINP-II).

The monthly weighing was found to have been carried out regularly with
a high degree of participation. More than 90 per cent of enrolled children
were weighed each month, and participation in feeding was almost 97 per
cent of those eligible. The proportion of children participating in feeding
who were actually 'ineligible' was 2 per cent. Almost all mothers interviewed stated that the food supplement was palatable and readily acceptable to their child. Most reported little sharing of the supplement or
substitution of home feeding. This was probably due to the close attention
paid by CNWs, the on-site feeding modality and the provision of the food
supplement in the form of *ladoos*, a traditional snack.

Although growth monitoring by CNWs was found to be regular and
accurate, maintenance of growth cards by mothers was less satisfactory.
Only 45 per cent of surveyed mothers had received their children's growth
cards; 73 per cent of these retained them but only half had them properly
filled with all weight entries.

Among the project's disappointments was the poor enrolment of pregnant and lactating women in supplementary feeding—only 50 per cent of
those eligible. This low enrolment has been attributed to the inconvenience
of daily feeding and to the fact that the health worker was made responsible
for selecting pregnant women for supplementation. Cultural factors undoubtedly also played a part. The follow-on project allows selection by the
CNW and take-home feeding for eligible mothers.

Shortly after TINP began the State Government initiated a noon-day
meal scheme to provide food to every child from age 2 through 15. This
does not appear to have had an impact on the extent of severe malnutrition
in the TINP areas as baseline samples drawn in the first three years of the
project (1980–83) showed virtually the same levels of severe malnutrition.
The evaluation figures demonstrate a greater reduction in malnutrition in
the 6 to 24 month age-group than in the 25 to 36 month age-group who were
also covered by the noon-meal programme. In 1988 a TINP district, Pudu-
kottai, was covered by the national Integrated Child Development Services
(ICDS) programme. Feeding of the 25 to 36 month age-group was discontinued as they were expected to receive food from the noon-day meal
scheme. A special study showed that malnutrition rose among the 24 to
36-month-olds in this population. Thus, the overall impact of TINP appears
to have been substantial, although undernutrition of a moderate degree remains a major problem to be addressed in TINP-II.

Evaluation also showed that while infant mortality fell throughout the project period, this was no more significant in TINP areas compared with the rest of Tamil Nadu. There was a clear decline in hospitalization for diarrhoeal illness, which seems to have been associated with earlier and better use of home sugar–salt solution. Immunization levels climbed to over 80 per cent throughout the state, associated with the national Universal Immunization Programme. Other health services were found to have rather low coverage. Coverage of children with six-monthly deworming was estimated to have been nearly 50 per cent while vitamin A supplements reached only one-quarter of children. This too was the responsibility of the health worker initially and was plagued by uncertain supply of the liquid vitamin. It will now be given on a regular basis by the CNW herself. The referral of children to the primary health care system if they failed to gain weight during supplementation was poorly implemented and remedial actions were rarely, if ever, taken.

Health service delivery in Tamil Nadu is made difficult by the control of key functionaries by several independent directorates, a large number of staff vacancies, frequent transfers even of peripheral staff, and a lack of adequate training and supervision. The state government has appointed an expert committee to address these structural problems and it is likely that significant changes will be made. TINP-II will include modifications in the health component, including joint coordinated training and supervision of health and nutrition staff and a closer working relationship at the village level.

The communications component was evaluated largely through qualitative techniques. Substantial improvements were noted in mothers' knowledge and home treatment of diarrhoea as well as in their appreciation and acceptance of immunization. Unfortunately, little information was collected on the frequency and timing of breast-feeding or on weaning although it appears that child feeding practices improved throughout the project. Workers acknowledged the usefulness of the wide range of attractive and appropriately targeted communication materials. The training of project functionaries in communication skills was particularly noteworthy. In the future, the project will attempt to document nutrition and health behaviour more clearly and measure changes associated with communication efforts.

THE LESSONS LEARNED FROM TINP

On Project Design and the Implementation Process

Project design was facilitated by an excellent nutrition information base in the form of the Tamil Nadu Nutrition Survey.[6] The study was a systematic effort to analyse the nutrition aspects of food production, distribution and consumption with a view to developing strategies for improved nutrition in the state. There was also a clear understanding of why the existing 25 nutrition projects had failed to have the necessary impact. The Institute of Child Health at Madras had established morbidity patterns in the state and their relationship to malnutrition.

The involvement of World Bank Staff in the project design process helped to incorporate successful international experiences from other Bank financed projects. The use of community-based nutrition workers as the main change agents, a strong nutrition education component, focus on the 0–3 age group, etc. were based on the Bank's Indonesian project experience, while the training and visit system of agricultural extension suggested frequent, decentralized in-service training and well defined work routines for field staff.

Phased implementation of the project with a pilot phase in the first year which permitted testing and refinement of project design were important reasons for successful implementation. A separate project coordination unit headed by an officer of the Indian Administration Service (IAS) in the rank of Head of Department and the constitution of an Empowered Committee chaired by the Chief Secretary and Secretaries of the relevant departments helped to speed up the decision-making process and facilitated implementation. A Project Management Fund provided modest means for testing innovative ideas and conducting research studies. Local communities were prepared to receive the project at a briefing on project activities and objectives by the workers and supervisors before project services were introduced.

'Catch them Young'

TINP was one of the first nutrition projects anywhere in the world to emphasize the need to improve the nutritional status of infants and very young children and to design a project exclusively for them. However, it did not focus adequately on 0 to 6-month-old infants. Project experience has proven that inputs must begin prior to the age of 6 months to leave significant impact on child malnutrition and morbidity. A study by a private researcher showed that the average age at entry into feeding was 7.87 months, suggesting that growth faltering and malnutrition are problems by 6 months of age. Another study showed that of all children becoming severely malnourished, nearly one-half had been so when first enrolled at 6 months of age. Although project design included supplementary feeding for pregnant mothers, antenatal care, and growth monitoring of infants from birth, performance of these tasks was poor. Further, there was no management of low birth weight babies. Only by initiating growth monitoring at birth will the project be able to detect infants who are clearly failing to thrive and focus on their health, breast-feeding and possibly even provision of supplementary feeding before the age of 6 months. Project experience also suggests that much more emphasis needs to be placed on maternal health and nutrition. This in turn may necessitate strategies to improve the health and nutrition of adolescent girls and younger girl children.

THE CHALLENGE

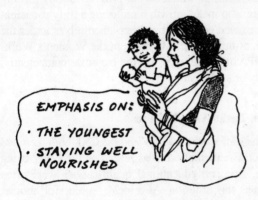

EMPHASIS ON:
- THE YOUNGEST
- STAYING WELL NOURISHED

RATHER THAN...

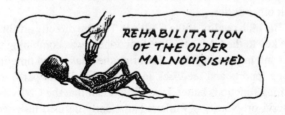

REHABILITATION OF THE OLDER MALNOURISHED

Stephen

TINP turned the emphasis of nutrition from rehabilitation to prevention and promotion.

Growth Monitoring Can Work

TINP has demonstrated that growth monitoring can be done successfully in large-scale nutrition projects, provided workers perceive it to be the centre-piece of the project.[7] Moreover the project must be able to prove to mothers that regular weighing will promote the healthy growth of their children by early detection of problems and by demonstrating the ways in which such problems can be overcome. The mechanisms that helped growth monitor-ing to work in TINP were the selection process and the short-term food supplementation. The selection process compelled workers to monitor the growth of children regularly. The weighing and supplementation demon-strated to mothers that there was a simple means to ensure the healthy growth of their children. It is interesting to note that sustained growth moni-toring has been less successful in projects which either permit universal supplementation (ICDS in India) or which do not provide for any feeding (Indonesia). The challenge is to make growth monitoring a truly participa-tory exercise, preferably carried out by the mothers themselves under the guidance and supervision of the worker. Members of the Women's Work-ing Groups in many TINP villages already use the bar scale competently, testifying to the feasibility of such a strategy.

On Workers' Selection, Tasks And Routines

The key players among the staff were the CNW and the CNI, both recruited exclusively for the project. Great emphasis was placed on the CNW being a resident of the village. Age and educational qualifications were often overlooked in order to meet this criterion. As a local, 'successful' mother the CNW enjoyed considerable credibility in the community and her own motivation to serve was high. Her presence in the village made it possible to establish contact with mothers whenever available or not preoccupied with other duties.

The high quality of the CNWs in TINP is directly attributable to the CNI. The key to the CNIs effective functioning was combining training, supervi-sion and monitoring tasks. Ensuring the quality and timeliness of the moni-toring reports and feedback in turn helped her to perform the review and training functions better. It was important that the CNI was not a first-level supervisor. Nutrition workers had clearly defined tasks and priorities and their daily and monthly routines were specified. Mornings were devoted to feeding and record-keeping while afternoons were reserved for home-visits and nutrition education. There were fixed dates for weighing, sectoral meetings, block-level and district-level meetings, and in-service training sessions. The high level of motivation among CNWs and CNIs can be attributed to the support that they received from the training, monitoring and communications wings of the project, which were responsible for much of the project's success.

In contrast, health workers were recruited most often from outside the villages they served, even from urban areas, and trained in institutional settings with little reference to actual rural health facilities or resources. Their tasks were many, varied and not prioritized (except for the priority given to recruitment of family planning acceptors). Their supervision was sporadic, usually 'bureaucratic'—relating to reports and procedures, and lacking in supportive and motivating components. Absenteeism, frequent transfers and neglect of community work were all-too-often the result.

Supplementary Feeding

The pre-mixed food supplement used in TINP was nutritious, widely acceptable, palatable and digestible. Mothers commonly expressed satisfaction with the food and believed in its impact on their children's growth. They had seen this and other food prepared in cooking demonstrations held by the CNW every fortnight, and many prepared the food at home when their children graduated from feeding at the centre or for their other children. The problems encountered included: children's difficulties in consuming the entire ration at one sitting; failure of some CNWs to insist that the food supplement should be consumed on site and to provide the food as a gruel for children under one year; and a diversion of food from the beneficiary to others in the family, particularly elder siblings who brought the young children to the centre and were tempted to eat some of the *ladoo* themselves. Better education of mothers on the role of supplementary feeding in stimulating growth, addition of milk powder to enhance the density and quality of protein in the food, and reduction of bulk by malting or the addition of amylase-rich flour (ARF or powdered malt) are the improvements being contemplated for the next project.

Most of the food used in TINP came from a public sector undertaking of the Government of Karnataka. The product was marked by high quality and consistency, and supply was uninterrupted and at a steady cost. Although the project's experiment to produce food locally through women's cooperative societies posed some problems in supervision and quality control, this approach will be continued and perhaps expanded in view of its demonstration effect as well as its economic benefit to local women.

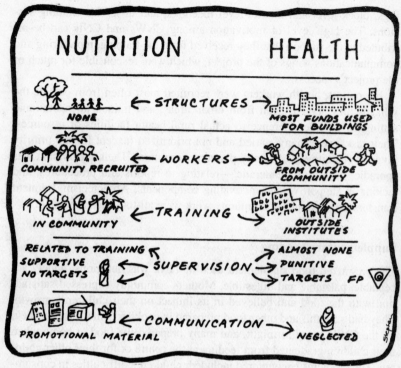

The relative success of the nutrition activities in comparison to health is reflected in the contrasting approaches of the two sectors.

Reducing Moderate Malnutrition

While the project reduced severe malnutrition by over 50 per cent, moderate malnutrition was reduced by only 14 per cent in the first project block. It still affected 30 per cent of children. At the start of the project about 20 per cent of the child cohorts were in Grades III and IV. Half of these children had improved to Grade II by the end of the project. Adjusting for this inflow into Grade II, the net change in this grade shows a considerable reduction in moderate malnutrition.

However, it is evident now that the Project's impact on malnutrition could have been greater had the criteria for feeding allowed moderately malnourished children to be fed. High rates of relapse into feeding after the first 90-day period also suggest the need for revision of the exit criteria. For TINP-II it was necessary to modify the entry and exit criteria to deal effectively with both problems. Thus, it was decided to include Grade II children in feeding, removing them from feeding only on their graduation to Grade I. This would considerably increase the period in feeding of children in Grades II, III and IV.

To test the effectiveness of these revised criteria, an experiment was carried out in one CNS circle (10–12 villages) in Thirukazhikundram block beginning in June 1988. All children in Grade II were fed, in addition to Grades III and IV and growth falterers. The results of this experiment exceeded the most optimistic expectations. First, a remarkable decline occurred in the number of children in Grade II, from 26 to 13 per cent with a corresponding upward shift in numbers of Normal and Grade I children. Second, the percentage of children requiring feeding declined from about 50 per cent at the start of the experiment to 25 per cent at the end of one year—i.e. a 'feeding level' comparable to the 'steady-state' level achieved in TINP-I after much longer periods under the old criteria. The experiment has now been extended to other blocks to ensure the consistency of such remarkable results.

The project had earlier (1986) begun an experiment in a different CNS circle of the same block to examine the effects of 'universal' feeding of children under two. The results of this experiment contrasted in an interesting manner with those of the later experiment (Fig. 2).

In the universal feeding area, grade shifts were very gradual and there was even some deterioration in nutritional status. Grade II malnutrition never declined below 25 per cent in spite of continued feeding. The selective feeding area improved far more than the universal feeding. With the active recruitment of children for feeding which is practised in TINP, the percentage of children who came under universal feeding was as high as 80 to 90 per cent. The cost implications of this are quite serious as the programme covers several hundred thousand children a year. Selective feeding achieves greater effectiveness at lower cost. Thus, the Project will use the revised criteria, including Grade II children in feeding. Early feeding of all Grade II children might help to avert stunting also. Most important, we expect a rapid decline in the number of children requiring the supplement as occurred in TINP-I. With a strong nutrition education component, a community-based nutrition surveillance system could eventually replace the government-sponsored programme.

In Health

Project experience showed that investment in health infrastructure and sup-

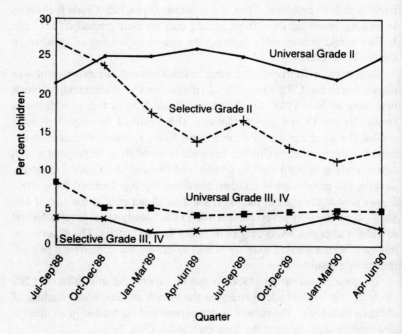

Fig. 2. Change in nutritional state by 'universal' or 'selective' feeding.

plies alone, even on a substantial scale, is not enough to improve the delivery of health services to those in need. The problem was complex, related to weaknesses in the health system and to poor coordination. The health department staff did not readily accept the Department of Social Welfare as the lead agency. It is important to ensure that the primary health care system is designed to meet the needs of the target group and is responsive to difficulties they encounter in its use. Health personnel, their skills, training, motivation and accountability are the keys to a well-run, successful health system and their ability to cooperate with other delivery systems that have impact on health is crucial.

Family Planning Targets

The target approach to family planning has been a major deterrent to the establishment of an effective and comprehensive MCH service delivery system. Achievement of family planning targets, especially sterilization, is a prime indicator of performance at all levels of the Health Department and failure to achieve these targets invites punishment. The involvement of agencies beyond the health system and provision of incentives has made the programme fiercely competitive at the field level. Moreover, the emphasis is on quantity rather than quality. The MPHWs therefore have real and opportunistic reasons to be absent from their work-stations and to deviate from work routines. Unless the family planning strategy is modified to allow the establishment of a first-rate MCH system, it will be difficult to achieve any of the related objectives satisfactorily, much less real planning of families!

Referral

Referral of cases failing to respond to food supplementation was a special health input of the project. For the referral process to be effective, a chain of activities is required: identification of a case by the CNW and referral to the MPHW; diagnosis by the MPHW with screening for medical and non-medical causes; treatment by the MPHW or referral upward to the Primary Health Centre or a hospital if necessary; travel of the referred patient to the treatment facility; and complete diagnosis and treatment of the illness at the higher level facility with feed-back to the originating level to allow follow-up. In the Project the process met with difficulties at every stage. The CNW lacked basic health training and was neither perceived to be nor allowed to perform as a front-line health worker. Although referral by the CNW to the MPHW was usually completed, the combination of infrequent visits by the MPHW to the CNC and her limited ability to diagnose and treat illnesses seriously constrained referral even at this stage. Of the cases referred upwards, few could afford the lost wages, time and transportation costs to make the trip to the referral hospital. At the PHC or hospital, no special efforts were made to handle the referred cases and visits usually ended by reinforcing the general lack of credibility of the primary health care system. Thus, strengthening the referral system will involve upgrading the skills and resources of the CNW, the MPHW and the Medical Officer at the referral centre, removing the social and financial constraints of those referred, re-ordering the priorities of the Medical Officer, revising procedures at the referral centre for dealing with referred cases and improving facilities at the referral centre. Unfortunately, this is a very tall order.

Communications

The complex design of TINP necessitated acceptance of the Project by the community and their full cooperation in implementation. At least three activities that flouted convention and were initially highly unacceptable to the community were basic to project design. The first was weighing, which was thought to attract the evil eye; the second, selection of children for supplementation, was contrary to the approach of universal feeding in all other feeding programmes; and third, nutrition education by the relatively young CNWs often went against the conventional wisdom and traditional practices recommended by village elders. The success of TINP can be judged by the extent to which these three activities have become fully institutionalized. It is remarkable indeed that project staff were able to persist within an unpopular design and subsequently win full acceptance and participation in the project.

While TINP undoubtedly had the greatest impact among on-going efforts in the state for health and nutrition education, and the CNW became an outstanding communicator, a more systematized and consistent social-marketing approach would have yielded better results in modifying the knowledge, attitudes and practices of the target group. A considered mix of media including mass media support also would have enhanced the communication effort of the front-line workers.

Training

TINP's training system for nutrition workers was innovative, highly effective and economical. An outstanding innovation in the Project was the method of training CNWs. Instead of the usual residential programme in a distant training institution, CNWs were trained at the block headquarters. This arrangement enabled the CNW to commute from her village home daily, usually by foot or cycle, and obviated the need for these village mothers to stay away from their families for long periods of time. Secondly, the syllabus and training plan were designed by the CNIs—who were both instructresses and second-level supervisors—during their own training. This had the double advantage of training that was familiar with field situations and which enabled the instructress to continue to support and monitor trainees in the field after the formal training was over. The emphasis placed on developing the communication skills of CNWs, production of excellent training-support materials by the communications unit, and the use of a variety of training methodologies to make the programmes participatory and interesting were all important elements of success. In addition, teaching the workers to adapt project objectives to their own villages, including a meeting of CNWs with their village leaders to explain and win endorsement for the programme, and training them jointly with the MPHWs were important strategies which ensured relevance in the project.

The CNI made continuous in-service training of the CNW possible throughout the project. Bimonthly review sessions were used to sharpen skills in weighing, plotting growth charts and keeping records. Special attention was paid to workers whose performance was identified as weak.

In sum, the trainees learned in a situation with which they were familiar instead of in an alien environment in an institutional setting. This paralleled the situation in which they themselves would train mothers. Being trained with other workers from the local area gave them a chance to share and solve local problems. The trainer built up a long-term relationship with the workers, enabling her to modify her training plan to suit the trainees' needs and making training evaluation automatic. Training was cheap because there were no overhead or institutional charges. In-service training was possible because it was also local and cheap and there were numerous opportunities for extra training, especially for workers who needed it.

Organization, Management and Coordination

The project proved unambiguously that coordinating different departments of government is a difficult task. Bureaucracies may not work together even when there are natural complementarities of function. It is significant that the Project Coordinator was able to communicate directly with the nutrition staff who were employed exclusively for the project without conflicting instructions from any other department. However, such direct communication was not possible with staff controlled by another department (Health) making for the weak coordination of functioning seen at the field level in the Project.

Moreover, when tasks are added on to the existing jobs of functionaries of other line departments they may not accord the 'new' tasks the necessary priority. Thus, projects which place an additional burden on existing structures must study the structure of the implementing organizations carefully in the pre-project stage and, if necessary, re-order them to meet the new challenges posed by the project. The priorities of the project and of all concerned departments must converge. Appropriate organizational arrangements are crucial for successful project implementation.

A FINAL WORD

By doing things differently and doing things well, the Project has not only taught valuable lessons on how to get the job done but has also set the stage for initiating certain policy changes, creating certain value systems, pursuing certain management techniques, and re-organizing and restructuring government bureaucracies. These will provide a momentum to efforts to improve health and development in Tamil Nadu in the future.

References

1. Berg, A. (1987). *Malnutrition: What can be done? Lessons from the World Bank experience.* The World Bank, Washington, pp. 139.
2. Office of the Registrar General, Vital Statistics Division. *Population of India; 1991 Census Results and Methodology.*
3. National Nutrition Monitoring Bureau. (1990). *Interim report of repeat survey, Phase I, 1988–89.* National Institute of Nutrition, Hyderabad.
4. Shekar, M. (1991). *The Tamil Nadu Nutrition Project: A review of the project with special emphasis on the monitoring and nutrition policy programme.* Working Paper 14, pp. 95.
5. Department of Evaluation And Research (DEAR). (1989). *Evaluation of TINP.* Government of Tamil Nadu, Madras.
6. Cantor, D. D. (1978). *Tamil Nadu Nutrition Study.* USAID, Madras.
7. Shekar, M., Latham, M. C. (1992). Growth monitoring can and does work! An example from the Tamil Nadu Integrated Nutrition Project in rural South India. *Indian Journal of Pediatrics*, **59**:5–15.

CHAPTER 9

Mobilization for Nutrition in Tanzania

URBAN JONSSON, BJÖRN LJUNGQVIST AND OLIVIA YAMBI

The authors describe the community action and nutrition improvement effort in Iringa, Tanzania, which has grown into a national programme. All the authors participated in the design and implementation of this programme which is now an international model of community development for improved nutrition.

Urban Jonsson, Ph.D., a nutritionist, was the Representative of UNICEF in Tanzania before assuming the position of UNICEF Global Adviser in Nutrition.

Olivia Yambi, Ph.D., is a nutritionist with the Tanzania Nutrition Council, Cornell University Division of Nutrition Sciences. She is currently Nutrition Officer in UNICEF, New Delhi.

Björn Ljungqvist, Ph.D., a nutritionist, has worked extensively in East Africa where he assisted in the design and implementation of the Iringa nutrition project. He has recently left Iringa to become Coordinator of UNICEF programmes in Uganda.

INTRODUCTION

There is a new development paradigm emerging which reflects the changing view of the role of the poor, in particular poor women, in poverty alleviation. Poor people are increasingly seen to be essential actors in poverty eradication strategies, setting priorities, assessing and analysing their own situations, and designing appropriate, affordable and sustainable activities. This is particularly evident in the field of nutrition where, in the wake of the World Food Conference in Rome in 1974, the direct interrelationship between poverty and hunger was at last acknowledged.

Economists, political scientists, anthropologists and sociologists have now moved action on malnutrition out of metabolic laboratories and Third World experiment stations on to the main agenda of planners and political decision-makers. Initially multisectoral nutrition planning came into vogue, but its complexity and political intricacy eventually led to its downfall.[1]

Meanwhile, greater experience in community-designed and implemented nutrition programmes which emphasized the involvement of women gave new directions to practical nutrition efforts. The most positive results were achieved in programmes using a community-based monitoring system with particular attention to the growth of individual children and a clear conceptualization of the multiple causes of inadequate growth and malnutrition.

This chapter describes the application of one such community-based approach whose conceptual framework attributed malnutrition to a complex array of situations. When these situations were analysed and understood locally, practical community-based actions emerged and a measurable change occurred in undernutrition. We describe the antecedents, planning and implementation of the programme in the Iringa region of Tanzania and its expansion to other districts in that country and beyond. We conclude with an analysis of the factors which made Iringa a success and transformed it from a single field nutrition project to a large movement in development which used nutrition as an indicator of developmental progress.

THE IRINGA NUTRITION PROJECT (INP)

Throughout the 1970s the Tanzania Food and Nutrition Centre sponsored surveys and small research projects in an effort to understand and address the large problem of malnutrition in Tanzania. In numerous discussions and workshops it was concluded that there was no pre-packaged set of technical interventions that could solve the nutrition problem. Instead, it was necessary to develop a conceptual framework which explained the factors underlying malnourishment and, therefore, pointed to potential interventions. It was believed that if these were based in the community, they could lead to effective action. The resulting community programmes were to conform to six criteria:

— they should bring about improvement in the condition of women and young children, including a reduction in the heavy workload of women;
— they should encourage self-reliance and the use of local and national resources;
— they should enhance social equity reaching the poorest;
— they should achieve integration and convergence of services on the same target population;

— they should give priority to services and activities at the household and village levels; and

— they should carry out planning and implementation with the participation of villagers.

A detailed proposal was prepared for field intervention in the Iringa region in Tanzania's southern highlands and was submitted for international funding to the Joint WHO/UNICEF Nutrition Support Programme (JNSP) funded by the Italian Government. The project aimed to reduce infant and young child mortality, ensure better child growth and development and improve maternal nutrition. Priority activities were related to family/village food production and conservation, improving the food intake of young children, various health sector activities, and support to household and village institutions related to these goals. Project preparation had taken place in Iringa, not in the capital, and had involved a large number of regional and district level staff, not only from health but also from related development services in the rural areas.

Structures and Strategies

The INP utilized existing administrative structures, starting at the regional level and involving districts, divisions, wards and, most peripherally, 168 villages.* At the village level, activities were initiated and coordinated by the Village Health Committees answerable to the Village Council and comprising the Village Chairman, Secretary and other individuals chosen by the Council. Comparable participatory committees existed at the ward, district and regional levels, ensuring access to the government offices and resources available at those administrative levels. Full time government administrators were charged with coordinating and ensuring access of these nutrition committees to the various sectoral resources, both human and financial, such as extension workers from the departments of Health, Agriculture, Community Development and Education. A National Steering Committee with representatives from the Prime Minister's Office, the line ministries, the Nutrition Centre, UNICEF and WHO provided overall policy guidance. This function was eventually delegated to the Regional Steering Committee at Iringa and later to other regions which took up this approach to development.

*Each village is divided into blocks, consisting of ten households represented by an elected leader, established initially for political purposes. The village sub-unit structure has been successfully used for many development efforts.

The proposed programme had 11 projects and 38 sub-projects including support to the health sector, environmental health-hazard control, education and training, child care and development, technology development support, household food security, food preparation, communications, monitoring and evaluation, research and management. A 220-page Plan of Operations outlined all the activities in detail. The centre-piece of the programme was community-based growth monitoring in which each village would conduct a quarterly Nutrition Assessment Day. Political support ensured large levels of participation in the measurement of children's nutritional status. There was also high participation in the related analysis of the findings and community discussion of actions to be taken to improve nutrition (as well as to resolve other problems identified). This 'Triple-A cycle'—assessment, analysis and action—became the hallmark of the INP. It describes the procedure followed at each level—household, village, ward and district—in dealing with the issues emerging from the three-monthly assessment procedure. The community actions that emerge ranged from capital-intensive

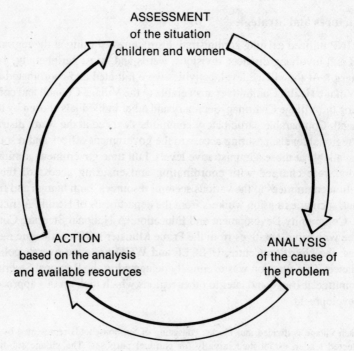

ASSESSMENT
of the situation
children and women

ANALYSIS
of the cause of
the problem

ACTION
based on the analysis
and available resources

The Triple-A cycle: assessment, analysis, action.

infrastructure projects such as piped water or construction of health centres to income-generating activities, establishment of child-care centres and a host of agricultural, animal husbandry and environmental interventions.

Social Mobilization

High-level political support and action was the hallmark of the programme from the outset. The INP was launched in December 1983 by the then Prime Minister who spoke for nearly one hour to a gathering of thousands of people in a stadium in Iringa town. The inauguration was itself a major act of social mobilization. It was followed by mass meetings in each of the INP villages facilitated by trained workers, and the screening of a carefully made film 'The Hidden Hunger.' The film highlighted the wide prevalence of 'invisible' or 'hidden' forms of malnutrition and the major underlying causes. Shown in each of the 168 villages before the first scheduled 'health day', it initiated the regular quarterly day during which all children were weighed, immunizations provided and ORT demonstrated. On this day, extension workers described and discussed alternative intervention responses to the village-wide growth monitoring results. More than 1000 leaders were 'trained' during these campaigns—three times for one day each. Administrators and politicians from the village to regional levels were taught how to analyse the causes of malnutrition and the options for action at their level. The Triple-A approach was emphasized in the training.

Following the initial village orientation, two volunteers were trained as temporary village health workers (VHW). They learned to conduct growth monitoring and record growth information. Mothers were given weight charts and taught to plot the weights of their children at the regular weighing sessions. A simple village summary of the measured nutritional status was prepared and submitted quarterly to the Ward Implementation Committee. Importantly, in addition to the data, these reports contained specific descriptions of the analysis and action to be taken as a result of these findings.

After the crash training programmes in each village and the initiation of health activities, village day-care centres were established. Attendants were given a brief two-day orientation on child care prior to initiation. These village workers later received one to three months of more formal training from the Social Welfare Ministry or in training centres established by the project.

Training

Village committees chose volunteers to participate in the six-month training of village health workers. Training was conducted in batches of 20 to 25 over a period of nearly three years. Most of these workers were chosen from amongst the original volunteers. The VHWs became the village-based outreach of a health care system, providing a wide range of services to previously-unserved villages. At the time of the villagization programme in Tanzania it had been planned to establish a health post in each village. It became apparent that this was a financial impossibility and the VHWs trained in the INP were the first step towards developing an alternative form of national primary health care. The VHW training comprised two months of classroom instruction followed by three months of field experience and a final one month in class. On graduation, the workers were provided with first-aid kits containing basic medicines, weighing scales and bicycles. The kits were issued free of charge and their contents replaced through the health system. Later in the project, VHW training was reduced to two months, with greater attention to brief refresher training and closer supervision in the field.

In addition to day-care attendants, VHWs and the village orientations, there were a wide variety of other training courses, seminars and orientation for personnel at all levels of the system. These were designed to improve technical knowledge as well as organizational capacity and foster commitment to the multisectoral, community-based, problem-solving approach. This helped those involved to recognize the links between malnutrition and its contributing causes. The search for solutions extended from the obvious activities of food production and health care, to attempts to mobilize resources at every level of the administration to support community actions that would improve child nutrition. The recognition that child growth was the outcome of environmental, economic and social factors permeated the entire project, a strong tenet of the INP philosophy.

The Information System

The community-based growth monitoring activity which served to focus attention on the nutritional status of children and provided villages with a tool to examine their nutrition problems was also the basis for an information system which was used to motivate and activate higher levels of government to take action at the community level. The system was primarily motivational. Programme activities were measured in terms of their nutritional impact rather than simply as 'inputs'.

The village weighing days, often held monthly, were attended not only by all children and their mothers but also by most members of the village committee. There was generally little effort to counsel mothers of individual children during these sessions but weights were charted and subsequent home visits were made to each undernourished child. Group health and nutrition education sessions were held and mass services such as immunization, demonstration of ORT, treatment of malarial fever were provided by health workers from nearby dispensaries. The simple one-page report submitted quarterly to higher levels described the weight-for-age of all participating children and reported on any deaths occurring in the previous quarter along with the presumed cause. Of even greater importance was the written record of actions being taken at the village level. The minutes of village meetings described requirements from government sectors at higher levels. They represented an on-going dialogue from the village to higher levels of all participating ministries.

Home Visits

The VHW was often accompanied by other members of the village health committee or the neighbourhood leader on visits to the homes of severely malnourished children. Families were interviewed regarding feeding practices, illness, hygiene and other factors in the home which contributed to the child's malnourishment. Discussions of resource constraints or problems in child care were frequent. A family action plan was made and a discussion held occasionally by the village council in the case of extenuating circumstances such as family illness or unemployment. Family actions were usually simple such as increasing the frequency of feeding, changing the child's diet, taking her more regularly to the day-care centre, improving hygiene practices or consulting a health worker at the dispensary. Sometimes actions went beyond normal family means to involve agriculture, provision of credit or some other employment opportunity. Not only the mother but also the VHW and community members watched with interest as the child was weighed at the next monthly health day to see if their actions resulted in growth.

The concern for the individual child on the part of the village health worker and the other village members is an important motivational factor. Sometimes even a ward secretary or divisional or district official may accompany the worker to a household to see conditions for themselves and be actively involved in practical suggestions. Thus, the home visit is a mixture of education, social persuasion, peer pressure and political persuasion or even intimidation, designed to influence household behaviour and result in clear action for improved nutrition.

Village-level Activities

Plans at the village level include the establishment of day-care centres, gardening and other agricultural activities, and efforts to improve water supply and latrines. A given project may take months or more for im-

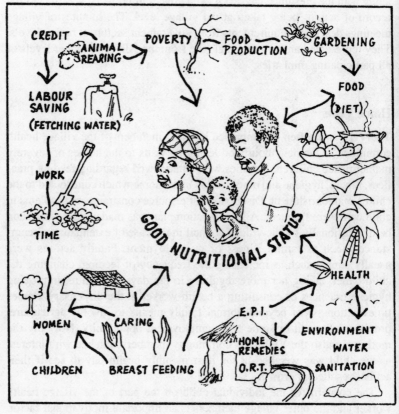

A wide array of village-level activities contributes to improving nutritional status.

plementation, but the quarterly reports reflect progress and keep the commitment clearly in front of the village council for their attention and continuing action. Although the projects chosen generally came from a long list of possibilities developed by the central management, numerous alterations in design and implementation have resulted in a wide array of activities.

Supervision

Support and supervision from the ward level covering a number of villages was extremely important. It ensured continued attention to village activities, provided the summary of growth monitoring results to higher levels along with the status report of activities being undertaken in the villages. It was at this level that mobilization of government resources for individual villages was most critical. The Ward Secretary was provided with a motorcycle by the project which facilitated communication with the villagers. Similarly at divisional and district level the provision of vehicles was an important step to ensure good supervision and regular communication and also the access of extension workers from various departments to the village. Without support from the INP for transport and related allowances the high level of participation of numerous development sectors would most likely have been substantially lower.

Mid-term Evaluation (1986)

In 1986 the Iringa Nutrition Programme was evaluated through an internal review involving more than 50 people from regional to village levels, as well as by an international team.[2]

The participatory evaluation was itself a Triple-A process and confirmed the value of the participatory approach. Increased awareness of nutrition, the excellent functioning of the village monitoring system, integrated health activities at the village level such as EPI, and some innovative project activities such as the production of efficient stoves and use of germinated flour were all recognized as major positive achievements. The external review felt that Iringa was too well-off to be representative of all Tanzania, that the cost of the project per child was high, and that many of the projects fell far short of expectations.[3] The team did not seem to understand or accept the value of the Triple-A approach, so much a part of the regular activities in Iringa.

These and other criticisms of Iringa helped to sharpen the underlying conceptual framework and the action programmes. The array of underlying causes of undernutrition were regrouped into three critical areas: household food security, health services, and child care. By far the most important were child care practices strongly related to the knowledge and attitudes of the child care taker, normally the mother, and the time available for care. The reduction of the worker's load to enable mothers' education therefore became a major prior.ty in INP.

Expansion and Modification

A decision was taken to decentralize INP management and the District Implementation Committees were strengthened, taking over the responsibilities of regional and national authorities. Individual situation analyses were prepared and the programme was expanded to cover the entire Iringa region, with some 450 new villages added to the original 168. The addition of 150 000 children to the programme was managed almost entirely by the existing staff with very little outside support. The expansion was on lines similar to the original project, with a campaign in each village. Recruitment of health workers, establishment of the village-based monitoring system and provision of some key health services, such as immunization and ORT, were undertaken.

The immediate impact was impressive. In a short time the Iringa region reached 80 per cent coverage with immunization, the highest in Tanzania at that time. Participation in the monitoring system was even higher and the prevalence of malnutrition declined rapidly. Project activities were regrouped into six areas related to the factors underlying malnutrition:

— Systems development and support (including policy and programme communications, monitoring and evaluation, integrated training and infrastructure support);
— Maternal and child health (dispensaries, MCH services, VHWs programme, training of traditional healers and birth attendants, CDD, EPI, ARI, malaria, nutrition rehabilitation, maternity care and control of micronutrient deficiency disorders);
— Water supply and environmental sanitation;
— Household food security (food and nutrition planning, agro-forestry, crop promotion, home gardening, small animal husbandry, food processing and preservation, and food preparation);
— Child care and development (village child care-taker organizations, child-to-child actions, technology development support and studies); and
— Income-generating activities.

The unit cost of expansion of INP demonstrated a decline in the per child cost which fell to US$5 from the $12 per child per year in the original project areas. Increasing attention to INP throughout Tanzania led to considerable mass media coverage. In March 1987 a workshop on social mobilization was organized in Iringa in which a large number of national and regional government and party staff from all over the country participated. They defined the key elements of the Iringa experience as :

— Advocacy;
— Information/Communication;
— Training/Education;
— Provision of some key services;
— Mobilizing agents ('strategic allies');
— Social organizations and relations; and
— Programming for social mobilization;

These became the guiding principles for the programme's expansion to the rest of the country.

The Final Evaluation

The INP was evaluated again in mid-1988 by a team of experts. Severe malnutrition had declined from 5 per cent to under 2 per cent, and overall undernutrition had declined from 50 per cent to about 37 per cent.[3] A fall was seen in severe malnutrition in all expansion areas, the minimal predictable outcome of the project wherever it was implemented. Process assessment showed that 85 per cent or more of the target group had been reached and that 80 per cent of mothers fully understood the growth chart and were adhering to suggested child care practices such as frequent feeding.

Increased human and institutional capacity had been an important goal of the programme. The evaluation showed that all levels of institutions in Tanzania had benefited. More than 50 research and action studies in the Iringa region had stimulated national and regional research and training institutions to carry out practical operations research. While political forces had supported the effort, the Party also benefited from the social mobilization and increased participation. The INP also introduced a new style of integrated planning and management extending downward from the regional level to each village committee. It had demonstrated that decentralization below the region was not only possible but desirable and had strengthened district divisional and ward capacities. Several technical innovations look place as well, such as the construction of low-cost multipur-

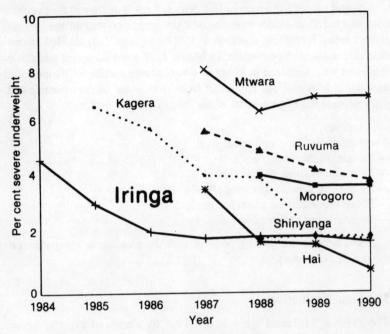

Fig. 1. Severe child malnutrition in seven Tanzanian regions, 1984–90.

pose training centres, improved ventilated pit-latrines and reduction of dietary bulk through germinated flour. Village-based child care, nutrition rehabilitation activities and the national immunization effort had also benefited a great deal. There was wide appreciation of the Triple-A process and of the clearly-formulated conceptual framework. Their use and the wide-scale social mobilization were identified as the key elements contributing to the success of INP.

The uniqueness of Iringa as a nutrition effort lies in the development of the process rather than in any particular element of the project. It is an understanding of this Triple-A process that will determine how the project's success can be transferred to other situations and conditions. The growth monitoring activity is ultimately a communication strategy operating at all levels from household through village and upward to the region. It facilitates communication between mothers, with village leaders and other personnel, government resource persons and political leaders. The attention to child malnutrition and death, enabled by the INP information system, brought all levels into a common communication relating to these issues. It increased the participation and accountability of government authorities and provided an objective means to assess their performance.

The attention of the INP to the measurement of nutritional status and the repeated assessment and charting of growth started as a strategy to mobilize communities. Thus, third-degree malnutrition was characterized as a condition next to death. Regular weighing of each child was possible, and villages could see progress even if they could not measure fall in the rates of mortality. The visualization of growth on the weight card was a tangible means for mothers to see the effect of their own actions. The cards of all children taken together gave a similar picture to the entire village. The fact that villages could organize and sustain this monitoring activity on a regular basis was an indication of the independence this project engendered and a key element of its success. With the elimination of third-degree malnutrition it is now becoming more difficult to sustain interest. This demonstrates the value of a focus on growth rather than on nutritional status, as every child should grow every month. It is likely that Iringa will increasingly shift attention from established malnutrition and its elimination to the promotion of healthy regular growth in each child, thus ensuring a greater degree of involvement among all families in the assessment and analysis of nutritional status and action to improve the overall health and nutrition of each child.[4]

Costs

A detailed cost analysis included both external and internal inputs at national, regional, district and village levels. For the estimated 46 000 children in the original programme, the annual cost per child was $3.60 for start-up, $5.30 for expansion and $8.05 for continuation. The start-up cost of $14 per child in the original area was weighted heavily by the costs of personnel and initial training. Staff costs were the largest expenditure category (nearly 40 per cent) and vehicles and transportation accounted for a further 26 per cent. While many of the start-up and expansion costs could be reduced, those for training, supervision and ongoing operations and supplies were a minimum for the project. Some 15 per cent of the total funds were contributed from national resources and two-thirds by the villagers themselves, mostly in the form of labour for construction projects. Thus, while the unit cost seems reasonable, the project would still strain national resources were the government to be responsible for all the costs of initiation, expansion and maintenance.

Expansion of the INP experience began as early as 1985 with modest funds from UNICEF and donations from abroad. Under the guidance of the National Coordinating Committee for Child Survival Programmes and the Planning Commission, additional regions in Tanzania were encouraged to formulate programmes. Resources were mobilized from the National Treasury and from abroad. The World Bank, EEC, IFAD, NORAD, SIDA and ODA have all expressed commitment or preparedness to provide assistance to the expansion of the programme. It is now expected that the entire Republic of Tanzania will have adopted the 'Iringa Approach' by 1995–96.

FACTORS CONTRIBUTING TO THE SUCCESS OF INP

Many observers of the INP have explained its success as being due to the favourable political climate and special circumstances in Tanzania. For example, of the five characteristics identified by Pelletier[4] as contributing to the good progress of the INP, three are environmental and only two are programme factors:

— the strong ideological and political support in Tanzania for improving human welfare;
— the sturdy political administrative system upon which the programme was based;
— the fact that Iringa is one of the few surplus food producing regions in the country;
— the efforts made to strengthen regional programme management; and
— the close involvement of the Tanzania Food and Nutrition Centre (TFNC) in operations research.

Although these environmental factors were important, we believe that several other programme factors were even more important.

THE TRIPLE-A APPROACH

The Triple-A approach recognizes that poor people constantly develop new strategies to cope with their situation. These coping strategies are often very carefully chosen to use available resources in the most efficient way. Some strategies serve to avoid crises, others to survive them. They all involve the crucial steps of assessment, analysis, action and re-assessment, i.e. Triple-A cycles. The recognition of existing Triple-A cycles reflects the view that poor people are *key actors* and not just passive beneficiaries of services. This in turn creates confidence, self-reliance and ownership of the pro-

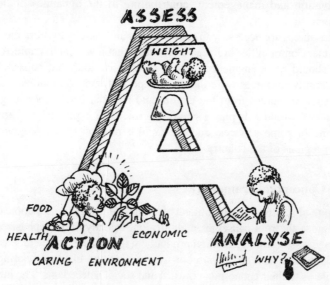

The 'Triple -A cycle' empowers people.

gramme by the people, and forms a basis for mobilization and participation. The Triple-A approach empowers people.

The Triple-A approach implies a *process-orientation* which programmatically means an avoidance of pre-packaged technical solutions. Instead, a method is communicated to empower people to find the best intervention, technical or otherwise, in a given situation. As this situation is changing constantly, programme interventions must be modified frequently. Such flexibility—a built-in capability to change—was an important characteristic of the INP. The entire programme was reviewed and re-planned every three months involving all who were instrumental in implementation. This also made it possible to use new opportunities that arose from time to time.

The Triple-A approach enables participants to focus on two important aspects: the need for information and the need for resources with which to act. Information is required for all steps of the Triple-A cycle. The INP created community demand for information at a very early stage, which explains the successful introduction of growth monitoring and promotion. Pelletier recognized that the *use* of growth information in the Triple-A approach in Iringa was much more important than efforts to increase the *validity* of the information.[4] Growth-information was primarily used for motivation and management, contributing to the dynamics of the programme.

Resources are necessary to enable action and thereby to 'turn' the Triple-A cycle. Communities in Iringa understood that it was *their* Triple-A cycles that should be strengthened, which made it obvious that household and community resources were the most important ones to mobilize, re-orient and use. Resources from the district and regional levels, including JNSP resources, would only play a supporting role. This explained the early cost-sharing of some services, and the rapid expansion of the programme to other regions of the country.

The Conceptual Framework

In spite of relatively high political awareness in Iringa, most people did not recognize the root causes of malnutrition. Initially they emphasized food storage losses, low agricultural production, inadequate protein (e.g. poultry) production, a lack of drugs, poor hygiene and the like, not relating these problems to their economic, political and social antecedents. The introduction of the conceptual framework which explicitly identified the immediate, underlying and basic causes of malnutrition and the interactions between them increased the analytical capability of those involved in the INP. After training, the people from all sectors and levels of society involved in the programme were able to use the framework as an analytical tool.

The framework facilitated multisectoral cooperation. It showed that everybody was important in attacking the problem. It also helped in understanding the different roles of the various levels of society. Its lack of detail allowed for gradual development. It became an important empowering instrument. People and their representatives could articulate their situation better and identify which particular constraints were to be attacked in order to improve their situation.

Process Targeting

Most often targeting means the identification of beneficiaries and provision of commodities (e.g. food) or services to them. In Iringa targeting was aimed at the poverty-creating process. It also involved all levels of society. The village identified households with malnourished children and provided community support to address the poverty-creating circumstances; the districts identified the most affected villages and provided district-level support; and the region identified districts which needed support. Education, empowerment, access, participation, involvement and sharing—all describe the effort to break the poverty cycle.

Training for Everybody

In one way the INP was a massive training programme. Everyone, from regional officials to district extension agents, committee members, village leaders, volunteers of all sorts and household members received training throughout this programme—some for as little as a day, others for as long as six months. Some of this training was typically 'top-down', but some was 'Freirian', aiming to empower through participation. People at all levels were involved and *Lishe* (nutrition in Swahili) became an internalized concept in the whole society.

It was proven repeatedly that people with very limited basic education could be trained to perform well provided they were motivated. Motivation came from a better understanding of the problem and of capabilities. The villagers could perform growth monitoring and analyse the data them-

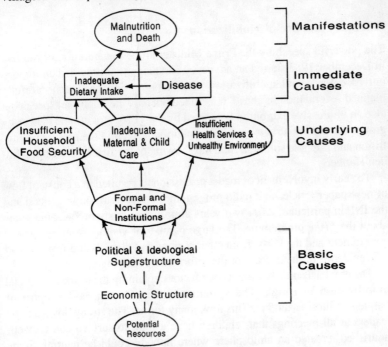

The conceptual framework: direct and indirect causes of malnutrition.

selves, very briefly trained VHWs could dispense important drugs, women could handle child care/feeding centres and villages could construct buildings and latrines. All this resulted in extraordinary mobilization of household and community resources, both human and organizational. These aspects of the programme were recognized as extremely important by Cerqueira and Olson who reviewed the 'nutrition education' aspects of six programmes including the INP.[5]

They found the INP very different from the other programmes in that it used a bottom-up, 'Freire-type' empowerment approach instead of the more common, top-down social marketing approach. Instead of aiming directly at changing behaviour, the INP increased understanding of the causes of the problem through the Triple-A approach, which then made changes in behaviour a decision among households. They found that the training in INP prepared people for both individual and collective action, depending on the resources required to solve a particular problem. The use of all available media channels, including traditional media, contributed both to efficiency and to the internalization of the programme.

Advocacy and Social Mobilization

The powerful speech by the Prime Minister at the inauguration of the INP in December 1983 started an advocacy campaign that provided an important base for social mobilization. The inauguration had been carefully planned several months ahead. It included not only the important speech but also an impressive exhibition organized by the TFNC, traditional dances by groups selected in a region-wide competition reflecting the problem of nutrition and possible solutions, and the showing of the first Iringa film, 'Hidden Hunger'.

The early involvement of media professionals resulted in a constant flow of newspaper articles and radio programmes about nutrition in general and the INP in particular. After two years almost everybody in Tanzania knew about the *Lishe* programme. The large number of visitors from the central government and the Party, from other regions and districts and from abroad was evidence of the success of the information campaign.

The emphasis on advocacy is one factor explaining the successful social mobilization in Iringa. The systematic identification and support of 'strategic allies' is another. This took many forms. The strong advocacy by leaders at all meetings that 'children have a right to survive and be wellnourished' created an atmosphere where nobody could be neutral. Some people expressed their agreement and commitment to this goal more strongly than others. They were immediately identified as strategic allies and were supported to become social mobilizers in their own communities or offices. The support most often consisted of extra training, participation in a workshop or selection/election for a particular task. Their work, which can never be documented fully, contributed to the transformation of the INP from a programme to a movement.

Community Participation

Almost all important aspects of the INP were characterized by a high degree of participation. A study that compared four well-known nutrition programmes (three of which are described in this book) on the basis of eight programme elements that would benefit from community participation found that Iringa scored highest overall and in each element separately (Table 1).[6]

The application of the Triple-A strategy was identified as the key to the good progress of the INP. This approach is fundamentally participatory and empowers households and communities. It results in a greater mobilization of local resources. For example, the establishment of centres to care for young children, financed by the communities, was the result of such participation. Community participation in Iringa did not primarily aim at increased efficiency, but rather at empowerment. Another tool was growth

Table 1. Level of community participation in four major nutrition programmes[6]

| Components | Community participation in | | | |
	Tamil Nadu TINP	Thailand	*UPGK* Indonesia	Iringa Tanzania
1. Needs assessment	1	1	1	3
2. Organization	2	1	2	4
3. Leadership	2	1	2	5
4. Training	5	1	1	4
5. Resource mobilization	1	1	2	5
6. Management	1	1	2	5
7. Orientation of activities	5	3	5	5
8. Monitoring and evaluation	4	2	5	5
Total score	21	11	20	36

1 – minimum and 5 – maximum community participation

monitoring which served the purpose of individual empowerment and was also a source of information used in community level discussions and decisions. Thus, growth monitoring played a role in social mobilization and enhanced participation. This gradually created an articulated demand by the communities at the higher administrative levels of society, i.e. districts and region.

The participation that the Triple-A strategy invokes in fact goes beyond the involvement of communities in project implementation. It creates an environment in which outsiders are accepted and allowed to participate in programmes designed and owned by the communities, rather than the reverse which usually prevails—where the community is expected to participate in activities designed and directed from outside.

Participation, however, was not seen as a goal in itself in the INP. The participants were expected to share some basic values such as the rights of children to survive and be well-nourished.

THE PROGRAMME'S RIGHT BEGINNINGS

Tanzania was among the first three countries to prepare a proposal for funding through the JNSP. In contrast to many other programmes, the INP proposal could be prepared with minimum 'interference' from WHO and UNICEF headquarters. The first stage of preparation occurred without any outside involvement. This created a positive attitude and feeling of ownership among Tanzanians and also allowed for sensitive political decisions (such as choosing Iringa) to be taken by the Government without considering the views of funding agencies.

It is often said that donor agencies do not allow adequate time for development programmes to be prepared and implemented properly; that they need results too early. The same is true for communities. When people get involved in a participatory process they want to see results. This was recognized by the INP Management Committee. Resources were therefore allocated to accelerate the immunization programme and to build a capability at the community level to rehabilitate children who had been identified as malnourished by the growth monitoring system. A little later the INP provided funds for a village kit of essential drugs. This decision was criticized by the donor of the Essential Drugs Programme which was providing monthly kits of essential drugs to all rural health centres and dispensaries in Tanzania. They did not believe that VHWs could or should dispense drugs. However, these elements of the programme enabled communities to feel that results would be achieved quickly.

A High-level National Steering Committee

The JNSP National Steering Committee was chaired by the Deputy Principal Secretary of the Ministry of Local Governments and Cooperatives. The Iringa Regional Development Director and all five District Executive Directors were also members of the Committee, along with regional extension leaders in health, agriculture and education and directors from some national institutions including the TFNC. The meetings were held in different villages covered by the INP and discussions at them were very open and frank. The meetings soon became an extraordinary forum for training each other. Many of the innovative steps of the programme were devised at these meetings, and because the Government was represented at a senior level, new ideas could immediately be applied in other regions of the country.

Information and Accountability

The early mobilization of village communities created a demand for information. This made it possible to establish the system of growth monitoring and promotion in all 168 villages within a very short period of time. The information was compiled at the village level and discussed in Village Council and Village Health Committee meetings. Decisions about support to households with malnourished children were made and tasks were assigned to specific people. They were made accountable to the village committee.

The compiled information was sent to the next administrative level (division) where growth data from all villages in the division were compiled. These data, tabulated by village, were then discussed both in district and regional development committee meetings. At each level, decisions were made about how best to support particular village or groups of villages identified as having problems. In the meetings of the National Steering Committee, Regional and District Implementation Committees, tasks were assigned to certain departments, staff or groups of people, with a clear expectation of accountability. The regularity of all meetings and the overall high quality of minutes from these meetings contributed to a high degree of accountability.

A People's Development Ideology[7]

No doubt Tanzania, and particularly the Iringa region, were well suited and prepared for a participatory project such as INP. The national political environment in which we were working is well described in the words of President Nyerere:

A decision for the children means that governments allow, encourage and help the people to act in support of the children, not that they try to do everything themselves. It means helping the people to understand the causes of their problems, and what they can do about them. It means providing them with the basic essentials which they will need for effective action. And it means allowing the people to control the implementation of the local decision they have made.[8]

Tanzania's basic development ideology was formulated in the Arusha Declaration in 1967.[8] Socialism and self-reliance were declared Party policy. This ideology puts people at the centre of all development: 'the aim is development of people, not things'. It espouses four fundamental principles: the absence of exploitation; control of the major means of production and exchange by peasants and workers; the existence of democracy; and belief in socialism. The strong belief in and advocacy for 'working together', first expressed in the establishment of 'Ujamaa Villages', penetrated the entire strategy. In practice this means a desire and willingness to work towards a consensus and to help each other. Even after the liberal policy introduced in the late 1980s, this ideology dominated the work of the Party and the Government. The INP was always explained as an articulation of this basic ideology. Survival and good nutrition of children were seen as concrete expressions of the development of people. These goals could be achieved best by working together.

In Tanzania, policies are proposed by the Government, reviewed and approved by the Party and executed by the Government under supervision of the Party. The INP started as a government initiative with reference made to the general ideology of the Party. After the important meeting at Iringa in March 1984 the Party saw the INP not only as a government programme but as an important articulation of their ideology. This ensured continuous support by the Party in programme implementation.

Villagization

At Independence, the population in Tanzania was scattered, as is still the case in many African countries. A scattered population cannot be politically mobilized and makes service provision very expensive. The idea to encourage and support people to move into villages gained momentum after the Arusha Declaration. The Village Act that outlined directives for the organization of a village was passed in 1975. Each village was to have a Village

Assembly consisting of all adults in the village. The Village Assembly elects a Village Council which is the 'Village Government'. A Chairman is elected by the Assembly and a Secretary appointed by the Party. The Village Council works through five standing committees, one of which is the Committee on Education, Culture and Social Welfare. This committee handles matters related to health and nutrition. The village is further organized into ten house cells, each with an elected cell leader. This organization had been fully established in Iringa when the INP started. The strong village organization facilitated social mobilization and community participation.

Decentralization of Power

In order to facilitate people's participation the Government adopted the Policy of Decentralization in 1972. Its goal was to decentralize and gradually delegate power at the grassroots level. The implementation of this policy, however, met with many difficulties. Local government structures had been abolished which meant that power remained at the centre. This was the reason why the INP was coordinated from the regional level in the beginning. The actual devolution of power came only in 1986 when the District Councils were re-established. The necessary decentralization of the INP was made possible by this step and after adequately-trained staff had been posted.

A Dynamic Health Sector

Health was the main subject at the 1972 Biennial Party Conference. A ten-year plan for development of the health sector was adopted (1972–82) which gave priority to rural preventive health services. The plan was to establish 25 new rural health centres and 100 dispensaries annually, plus train the required paramedical staff. This would provide one health facility for each of the 7800 villages. Donors, in particular the Nordic countries and USAID, provided strong financial and technical support.

By the end of the 1970s the result was impressive; the ambitious goal of training new staff had been achieved, 120 new rural health centres and 1000 new dispensaries had been constructed.[9]

An evaluation of the health sector in 1979, however, concluded that the goal of one dispensary in each village was financially unrealistic. The policy was changed to one dispensary per ward consisting of four or five villages. This opened the way for the Village Health Worker Programme to which the INP contributed extensively by showing the capacity and usefulness of trained VHWs.

EXPANSION AND REPLICATION OF THE IRINGA APPROACH

Most area-based nutrition programmes are designed as pilots with the hope that they can be expanded or replicated elsewhere. Often, however, such programmes turn out difficult to replicate. The most important testimony to the success of the INP is that it was expanded and replicated to cover half of Tanzania in a few years' time. The INP has been criticized by outside observers as being too expensive, too 'Iringa-specific' and too dependent on donor agencies, in particular UNICEF. It is also important to note that the expansion and replication took place during a period of severe economic austerity when most other socially-oriented programmes did not progress at all.

The explanation for this progress can be understood best from the fact that many aspects of the INP reflect the emerging 'new development paradigm' mentioned at the outset of this article. Some of the more important factors which contributed to the transformation of the INP from a project to a national movement are described below.

Both 'Top-down' and 'Bottom-up'

The Iringa approach is a combination of goal-oriented, normative, top-down advocacy and social mobilization *and* empowerment of people for bottom-up actions. The recognition of coping strategies existing at the community level was most important for this empowerment.

Cultural sensitivity and a listening attitude enabled participation, while committed leadership was required for advocacy and social mobilization.[1]

Although the Triple-A approach has been criticized as being mere common sense, it was its *combination* with the conceptual framework evolved at Iringa that empowered the people.

Both 'Short-term' and 'Long-term'

The conceptual framework ordered the causes of malnutrition into immediate, underlying and basic levels. It therefore encouraged people to find the politically-optimal mix of short-term interventions to address the immediate causes, and longer-term interventions to address the more basic causes.

It was never either/or but both. This pre-empted any unproductive discussion about questions such as 'either ORT and immunization, or empowering women'. Most people saw the synergistic linkages between the two types of interventions. The short-term activities were very important because they gave immediate visible results which made people enthusiastic. The long-term actions have ensured more sustained improvement in health.

Pluralism

Tanzania is a one-party state with one declared ideology. This does not mean, however, that there are no political differences among people or groups of people. The emphasis on 'a first call for children' and their right to survive and be healthy helped in overcoming these differences. An alliance was created among groups of many different backgrounds, interests and power-bases, including government, party, religious organizations, mass media, NGOs, other local groups and youth. They all joined together in a common cause—the survival of children.

Nobody 'Neutral'

In the process of advocacy and social mobilization nobody was allowed to be neutral. A perception that 'something is basically wrong, unfair and unacceptable' was created. Leaders were challenged to demonstrate what they were doing to help children survive and some, who could not provide a convincing answer were replaced in the next election. In this new environment of 'having to show where you stand', most people chose to join the movement.

Ownership

Community empowerment leads to community ownership. But in the INP, community ownership was never seen to be in conflict with the government. A deliberate effort was made to strengthen and establish linkages between the communities and the government. Just as communities need to feel ownership of community-level interventions, the government needs to feel ownership of the community experiment. This occurred at Iringa, facilitating expansion, replication and sustainability.

Voluntary Work

As with all other movements, the INP involved a lot of voluntary work, with very few people receiving any remuneration for their work. Primary school teachers, for example, assisted in the production of songs and drama; many politicians got involved in practical work and villagers assisted in the construction of dispensaries and in water programmes.

Slogans

The understanding and internalization of basic concepts are important in the creation of a movement. Simple slogans, such as '*sharing the burden*', '*hidden hunger*', '*the right to survive*', help in this process. These were built into the traditional media and communicated everywhere. It created a feeling that 'something is going to happen here'; it created expectations and hope for the future.

Women and Youth

Women and youth have been in the forefront of all movements, often representing the more powerless in society. The unleashing of their potential not only contributes to new leadership but also creates a strong commitment and enthusiasm, which was the case in Iringa.

The critical voices about the difficulties of replicating the INP in Tanzania have now ceased. The debate has moved on to the question of whether and to what extent the Iringa approach can be used in other countries. In this context it is important to realize that there are many successful community based programmes that have improved nutrition in other countries. The interesting observation is that many of these have characteristics very similar to the Iringa approach. This was realized during the preparation of a new nutrition strategy for UNICEF in 1989, when a thorough review of a number of successful nutrition programmes was made.

The Iringa Nutrition Programme received well-deserved recognition in April 1991 when the People of Iringa were given the Alan Shawn Feinstein World Hunger Award by Brown University. This award is intended

... to identify and recognize organizations and individuals who have uniquely enlarged public or scientific understanding of hunger, its causes and significant preventive measures; affected many through sustained efforts over a period of time to significantly reduce the number of hungry people; and/or pioneered new approaches to the reduction or the prevention of hunger.

It is significant that the recipient of this award was the people of Iringa and not any particular individual. The person who proposed the Iringa Nutrition Programme for the award had understood the essence of the programme.

References

1. Field, J. O. (1987). Multisectoral nutrition planning: a post-mortem. *Food Policy*, February, 15–28.
2. Government of Tanzania, WHO and UNICEF. (1986). Iringa Nutrition Programme (JNSP) Internal Review Report. Dar es Salaam, March.
3. Government of Tanzania, WHO and UNICEF. (1988). JNSP Iringa 1983–1988 Evaluation Report, October.
4. Pelletier, D. (1991). *The uses and limitations of information in the Iringa Nutrition Programme, Tanzania.* Cornell Food and Nutrition Policy Programme, Working Paper No. 5, February.
5. Cerqueira, M. T. and Olson, C. M. *Nutrition education in developing countries: An examination of recent successful projects.* Division of Nutritional Sciences, Cornell University, (forthcoming).
6. Shrimpton, R. (1989). *Community participation in food and nutrition programmes: An analysis in recent governmental experiences.* Cornell Food and Nutrition Policy Programme, May.
7. Yambi, O., Jonsson, U. and Ljungqvist, B. (1989). *The role of government in promoting community-based nutrition programmes: Experience from Tanzania.* PEW/Cornell Lecture Series, October 24.
8. TANU. (1967). *The Arusha Declaration and Tanu's Policy on Socialism and Self-reliance.* Dar es Salaam, National Printing Company.
9. Jonsson, U. (1986). Ideological framework and health development in Tanzania 1961–2000. *Social Science and Medicine*, 22(7): 745–53.
10. Chambers, R. (1983). *Rural Development: Putting the Last First.* London, Longman.

CHAPTER 10

Scaling-up in Health: Two Decades of Learning in Bangladesh

CATHERINE LOVELL AND F. H. ABED

The authors show how the Bangladesh Rural Advancement Committee—BRAC—has expanded its health programme from home-based oral rehydration therapy to a full range of health and development activities focusing on the poorest women in the community. BRAC remains a dynamic programme, ever-evolving to meet the needs of the people of Bangladesh.

Catherine Lovell, *previously Professor of Management at the University of California, served BRAC as a Management Adviser and has written extensively on BRAC programmes in education development as well as health. Her book* **Breaking the Cycle of Poverty: The BRAC Strategy** *was completed just prior to her death in November 1991.*

F. H. Abed *is the founding Director of BRAC. He has been awarded numerous international prizes including the Magsaysay Award and UNICEF's Maurice Pate award in recognition of BRAC's innovative approaches to rural development.*

INTRODUCTION

The Bangladesh Rural Advancement Committee (BRAC) was born in 1972 as a small charitable group whose aim was to help reconstruct Bangladesh after the Liberation War. Following the terrible upheavals of 1971, ten million refugees had returned to destroyed homes and crops. By 1991 BRAC had grown into one of the largest indigenous non-governmental organizations (NGOs) in the world. It is staffed by some 4250 regular employees plus 4000 part-time primary school teachers and has an annual budget of approximately US $20 million. By the end of 1990 BRAC had organized some 600 000 of the poorest rural men and women into more than 10 000 grassroots organizations in over 9000 villages. Growing at the rate of 2000 new village groups and 100 000 new members each year, BRAC is evolving a strategy which it hopes can lead its members to sustainable self-reliance.

BRAC is a large, complex and multi-faceted organization which is evolving continuously—adapting, learning, changing, growing. Health has always been one of its important programme areas. Health programmes have often run parallel with BRAC's other development activities rather than being integrated with them. Nearly two decades of learning in the health field have taught BRAC important lessons about the possibilities of and constraints in reaching the poorest in rural Bangladesh. BRAC continues to experiment with health interventions and implements the most promising on an increasingly large scale. BRAC has been characterized as a 'learning organization', its success being attributed to this basic feature of its institutional strategy. Korten[1] and Chen[2] observed that BRAC 'learns as it does' through a responsive, inductive process. Lessons from past and current field activities are translated into revised or new programmes or implementation strategies for the future. Programme planning, design, implementation, learning and redesign are mutually-reinforcing and simultaneous processes. In practice the 'learning organization' concept means flexibility in programming, adaptation in the field, 'high-risk' experimentation and a willingness to fail—and thereby to learn how to succeed. Flexibility has been necessary on the part of staff as well as of donors.

BRAC's openness to risk and change emanates from a basic self-confidence which is anchored in a few guiding precepts. The organization's primary principle is a belief in people's ability to learn and to manage their own affairs if given the opportunity, methodology and skills to understand their particular circumstances in the larger setting. Thus, BRAC encourages people to understand their own situations and helps them to acquire a framework which permits the rejection of fatalism and to seek action for self-help. A second guiding principle is self-reliance. BRAC believes that people can be self-reliant if empowered through an understanding of their circumstances and supported by others in their group. Dependency relationships are not set up. BRAC sees itself not as a patron but as an assisting agency, a participant in a community-driven development process. Its long-term contribution will be measured in terms of the enhanced capacity of the village people to determine their own futures.

BRAC'S HEALTH PROGRAMMES

BRAC entered the health field early in its history, continuously expanding health programmes in one form or another ever since. Over two decades

BRAC has learned that for lasting impact on their health and nutritional status, the income-generating capacities of villagers must be improved and their health consciousness developed, so that they can look after some of their own health needs. Also, villagers must develop an ability to utilize and make demands upon the existing government health infrastructure.

Over the two decades BRAC moved along from its early efforts to deliver health services to its current emphasis on enabling people to address their own health concerns. Work at the village level was reinforced by efforts to assist the government health system to improve its services. The programme focused increasingly on measures to help build the capacity of villagers to demand basic government health services intelligently.

THE EARLY EXPERIENCE

The evolution of BRAC's learning in the health field is similar to that in other developing countries in the same period. Along with others, BRAC moved from an emphasis on curative services to increased focus on preventive measures, with primary health care at the forefront.

BRAC's earliest health programme, begun in 1972, was essentially curative. The first BRAC project at Sulla Thana* was a 'community development programme' with health as one component, rather than a programme targeted to the poorest in the villages. Project workers found disease rampant and therefore introduced health services by establishing four clinics with attending doctors. The doctors soon found that 10 to 15 diseases accounted for 95 per cent of health problems. By the end of the first year of its health programme, BRAC decided to train locally-recruited paramedics similar to the Chinese barefoot doctors who had been discussed so enthusiastically worldwide in the late 1960s. BRAC's health professionals prepared a list of 'essential drugs' that could be administered by the paramedics, thus undermining doctor dependency. After several months of training the paramedics were to treat simple illnesses for a very small fee and refer more complicated cases to the clinics. Family planning was also stressed on the basis of the observed 'need' of the villagers.

In order to make this health system self-sustaining, BRAC experimented with an insurance scheme in which households prepaid with five kilograms of paddy per person per year. However, evaluation of this effort revealed that, although about 30 per cent of costs were recovered, health care was not reaching those most in need. The beneficiaries were primarily well-to-

---

*In 1972, a thana was a government administrative unit of 100 000 people.

do villagers. The poorer villagers felt that 'future' illness was less important than the current benefits of five kilos of paddy, and hence they did not join the scheme. The scheme operated for about two years and then was abandoned; but the lessons from this failure were internalized.

BRAC then experimented with a system in which the paramedics worked for a group of villages, charging set fees for specific services. However, some of the paramedics began to expand their range of treatments and drugs as though they were qualified doctors. Some started their own practices, adding to the number of quack doctors already operating in many villages. The village communities were unable to exercise control over them. Ultimately, BRAC decided to retain only the best of these paramedics on its own staff and disband the others. In sum, these early efforts to establish a self-sustaining curative system had failed.

However, the efforts at Sulla were successful in other ways. In 1975 the Sulla area had a high contraceptive prevalence rate with about 20 per cent of couples using contraceptives. It had the highest continuation rate in the country with more than 50 per cent continuing beyond six months, largely because the clinics were able to take care of the side-effects of contraceptive use. Through its successful family planning experience in Sulla, BRAC was able to identify the main constraints to further increasing the contraceptive prevalence rate—the low status of women, lack of income and illiteracy.

Secondly, the Sulla project became a field base for testing home-made oral rehydration solutions to prevent deaths from the diarrhoeal diseases which were rampant in the area. This experimentation was undertaken in cooperation with scientists, particularly with Dr Lincoln Chen at the International Center for Diarrhoeal Disease Research, Bangladesh (ICDDR,B). It helped to develop a home-based method for treating diarrhoea which was later to become important to the entire country. Although ORS packets were beginning to be widely distributed or sold in other parts of the world, infrastructural constraints made distribution of these packets to most Bangladeshi villages all but impossible. In 1977 BRAC switched to its 'target group' approach, working with the landless, the poorest segment of villagers, rather than with the village community as a whole. Another curative health model was attempted at Sulla and in the Manikganj laboratory area where BRAC had by this time some 250 village organizations. Under this new health plan, one woman was chosen from among the poorest families in each village to be a health worker. Unlike the paramedics who were earlier selected and employed by BRAC, the *shasthya shebikas* were selected by their respective landless village groups. They were accountable to their own groups for their activities and would not leave their villages to become quacks. They were given simple health and family planning training and supplied with a few basic drugs which they dispensed to other villagers. To enhance their interest in this job, the *shebikas* were allowed to charge a small fee from every patient seen and to sell medicines with a small mark-up. Also, BRAC supplied credit to these women so that they could undertake small income-generating activities such as poultry-raising. Several hundred of these *shebikas* have now been trained and continue to work in Sulla and Manikganj, two of BRAC's most integrated project areas.

In the beginning, the *shebikas* also supplied contraceptives. However, later that year the government restricted the distribution of contraceptives by NGOs. At that time BRAC started its first important efforts to cooperate with the government health system. It trained its *shebikas* to encourage villagers to go to the government clinics for contraceptive services and for treatment of the diseases which they could not handle.

During this period BRAC had become aware of and wanted to tackle tetanus, one of the biggest killers of mothers and their newborn. However, the government was not prepared to supply sufficient tetanus vaccine and, even if vaccines could be found, the problems of maintaining adequate refrigeration precluded their distribution and use. BRAC recognized that large-scale immunization was beyond its own capacity. Ultimately, it decided that unless the government health infrastructure could sustain the programme, a single NGO should not take on this kind of health effort.

THE NATION-WIDE ORT PROGRAMME

Based on these initial health programme experiences, BRAC turned its attention even more actively to things that the villagers could do to improve their own health status. BRAC had been following and learning also from events and policies at the international level. The International Year of the Child in 1979 provided an impetus to think about programmes focused primarily on children which would significantly contribute to their survival. Diarrhoea claimed more young lives than any other condition. BRAC's early experiments at Sulla with oral rehydration during diarrhoea had been successful in saving children's lives. Field-testing of ORT by ICDDR,B had shown its potential. Also, the work with ORT among the Bangladeshi refugees in the Calcutta area during the 1971 Liberation War had shown what ORT could do in epidemic situations. All these considerations led BRAC to embark on a nation-wide ORT programme. The decision to undertake a large-scale ORT programme forced BRAC to choose carefully between ORS packet distribution and teaching mothers how to mix and use a home-made solution. Research at Sulla and ICDDR,B had found that a pinch of salt and a fistful of unrefined sugar (locally called *gur*) mixed in half a litre of water produced a solution with most of the qualities of the scientific ORS powder being distributed in packets. BRAC had found that it was possible to teach village women how to make the solution and at the same time to teach them a short, seven-point message about diarrhoea prevention and treatment. The Scientific Director of ICDDR,B, Dr Chen, felt strongly that, even if sufficient quantities of ORS could be produced, packaged and marketed, poor people, particularly in remote areas, would not have access to it. BRAC thus decided that its nation-wide effort would be based on teaching mothers the home-made solution method. In the early months of 1979 BRAC started to teach the home-based oral rehydration method to 30 000 families at Sulla. This became the testing ground for effective teaching methods and for working out the management and logistics necessary to scale-up such a programme and maintain quality control. In early 1980 BRAC launched its nation-wide effort to teach oral rehydration therapy to every one of 13 million village households in the country. This major undertaking was largely a curative effort but the cure was one which every village family could do for itself.

Backed by an experienced group of managers and a well-developed management information system, teams of trained female workers went house-to-house to teach village women how to make the solution properly and give it to their children. The teaching method and materials were carefully structured and based on the intelligent use of local belief systems. The ORT teachers, recruited from villages in the same regions of the country and trained by BRAC, worked under an incentive salary plan in which they were paid according to the quality of their teaching. Monitoring teams followed them into villages a fortnight later, interviewing a random sample of five per cent of village women to find out how well they had understood and learned the messages. Samples of solutions mixed by the village women were taken to laboratories for testing on a regular basis. A worker's pay was determined by how correctly the sampled mothers could prepare the solution and the number of messages they could recall spontaneously from the basic seven. Supervision of the teachers as they moved from village to village was strict but supportive.

An active management information system (MIS) remained in place throughout and an able evaluation division studied the programme as it progressed. It provided feedback to management on aspects of the programme which needed further research or improvement in implementation.

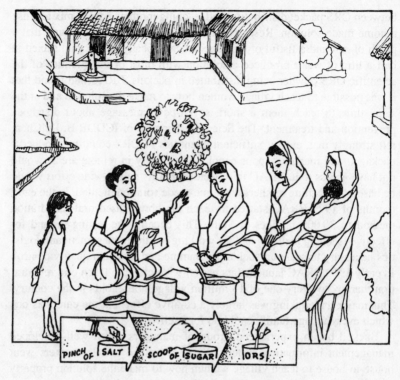

More than 2000 trainers visited 13 million households to teach all women how to prepare and use oral rehydration solution at home.

Teaching materials and training were modified and improved constantly. After the first 50 000 mothers had been trained, surveys found that although message retention and mixing skills were over 80 per cent, the oral rehydration solution was used in only five per cent of diarrhoeal episodes. Analysis of the situation revealed a major deficiency in the implementation strategy. The programme had focused on women alone, teaching them about dehydration from diarrhoea and the ORT method. However, as men were important decision makers in the family, it was difficult for the women to use ORT without the concurrence of their husbands, fathers or other men in the family. Accordingly, the teaching programme was modified to include male teachers whose job was to hold meetings and seminars with men in mosques, market places and schools. The inclusion of men in the target group very quickly increased ORT use to 20 per cent.

Anthropological research revealed further problems. In some parts of rural Bangladesh, four types of diarrhoea were recognized for which they had different names and treatments. Only one of these types—a severe, watery diarrhoea—was known to the women as the Bengali equivalent of diarrhoea. Since the delineation into four types had been unknown to the teachers, in the initial teaching they had used the Bangladeshi equivalent of the term diarrhoea. As a result the mothers thought the solution was for that type only. In the early stages of the programme over 55 per cent of women were using ORT for that type of diarrhoea, but not for the other types. This discovery led to a change in terminology and a major change in the seven points to remember. Altogether some three dozen evaluation studies of the project were carried out. Many have been published in national and international journals;[3,4] all have been useful in modifying and improving the programme.

In November 1990, a decade after the nation-wide ORT teaching effort began, BRAC completed teaching the therapy to the last of the 13 million village households. ORT is now an accepted part of the treatment of diarrhoeas throughout the country. Most recent evaluations have shown a high retention of knowledge about ORT (80 per cent) and widespread effective skills in mixing and administering it. During the ten years, BRAC had supplemented the face-to-face village teaching with radio and television advertising, posters, billboards and other forms of mass communication designed to reinforce the message.

The mammoth ORT programme provided several important lessons for BRAC, donors and health professionals. First, it dispelled the perception that NGOs were only capable of small, localized activities and of little consequence nationally. Secondly, it dispelled any notions that health programmes must necessarily lose quality if they are on a very large scale. It taught BRAC managers and field staff to think nationally, and inspired confidence to go to scale on other programmes. It confirmed the potential of lay workers to convey useful health information and change health behaviour. It was responsible for increasing the size of BRAC. In the first half of the 1980s the number of BRAC staff grew five-fold to reach 2268 by 1985; over two-thirds of the new staff members were part of the ORT programme. By 1990 BRAC employed 4290 people in its various development programmes in addition to over 4000 teachers in its education programmes. The size and dynamism of the programme required BRAC to develop its logistics, training, research and management capacities in major ways.

BRAC'S CHILD SURVIVAL PROGRAMME

In 1986 BRAC launched another major rural health initiative, a four-year Child Survival Programme (CSP). In addition to the ORT effort which was covering the last third of the country, it included preventive health measures chosen by the government, bilateral donors and UNICEF: immunization and high-dose vitamin A. In this programme BRAC staff members did not immunize or distribute the vitamin A capsules themselves but worked instead with the government to improve its abilities to perform and sustain these services. BRAC's CSP covered a third of the country—155 *upazilas* with 28 853 villages.* BRAC field staff assisted the government's district, *upazila* and union health officials to strengthen their management and improve their technical capabilities to provide mass immunization services and to improve their long-standing bi-annual vitamin A capsule distribution programme. BRAC played two major roles. It served as consultant and trainer to the government's rural health managers through a management development programme and provided on-site help with setting up the immunization system. For these the government's field-level workers had to be trained in immunization techniques, which BRAC facilitated. During the house-to-house ORT teaching, BRAC also mobilized village communities to cooperate with the immunization drive and organized them to demand sustained immunization services after the first round of vaccinations was completed.

By 1990 BRAC's four-year Child Survival Programme had helped the government immunization programme reach some 4.5 million households and 30 million people, and was deemed successful. In the third of the country where BRAC's CSP assisted the government, universal child immunization (UCI) was achieved. As Fig. 1 indicates, immunization levels in the BRAC-assisted area (Rajshahi) were 41 per cent higher than in the area of the country where the government's programme was assisted by CARE (Khulna), and 63 per cent higher than in those parts of the country where the government did the programme on its own (Dhaka and Chittagong).

However, in spite of this initial success, the sustainability of the government's immunization programme remained a question. As a result, the government Health Ministry asked BRAC to continue its help with on-going management development and community demand creation in a large number of the *upazilas* covered. BRAC calls this its[6] government facilitation

---

*An *upazila* is an administrative unit with 200 000 to 300 000 people. There are 460 *upazilas* in the country.

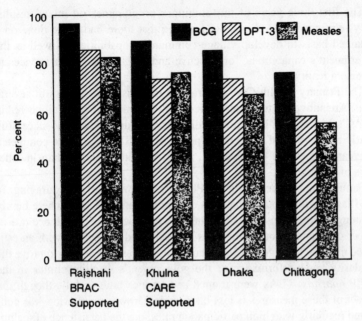

Fig. 1. Source: Bangladesh, WHO Coverage Evaluation Survey, February 1991.

programme. Under it, cooperation is continuing for another three years in the 60 *upazilas* which had the lowest coverage rates.

THE PRIMARY HEALTH CARE PROGRAMME

A sub-project of the Child Survival Programme was a significant, multi-component Primary Health Care Programme (PHCP) conducted in 15 of the 155 *upazilas* covered by the CSP. About three million people live in these 15 *upazilas*. The PHC programme added health and nutrition education linked to growth monitoring, traditional birth attendant training, clean water and sanitation development, and family planning to the CSP interventions (ORT, immunization and vitamin A capsule distribution). Like the CSP, the PHC programme had an explicit goal to strengthen the capabilities of the government health care delivery system. In these 15 *upazilas* the goal was to help the government to upgrade its capacity to deliver a larger range of health services than immunization and vitamin A tablets to the villagers.

The first three years of this ambitious programme had mixed results. They reinforced BRAC's earlier learning that more had to be done on a sustained basis to develop village community capabilities, as well as the government's capabilities, for effective and sustainable health services to become a reality.

The Primary Health Care Programme demonstrated success in several areas. An innovative tuberculosis treatment scheme, originally pioneered in BRAC's Manikganj 'laboratory' villages was found to be very successful. Nearly 80 per cent of those participating in the TB programme completed the year-long course of treatment, some four times higher than in other areas of Bangladesh.[5]

Family planning results in the PHCP were particularly encouraging. In 45 villages, with a total population of approximately 65 000, where family planning interventions were undertaken, a contraceptive prevalence rate of 51 per cent using modern methods was achieved (compared with an estimated national average of 23 per cent). BRAC was also able to improve the regularity and performance of the government's satellite clinics in the PHCP *upazilas*. TBAs were trained and latrines built widely, though the impact of these measures is less discernible. Growth monitoring was conducted regularly with high participation rates, but the persistence of malnutrition in spite of repeated educational efforts was frustrating to workers and mothers alike. Mothers' clubs were organized for the poorest women. Well attended monthly meetings proved to be a useful means of increasing villagers' awareness of health and nutrition issues.[6]

Attempts to activate village-wide health committees were not so successful. The activities begun by the PHCP and evaluated as successful are being continued either by BRAC's Rural Development Programme branches or under its recently-restructured health programme.

THE WOMEN'S HEALTH AND DEVELOPMENT PROGRAMME

In late 1990 BRAC restructured its health programme to integrate it more closely with the basic Rural Development Programme and with the extensive non-formal primary education programme which had been developed by BRAC over the previous decade. The new $8.6 million programme is being carried out in 10 *upazilas* for the first two years and in 15 *upazilas* in the third year. It will cover a population of approximately 2.4 million people in 1500 villages. Renamed the Women's Health and Development Programme (WHDP), this effort brings together the various village-based

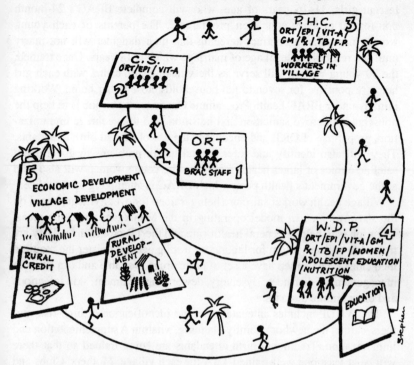

BRAC's health programmes have become increasingly comprehensive and, along with an expanded education programme, will integrate with the large BRAC rural development and credit programmes.

initiatives and government health system improvements which have evolved over time. Its goal is to reduce maternal and infant mortality by 50 per cent. Additional goals include the treatment and cure of a large proportion of tuberculosis cases using the methods tested earlier. The WHDP will conduct an experiment for the cure of other respiratory diseases, particularly pneumonia in children. The WHDP plan calls for integration of the health programme with BRAC's ongoing Rural Development Programme over a six-year period, eventually culminating in a self-financed Rural Credit Programme.

BRAC's long-term strategy combines literacy, health education, credit and income-generation with preventive, promotive and a small amount of curative health care. The over-arching goal is a health system that will be sustainable without BRAC. The first step in each village is to train 30 adolescent girls, 11–16 years of age, who will complete BRAC's 24-month non-formal primary education programme. The parents of each young woman must sign a contract agreeing that their daughter will not marry until she reaches the legal age of marriage which is 18 years. Once trained, the 30 young women will serve as the village health cadre, with each girl being responsible for seven to ten households close to her home. Working initially under BRAC health Programme Organizers, their job is to help the households improve sanitation and nutrition, and to encourage immunization, proper use of ORT, and encourage the use of trained birth attendants. They will also identify and refer special health problems to government satellite clinics or larger health facilities. The young women will also help at the government's health posts which BRAC is attempting to revitalize.

Village health workers also are being trained for every village, based on the *shasthya shebika* model operating in the Manikganj and Sulla areas. Their job is to help in general health care and the TB programme. They are trained to collect sputum for laboratory testing and administer the required medicines. The women have a set of basic drugs available and can assist in management of diarrhoea, dysentery, deworming treatment, skin infections and other simple diseases.

The WHDP includes antenatal care and identification of high-risk mothers, care of the newborn, family planning, vitamin A supplementation and immunization. Traditional birth attendants are being trained so that there will be at least one well-trained TBA for each village. Mothers' Clubs and Village Health Committees are being organized to link the community with the public health structure for immunization, vitamin A capsules, interventions in high-risk pregnancies, and for treatment of acute respiratory infections. The Village Health Committees will also maintain contraceptive depots until this function is taken over by the government. Membership in the Mothers' Clubs and Health Committees are primarily for women and the landless. The activities of the Village Committees are being carried out in close collaboration with the health staff at the government's union health post, the service closest to the village. Part of the job of WHDP is to continue to energize and upgrade the services of these health posts.

An important part of WHDP will also be a continuing programme of training in health management for the government's rural health administrators and continued work with these administrators to improve their management systems. BRAC's Management Development Programme provides training and field follow-up as it did under the Child Survival Programme.

A portion of WHDP resources is also devoted to the development of a new National Health Resource Centre (HRC) whose purpose is to build improved capacity within BRAC and other organizations to deliver higher quality preventive health services in rural areas. The Centre conducts monitoring, evaluation and research activities on health issues and provides training in the health field. It assists BRAC's own health programming and also that of other organizations in Bangladesh. Eventually, it will establish links with other regional health research and training facilities. The HRC will be a part of BRAC for the first three years, after which it is expected to become an autonomous, self-supporting institution.

At the present time Bangladesh has no system to collect reliable statistics on various development indicators. Statistics are collected on an *ad hoc* basis, so that comparisons over time are not possible. The HRC will establish sentinel sites in different regions of the country from which data, including births, deaths, migration, EPI coverage, school enrolment, nutritional status, disease incidence and other indicators will be collected on a regular basis. The Research and Evaluation Division of BRAC has already been experimenting for four years at six sentinel sites to develop a data collection system.

The HRC will also be a clearing-house for health-related information. A library of health studies will be established and continuously updated. The goal is to upgrade health research in order to find the right combinations of health interventions to reach the poorest of the poor in village contexts. The overall aim of the HRC is to provide scientific back-up to the government health system and to the people.

TWO DECADES OF LEARNING

BRAC continues to search for the right combination of health interventions that can move both villagers and the government health system toward higher levels of prevention and care on a sustained basis. Experiences with BRAC's health interventions over two decades have demonstrated that it is difficult to rely on the government's public health services to function effectively after an outside force such as BRAC departs. However, BRAC now feels that by helping the government's rural health system to improve its management, a higher quality of government health services will be available. By developing strong, better-educated and empowered village groups, capable of utilizing and making demands on government health services, a higher quality of preventive health measures will be practised in the community.

BRAC has begun integrating its health programmes with its core Rural

Development Programme rather than operating them as parallel efforts. Health education is an important part of the curriculum of the very large non-formal primary education programme (NFPEP). The NFPEP now comprises over 4000 schools, with the prospect of rapid expansion. Seventy per cent of those enroled are girls. Health issues are also an important part of the 30-lesson adult functional education-awareness course which every BRAC village-group member must complete. Health issues such as nutrition, sanitation, immunization, oral rehydration, breast-feeding, supplementary feeding and family planning are discussed regularly at the monthly meetings of some 10 000 village groups. Women's development remains a key focus of all BRAC's activities. BRAC has learned that progress cannot be made on health issues without the full involvement and leadership of women. It has also proved that, once empowered, the poorest illiterate women can become leaders in health improvements.

THE INGREDIENTS OF SCALING-UP RAPIDLY

Clearly BRAC has been able to scale-up its health programmes rapidly and effectively. This has been true of its nation-wide, single-purpose, oral rehydration teaching programme which reached 13 million households, and of the Child Survival Programme of assistance to government in immunization which covered a third of the country. It has also been true of its Manikganj and Sulla integrated programmes, of the complex Primary Health Care Programme conducted in some 2500 villages in 15 *upazilas* and most recently of its Women's Health and Development Programme which will reach 2.4 million people in 1500 villages.

BRAC has learned through these programmes that while the intensive involvement of an NGO is important, it can be only temporary. Health-aware villagers and effective government systems are essential for sustained results.[7] In situations where the government system is ineffective, NGOs must find ways to enhance the capacity of the government to provide sustainable services.[8]

BRAC continues to undertake a series of government facilitation programmes. It helps the government to enhance its capabilities in EPI, primary health care, non-formal primary education as well as in several economic sub-sectors: poultry, livestock, sericulture, irrigation and aquaculture. BRAC has learned that collaborative programmes with the government do work. Through commitment and hard work BRAC staff have been able to influence government workers to improve performance. How long improvements will continue after BRAC's withdrawal remains to be seen, but BRAC believes that system changes linked to community mobilization and demand will sustain improvements.

APPROACHES TO SCALING-UP

Five different approaches have been used by BRAC to scale-up so effectively: (i) replication, (ii) horizontal and vertical integration, (iii) supportive infrastructures, (iv) piloting and (v) model building. These modalities are not mutually exclusive but represent different perspectives on BRAC's scaling-up processes.

Replication

The most common way BRAC has scaled-up is by replication. The most obvious example of this was the spread of the ORT teaching method to households all over the country. After the development stage at Sulla, where the method was perfected, the ORT programme was replicated in village after village, incorporating improvements along the way. Replication was also used in the female paramedic (*shasthya shebika*) programme. The idea was first tested in the Sulla area, changed, retested, tried and changed again. When it was finally found reliable, it was replicated in the Manikganj area, and later in many other areas.

Horizontal and Vertical Integration

BRAC has also scaled-up through horizontal and vertical integration processes. Horizontal integration is illustrated by the development of the health programme in the 300 villages in the Manikganj area. Over a decade, the programme became multi-component in response to the most important needs expressed by the landless villagers themselves. Health components were added one by one to the core economic development programme so that today the villages have income-generating activities as well as a traditional birth attendant training programme, a government-linked immunization service, family planning services, a tuberculosis identification and treatment programme and a village-based paramedic cadre of curative service providers. Another example of horizontal integration was the addition of the immunization and vitamin A capsules to the oral rehydration teaching programme as it was covering the last third of the country. Thus, components are added to comprise an ever-widening range of services.

There are several examples of vertical integration in the development of

BRAC's programmes.* One example is the traditional birth attendant training programme which was integrated with the government health system by
encouraging TBAs to refer high-risk cases to the doctors at the nearest
health complex. Another example was the EPI effort in which BRAC added
EPI training and system development to the government's capacity to fur-
nish vaccines and maintain the cold chain. A third example was the government facilitation effort undertaken in the PHCP and WHDP. In these
programmes upgrading the quality of care at government health centres was
and is an essential part of the programme. Yet another example is the establishment of the new Health Resource Centre to meet the need for baseline
studies, professional monitoring, research and evaluation of health programmes and for improved expertise in health-worker training. Vertical integration implies added depth, a more complete approach to a given
problem.

Supportive Infrastructure

A third approach to scaling-up in BRAC has been the development of required support services. As health programmes were developed along with
other BRAC programmes, it became apparent that various kinds of training
were needed in large amounts. A Training and Resource Centre (TARC)
was created in the mid-1970s which has now been replicated to include six
residential training centres with some 70 trainers in residence as well as
available to give training in other locations. In 1990 the training centres
provided over 120 000 participant-days of training to BRAC staff, personnel from other NGOs and village-group leaders. About a sixth of that was
related to health programming.

A Materials Development Unit grew in response to the need for a host
of field materials including oral rehydration teaching booklets, posters and
flip-charts, nutrition posters and teaching aids, TBA training materials, immunization motivation materials, and printed matter on vitamin A and
breast-feeding.

A Research and Evaluation Division was established originally to do
baseline studies. But it was soon called upon to do field research and evaluation studies for programme managers and external observers. A Publications Unit also was needed to publish all the materials developed, including

---

*The term 'vertical integration' is used here in its economic sense and not as often used
in the health sector. It means addition of related, albeit hierarchical, elements of a
programme which are necessary to increase programme effectiveness.

GOVERNMENT HEALTH STAFF		*18,191*
TRADITIONAL BIRTH ATTENDANTS		*14,356*
VILLAGE HEALTH COMMITTEE MEMBERS		*3,399*
VOLUNTEER MOTHERS		*22,590*

Training at all levels has been a key strategy of BRAC's scaling-up process.

the functional education and non-formal primary education books and the best of the research studies done by BRAC. Now the Publications Unit also publishes a Bengali magazine directed at children which is devoted to health and other social issues. BRAC established a printing company which is now commercially profitable and does all of BRAC's printing.

A large Logistics and Purchasing Unit had to be established which arranges all transportation, purchases the bicycles and motorcycles used by thousands of field workers, and delivers all necessary materials to the field on time for training and programme implementation. Additionally, an Engineering and Construction Unit was set up to look after all construction of field offices and training centres.

A Computer Centre handles research and evaluation data analysis, accounting and other financial data requirements, and word processing arising from proposal and report-writing requirements. A Personnel Unit handles recruitment and other functions for the extensive staff requirements.

The 'Pilot' Approach

As in most effective development organizations BRAC normally develops its programmes by starting with a small pilot, which is enlarged when successful. Those activities that do not work at the pilot stage are abandoned. Those that are successful and seem particularly promising, and where constraints to expansion are not identified, are taken to scale.

Model-Building

A final way of thinking about successful scaling-up might be called 'model building'. BRAC has been a leader in developing various strategies for rural development and health programmes. In some cases other NGOs and the government have adopted the models and are now replicating them, usually with some modifications to suit their own situations and capabilities. The BRAC model is also disseminated by BRAC personnel who are much in demand by other NGOs, both national and international, because of their training and valuable experience in BRAC.

FACTORS ENABLING SUCCESSFUL SCALE-UP

Analysis of BRAC's experience also suggests that several factors were essential for successful scaling-up. The first is the ability to attract, train and retain a cadre of qualified, experienced and dedicated staff who are committed to the organization's fundamental philosophy. Without this core of people around whom expansion takes place, scaling-up would be impossible. An important component of this staff capacity is a large and effective training capability. However, it must be recognized that BRAC has had a special problem in retaining competent, primary health care-oriented doctors. It has had to recruit about ten doctors for every one that is willing to stay in the villages and concentrate on primary health care.

The second is management capability residing in the organization's systems and in a broad group of its personnel. Without management capability expansion is impossible. People do not come to BRAC as managers and rarely have they arrived with management training. All those who become managers start in the field, gain experience, receive training and coaching and are promoted when they have demonstrated talent. Effective management systems must be created, modified and expanded to keep pace with growth.

The third requirement, closely related to the second, is strategic management capability—the ability of top management to envisage a future for the organization and for individual programmes or projects, to know where the organization wants to go and what is required to get there, and to control the process. The fourth requirement for successful scaling-up is to be a *'learning organization'*, generating ideas from interaction with the field and encouraging learning in and between all levels of the organization. This openness must extend to the country and world as well, and entails a willingness to change in response to experiences within and outside the organization and to grow in response to needs.

Fifth, scaling-up is impossible without adequate financial support. Whether money is generated from BRAC's commercial enterprises or from donor grants, the ability to attract sufficient money to allow for experimentation, occasional failures and rapid expansion when opportunities arise is crucial. Until 1989 BRAC had received over US$11 million in grants made specifically for health programming. Many health components were also financed by broader rural development grants so the total spent on health activities was much larger than $11 million. The recent Women's Health and Development Programme has received an additional $8.6 million since late 1990. The principle donors to BRAC's health programmes over the years have been UNICEF, the Swiss Development Cooperation Agency, SFCA—Sweden, the Swedish International Development Agency, and recently, Britain's Overseas Development Agency (ODA).

A final requirement for successful scaling-up is to have concerned and dedicated leadership firmly grounded in the villages. They must be committed to helping as many people as possible, meet as many of their needs as possible. Small may be beautiful but big is necessary where needs are so widespread. Although programmes must develop carefully, incrementalism must not become an end in itself. The ultimate objective of every programme is to scale-up wherever possible. Anything less is inadequate performançe.

References

1. Korten, D. (1980). Community organization and rural development: A learning process approach. *Public Administration Review*, Vol. 40, No. 5, pp. 480–511.
2. Chen, M. A. (1988). *A Quiet Revolution: Women in Transition in Bangladesh*. Shenkman Publishing Co., Cambridge.
3. Chowdhury, A. M. R., Vaughan, J. P., Abed, F. H. (1988). Use and safety of ORT: an epidemiological evaluation from Bangladesh. *International Journal of Epidemiology*, Vol. 17, p. 655.
4. Chowdhury, A. M. R., Karim, F., Rohde, J. E., Ahmed, J., Abed, F. H. (1991). Home-

made ORT: a community trial comparing the acceptability of sucrose and cereal-based solution. *Bulletin of the World Health Organization*, Vol. 69, No. 2, pp. 229–34.

5. Chowdhury, A. M. R., Ishikawa, N., Alam, A., Cash, R. A., Abed, F. H. Controlling a forgotten disease: the case of tuberculosis in a primary health care setting. *Bulletin of the International Union Against Tuberculosis* (in press).

6. Chowdhury, A. M. R. (1990). Empowerment through health education: the approach of an NGO in Bangladesh. In: *Implementing Primary Health Care*, (eds. P. Streefland and J. Chabot), Royal Tropical Institute, Amsterdam.

7. Abed, F. H., Chowdhury, A. M. R. (1989). The role of NGOs in international health. In: *International Cooperation for Health*, (eds. M. Reich and E. Marui), Auburn House Publishing Company Dover, Massachusetts.

8. Streefland, P., Chowdhury, A. M. R. (1990). The long-term role of national NGOs in primary health care: Lessons from Bangladesh. *Health Policy and Planning*, Vol. 5, pp. 261–6.

III

The Experiences of Nations

NATIONAL COMMITMENT TO 'HEALTH FOR ALL'

'Health for All' requires the commitment of nations to provide health to all their citizens. Over 150 countries have made this commitment, and many have strived over the past decade to achieve the goals set out at Alma Ata or revised, individually-tailored goals. There have been some major successes such as that of Costa Rica but most nations have faced grave difficulties. Economic crises, political upheavals and new health problems such as AIDS have made many national paths to 'Health for All' more troubled than was envisioned at Alma Ata. For many nations the road during the next decade remains similarly uncertain. To reach 'Health for All' will require major reorganization of present health services, reorientation of staff and reallocation and substantial augmentation of resources. Nevertheless, experiences over the past decade are instructive, and the lessons learned have wider applicability in the continuing global struggle for health.

This section describes and analyses the experiences of six nations—China, Costa Rica, India, Nicaragua, Vietnam and Zimbabwe. All these countries joined in the 1978 commitment to provide essential health care to their entire populations. Socialist principles were manifest in their plans to make services available universally, affordable and equitable, as well as effective. However, amidst the few stories of success, the tales of failure to provide what was hoped or planned due to overwhelming economic constraints is all-too-frequent. It raises a question of paramount importance:

— How is equity in health care to be achieved amidst resource constraints and/or political differences that exacerbate inequalities and poverty?

The various experiences of these countries also raise other major questions:

— What is the most appropriate kind of health system, given the tremendous skewedness in socio-economic levels in most developing countries, the mixture of 'diseases of poverty' and 'diseases of affluence', and plurality among health care providers?
— What is the best mix of public and private health care in view of limited public resources everywhere but the great need for governments to provide for the poor?
— Are there ways of building resilience into health care systems (e.g. through self-care, private provision, public health activities) so that minimal levels of health survive changing economic situations?
— Are participatory modes of health development synonymous with particular forms of government or can they occur within a wide range of political systems?
— How can synergy be brought about between health care services and other development activities?

POLITICAL CHANGE, ECONOMIC REALITIES AND HEALTH

Zimbabwe illustrates the idealistic start of a newly-independent country. The story told by David Sanders is of an ambitious national approach to equitable development of both health and education, which falls on hard times as economic realities cause extensive cut-backs in services. This country sought compromises to preserve the most essential services, especially for the poor. While political commitment persists, shrinking resources diminish the effectiveness of health services. Community participation and support may not be able to fill the void left by the declining role of the government.

Richard Garfield recounts the tale of Nicaragua, a nation seeking compromise and improvement within an existing health system. The political nature of social commitment is demonstrated by the changing policies of the Sandinista Government through the 1980s. This socialist government's efforts to accommodate medical professionals created further dependency among communities on health workers and state finance. This led to a deteriorating level of primary health care as economic pressures reduced free services. Ironically, with a return to more centrist policies and politics, the community has turned to self-care in order to protect itself from the neglect of the government. While the government has developed, to a large degree, a philosophy of private medical care, it nevertheless remains committed to providing social services for the poor and to essential preventive health activities.

The experience of China's socialist system of health care was described in *Practising Health for All* and is updated here in two separate articles by Susan Rifkin and Carl Taylor. Through mass campaigns and a total involvement of the people, China achieved remarkable improvements in health during the 1970s. In the past decade, however, the country has undergone a sea-change in its political economy, scrapping the commune system which had supported the extensive primary health care network. With these economic underpinnings removed, a dramatic change has occurred in health services which are now based on fee-for-service private practice. Many of the practitioners are those who were compensated previously with 'work points' by their communities. This has led to a heavy curative emphasis and reliance on dispensing of medicines, and a loss of basic promotive health activities. The basic tenets of China's health care system, 'the Big Four', have largely disappeared. While the hospital system is still socialist and provides cheap, good quality care at the upper levels, its linkages with communities and peripheral workers have been largely eroded. The sense of community has been replaced by individual self-interest among practitioners and clients alike. Fortunately, the central government has maintained the most essential public health services, but privatization and the switch to capitalist goals has left medical care largely to the open marketplace.

Vietnam was, until 1975, a divided country. According to James Allman, the north evolved a highly-participatory, decentralized, community-based system of primary health care, in marked contrast to the Westernized hospital system prevalent in the south. The neglect of the rural population in the south was evident in the deterioration of health statistics at the time of its defeat in 1975. Following unification, the country remained true to the socialist system, expanding training of health workers and decentralized health clinics. However, economic stagnation over more than a decade has crippled the services, resulting in decline in health care activities. Earlier, there was no private system to replace the diminishing public one. However, in recent years, with the opening of free enterprise even in health care, a major increase has been seen in private consultation. Central public services such as family planning and immunization have continued with international assistance. Vietnam's high literacy level, especially among women, and dedication to universal education has helped in reducing infant and child mortality as well as fertility, despite the deteriorating health services.

During the 1980s, India demonstrated a steady decline in mortality, alongside continued government investment in health infrastructure and slow and steady economic development. But the decade also revealed that India would be hard-pressed to achieve even minimal levels of health for *all* on account of its widespread poverty and illiteracy, continuing high fertility and strained public resources. Meera Chatterjee reviews the significant developments in India's health in the 1980s and examines the implications of emerging trends for the 1990s.

In *Practising Health for All* four separate chapters had discussed India's earlier experience, placing hope in two major health sector developments of the time—the Community Health Workers' Scheme and the expanding role of 'voluntary' non-governmental organizations (NGOs). NGOs had led the nation in exploring technologies and methods to provide 'Health for All'. During the 1980s their efforts to provide quality care continued and were extended through training of government and other NGO workers. They continued to provide innovative approaches to important health problems as well as to integrating health and other development activities. However, the initial euphoria with NGOs has abated as it has become clear that their expansion to larger populations and the replicability of their approaches within the governmental system is severely limited.

On the other hand, it is recognized that the private commercial health sector already reaches a sizeable proportion of the population. As the inadequacy of government resources and managerial ability to provide health care to all becomes evident, policy and rhetoric focus increasingly on the role of this private sector. Trends in private sector involvement in public programmes such as diarrhoeal disease control, ARI treatment and family planning, and 'privatization' are being established. The growing recognition of the role played by the private sector could enable public programmes to better meet the needs of the poor and ensure wider coverage of the population with necessary public health activities. India's success in achieving high levels of coverage with immunization has paved the way for concerted attacks on other major health problems which could employ public–private partnerships.

Unfortunately, some trends in health point to the possibility that the poor in India may lose out as a result of inadequate public health budgets. The major effort to reach into village communities and provide basic health care to the poor—the village Health Guides' Scheme—was allowed to languish during the 1980s. Over this period, however, another village-level nutrition and health initiative—the Integrated Child Development Services (ICDS) Scheme—expanded rapidly to over 230 000 villages in the country. During the decade ahead, the potential of this scheme to provide quality care for young children and their mothers must be met. Malnutrition remains one of India's most intractable problems, steeped as it is in poverty exacerbated by rapid population growth. Particularly troubling is the situation in four large northern states where 40 per cent of India's population lives. These states lag several decades behind Kerala, whose early demographic transition was analysed in *Practising Health for All*. However, some other states of India provide hope that this vast country can achieve better health within its democratic and free market frameworks as rising political consciousness and demand play major roles.

The Costa Rican experience described by Edgar Mohs shows how careful analysis, social commitment and adequate resources can bring about good health. Through self-analysis and substantial modification of the classical medical care approach, the country emerged with a paradigm that enabled it to develop a viable health care system, truly offering health for all. In this socialist effort, Costa Rica was aided by a viable economy, although this has suffered substantially in recent years. The country used its money wisely, as shown in the allocation of funds to rural primary health care over urban hospital care.

In Costa Rica the roots of ill-health were felt to be related largely to social and economic inequality which caused a passive approach to health problems. Starting in 1970, a major reorientation of thinking about health care resulted in a more integrated network of decentralized essential primary health care services with a reduction in hospital and medical care services. Public efforts to ensure that everyone took greater responsibility for their own health led to greater acceptance of family planning, oral rehydration, higher levels of immunization, and substantially improved hygiene and sanitation. This changed paradigm—from dependency to an active, self-reliant attitude emphasizing self-help within existing constraints—led to a resilient and affordable health care system. Costa Rica's life expectancy and overall health are now among the best in the world.

Is this paradigm appropriate for everyone? What is the level of economic prosperity that is necessary for such a system? Would it be successful elsewhere? The absence of an army in Costa Rica and the extensive allocation of public resources to education and health, nearly 50 per cent of the national budget, are important elements. Costa Rica is a good illustration of an enlightened, 'top-down' approach: policy-makers recognized and implemented what was good for the people. While the Costa Rican model is not one of community development or participation, it is decentralized. The recognition that centrally-planned programmes based on sound epidemiological analysis and decentralized implementation can provide health for all underlies the hope that every nation can build and sustain an affordable health care system.

CHAPTER 11

The Potential and Limits of Health Sector Reforms in Zimbabwe

DAVID SANDERS

The author explains the idealism and initial success of a nation-wide emphasis on primary health care in Zimbabwe. This has been substantially curtailed and restructured as a result of economic hardships through the 1980s.

David Sanders, *M.D., is Associate Professor of Community Medicine in Harare and has been closely associated with the design and implementation of Zimbabwe's national health system.*

INTRODUCTION

Zimbabwe achieved independence from Britain in 1980 after a protracted and bitter liberation war by the black majority against white minority rule. It is a sub-tropical, south-east African country separated from the Indian ocean on the east by Mozambique and bounded by Zambia to the north, Namibia and Botswana to the west and South Africa to the south. In 1989 the population was estimated to be 9.2 million, the indigenous black population comprising almost 98 per cent of the total, with 73 per cent living in rural areas.

At Independence, resource ownership was highly unequal between blacks and whites: 45 million acres of prime agricultural land was allocated to about 5000 white settler farmers and a few large agro-industries owned by multinational corporations, while some 750 000 peasant families were crowded in a similar area of land. These 'Tribal Trust Lands' were much less favourable than the white farmers' lands in terms of soil type, rainfall and endemic malaria. The formal working class, which numbered just over a million, comprised agricultural, mining and industrial workers who earned poverty wages and often worked under harsh and unsafe conditions. Informal sector workers experienced even less secure and often more hazardous working conditions.

The liberation war further aggravated economic and social conditions through the combined effect of externally-imposed economic sanctions, increased military spending and social disruption. Peoples' health suffered not only as a direct result of injuries sustained during military hostilities but also from forced internment in crowded, unsanitary 'protected villages' and the manipulation of food supplies by the Rhodesian security forces. Simultaneously health and social services were greatly disrupted, resulting in the cessation of many preventive programmes and significant reduction in curative health services.

Zimbabwe's Independence saw the ushering in of a new and vigorous thrust in health care based on the primary health care approach which was designed to reduce these disparities. However, after a brief post-Independence economic boom there has been a decline in the economic well-being of much of the population. This increasing poverty has been caused by a combination of international recession, prolonged drought, South African-inspired and supported cross-border destabilization, and regressive domestic macroeconomic policies, including a recent structural adjustment programme. The relatively short period in which these processes have been operating provides an illuminating case of both the potential of effective health sector interventions based on primary health care (PHC) and their limitations in the context of a deteriorating economic environment.

This chapter will briefly review the changes in the macroeconomy which are most relevant to health as well as the most important developments in the health sector since Independence. It will examine in some depth two important programmes which illustrate the centrality of popular participation in the success of health initiatives and demonstrate that this component of the PHC approach is inseparable from the processes of popular involvement and democratization in society at large. Finally, it will assess progress being made by examining changes in child health and nutrition. An attempt will be made to analyse the factors responsible for this progress and their likely evolution over the coming decade.

THE ECONOMY AND SOCIAL SERVICES: WAGES, PRICES AND LAND

National minimum wages were introduced by the government in July 1980. At constant 1980 prices, wages for domestic and industrial (and other) workers rose significantly between July 1980 and January 1982 and were, in most cases, substantially greater than pre-Independence wages. However, in spite of regular increases since then, there has been an erosion of purchasing power since 1982. The gains made between Independence and January 1982 were undermined by a wage-freeze between January 1982 and September 1983 and by the 1982 devaluation and subsequent depreciation of the Zimbabwean dollar. These measures were part of an economic adjustment package imposed by the government in late 1982 under the stimulus of an International Monetary Fund stand-by credit scheme.* In early 1991 a new structural adjustment programme (SAP) was adopted which included measures to reduce government spending as well as to liberalize trade.

Another element of the stabilization package which undoubtedly had an important effect on nutrition was the removal in 1982 and 1983 of subsidies on basic foods. In these years prices rose by some 100 per cent for maize meal, 69–95 per cent for beef, 50 per cent for milk, 25–30 per cent for bread and 25 per cent for edible oils. Further price rises have occurred regularly since that time and have greatly accelerated since the introduction of the SAP in 1991. The combined effect of these price increases can be gauged from the movement of the consumer price index which more than doubled during the period.

The removal of subsidies contributed significantly to a rise in the cost of living. This was aggravated by the 1982 devaluation and subsequent depreciation of the Zimbabwean dollar and in 1991 by its precipitous decline in value. Thus the cost of a 'basket' of basic needs for an urban family with four children rose from an estimated Z$129.06 per month in 1980 to Z$337 per month in 1988.**[1] In 1991 it has increased even more.

Decline in real wages and food price increases have adversely affected many urban and rural dwellers. A significant number of rural households are unable to subsist on the land and depend increasingly on wages and food remitted by urban migrant workers. The National Household Capability Survey (1983–84) showed that about 60 per cent of households have no access to land; that 50 per cent of the land is controlled by about 20 per cent of households; that approximately 50 per cent of households have no cattle; and that about 10 per cent of households own half the cattle. The process of rural stratification developed with colonial land policies and is likely to have been accelerated by certain post-Independence policies, particularly credit schemes, as well as by the drought.

---

*The IMF agreement was suspended after approximately one year but most of its elements have been retained by the government.

**In 1980 US$1.00 was equivalent to Z$0.63, by 1985 it was worth Z$1.64 and by 1991 Z$5.08.

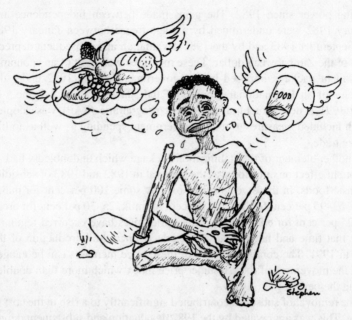

*Decline in real wages and increased food prices left many workers
on the margin of hunger.*

Land shortage is a fundamental factor affecting peasant well-being, and
negligible change has taken place in land distribution since 1980. By the
end of 1987 the government of Zimbabwe had acquired or set aside almost
three million hectares of land for purposes of transfer and settlement
schemes, 78 per cent in areas of limited agricultural potential. Some 52 000
households had been resettled, 32 per cent of the official target for the
resettlement programme, 14 per cent of households needing land in 1980
and 7 per cent of the 1980 peasant farming population. Like many other
social programmes in Zimbabwe, resettlement slowed down markedly in
the last half of the 1980s. In the late 1980s it was stopped altogether as part
of the government's attempt to reduce state spending.

EDUCATION

As education leads to better health behaviour, Zimbabwe's phenomenal
post-Independence expansion in school enrolment is highly significant.
Total numbers at school grew from about 892 668 in 1979 to 2 962 889 in

1989. The bulk of this expansion has been at the primary level. Its impact on health is likely to become evident only in the long run. On the negative side, increased schooling has imposed a financial burden on many parents, leading to reduced expenditure on other items including food. Until recently, primary education has been nominally free, but resources are required from parents for uniforms, transport, building funds and labour inputs. Such economic pressures appear to be contributing to an increasing drop-out rate. Primary school drop-outs numbered over 200 000 in 1988. The preponderance of girls withdrawing from school has negative implications for future maternal and child health, particularly among the poor where the drop-out rate appears to be highest. This will undoubtedly be aggravated by the re-introduction of school fees in 1992 as part of the recently-begun SAP.

WATER SUPPLY AND SANITATION

Since Independence there has been a major government effort to improve water supply and sanitation in the communal lands (formerly 'Tribal Trust Lands'). In 1984 about one-third of people in the communal areas had access to safe water sources. This proportion appears to have increased slowly and is continuing to do so. Water supplies are provided by three ministries: Local Government, Rural and Urban Development; Energy, Water Resources and Development, and Health, which has responsibility for small household supplies like shallow wells and protected springs. Donors, especially Norway, have played an important role in funding water development projects. In 1984–85 they provided some 58 per cent of the funding for water supply development in communal lands. Donor funding has increased as a proportion of total finance for water and sanitation while the government's contribution has decreased in real terms since about 1984.

A major difference between urban and rural dwellers lies in their access to adequate supplies of safe water. Within urban Zimbabwe there are differences between rich and poor housing areas. Wide disparities in access to water exist even within communal areas. These are based on economic status or geographical location, although these frequently coincide. For example, in Chiweshe Ward of the Save Communal Area, some 11 per cent of households were obtaining their water from unprotected wells and 52 per cent from rivers and springs.[2] In Zviyambe Ward the figures were 6 per cent and 27 per cent respectively. Forty-two per cent of households in Chiweshe Ward walked over four km to fetch water while in Zviyambe it was 54 per cent.

Sanitation programmes essentially involve the construction of ventilated improved pit latrines (VIPs). Very large numbers of these have been constructed in rural Zimbabwe since Independence. However, since recipients of assistance in building a VIP have to pay approximately 60 per cent (Z$151) of the total cost (Z$276) to purchase materials, poorer and female-headed households are discriminated against. The sanitation programme may thus be contributing to further inequalities in rural areas.

THE HEALTH SITUATION[3]

Health Status

In 1982 Zimbabwe's population growth rate was estimated to be 2.9 per cent; it dropped to 2.8 per cent by 1989.[4] The sex ratio was 96 males to every 100 females and the proportion of the population under 15 years constituted almost 48 per cent while that over 65 years was 3.2 per cent. The average number of persons per household was 4.7, but in the rural communal areas it was 5.4.

In colonial Zimbabwe as in other underdeveloped countries, the greatest burden of death and disease fell on infants, young children and women in the child-bearing period.[5] In addition, mortality varied substantially by geographical area, race and class. In 1980 there was a 1:3.5:10 ratio in the infant mortality rate (IMR) of whites, urban blacks and rural blacks, corresponding to a 39:5:1 ratio in incomes. While the IMR of 14 per 1000 for the white population approximated that of industrialized countries, for the majority black population it was estimated to be 120 per 1000.

While the better-off showed the disease pattern seen in industrialized countries, the majority of the population suffered nutritional deficiencies, communicable diseases and problems associated with pregnancy. Maternal under-nutrition contributed to low birth-weight in 10–20 per cent of all births. This and protein–energy malnutrition were the commonest forms of childhood malnutrition, predisposing the victims to more severe and often fatal infections. The most important of these were measles, pneumonia, tuberculosis and diarrhoeal diseases which, together with meningitis, neonatal tetanus and other infections of the newborn, accounted for most infant and young child mortality. Of the occupational diseases, industrial lung diseases such as asbestosis, silicosis (and tuberculosis) and coal-miner's lung, stress-related disorders such as high blood pressure, and plantation-related problems such as schistosomiasis and the toxic effects of pesticides and herbicides were all (and are increasingly) visible but undoubtedly under-reported. Mental ill-health and alcohol-related problems were also common, the latter being reflected in liver disease, indirectly in sexually-transmitted diseases and now increasingly in HIV infection and AIDS.

This disease pattern was rooted in the system of production which prevailed in Rhodesia, its distribution being reinforced by the structures of racial domination. Under-nutrition was particularly prevalent in the Tribal Trust Lands (TTLs) and among children of workers on commercial farms. Although the TTLs were termed the 'subsistence sector', with increasing land alienation and degradation due to a lack of inputs, peasants were unable to subsist from agriculture alone. Increasingly families were forced to supplement their unreliable agricultural production with cash remitted from the urban industrial or plantation sectors, while providing a growing supply of landless wage labour. Airborne infections spread easily in the cramped, often smoky housing conditions existing in both urban and rural areas. Poor sanitation and inadequate water supplies predisposed people to common and debilitating intestinal, skin and eye infections. In the white farming areas, where nearly 20 per cent of the black population lived, conditions were often worse.[6]

These environmental factors undermined much of the impact of the health care system. This system had all the features typical of an inappropriate, inequitably-distributed developing country service, compounded by inequalities based on racial discrimination. For example, in 1980–81 the average annual expenditure per head for private sector medical aid society members (subscribers to private health insurance) was Z$144 compared with Z$31 for the urban population using public services and Z$4 for the rural population. The latter concealed further disparities as only districts surrounding urban areas were relatively well served. In 1980–81, 44 per cent of publicly-funded services went to the urban-based sophisticated central hospitals serving about 15 per cent of the population while only 24 per cent went to primary and secondary level rural health services for the majority of the population.[7]

In line with the distribution of facilities, all categories of health personnel, especially professional grades, were concentrated in urban areas. In 1980 there were 1138 doctors, 4652 nurses, 2897 medical assistants and 393 health assistants. Of the doctors, 42 per cent were wholly engaged in private practice in 1981, with between 80 and 90 per cent of these being in Harare or Bulawayo, the two largest cities. According to the 1983 Ministry of Health manpower review, 67 per cent of public sector doctors were located at central level, with only 15 per cent in the eight provincial centres and a further 15 per cent in district or mission hospitals in the country's 55 districts.[8] Even the distribution of lower-level auxiliaries and medical assis-

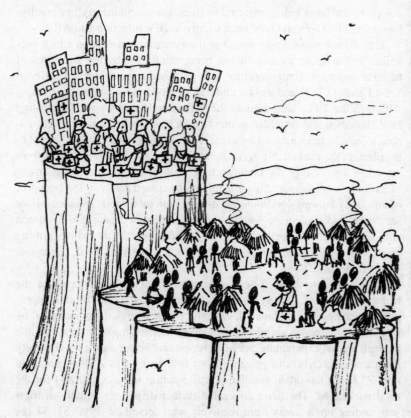

Most health services were found in the cities, inaccessible to the rural population.

tants was disproportionately urban, although this group and health assistants formed the core of the team at district-level and below.

Health Policy

Post-Independence health policy reflected the broader national objective to establish a society 'founded on socialist, democratic and egalitarian principles'.[8] The priority task in 1980 was stated to be the restoration and rehabilitation of the war-torn infrastructure.

With expressed recognition that the causes of ill-health lay in people's living conditions, the government guaranteed to transform health care so that all citizens would have access to a comprehensive integrated National Health Service. This health system was to be integrally linked to other development programmes, such as those in education, housing and food production. The adoption of the Primary Health Care approach demanded the direction of new resources towards previously-deprived areas for the improvement of nutrition and the control of preventable diseases. This policy stressed the conscious and active participation of communities in transforming their own health.

The state recognized the presence of multiple and uncoordinated providers of health care, and a maldistribution of personnel between urban and rural areas and between social classes. This threatened the establishment of a national unified health service. Various measures were proposed: the abolition of racially-discriminatory laws, a restriction on the expansion of private facilities, post-training bonding of health workers to the public sector, barring of immigrants from private practice, incorporation of the traditional health sector, rationalization of therapeutic procedures through the establishment of an essential-drugs list, and establishment of a universally-applied national health insurance scheme.

Health Programmes

Free Health Care. Health care has been provided free of charge since September 1980 to those earning less than Z$150 per month, a level designed to include all common wage labourers. However, the minimum industrial wage of Z$243.50 now exceeds this limit, which has not been revised since 1980. Notwithstanding the erosion of this benefit, the majority of Zimbabwe's population still qualify. However, because the responsibility of proving eligibility for free health care rests with users, many of whom experience great difficulty in furnishing the necessary evidence, many remain deprived. This has been greatly aggravated by the recent introduction of revised and substantially-increased user-fees for all components of curative care as well as ante-natal care, together with much more stringent implementation of their collection. This aspect of 'cost recovery' within the SAP threatens to undermine some of the improvement in access to health care achieved since 1980.

The Zimbabwe Expanded Programme on Immunization (ZEPI). The ZEPI was initiated in 1981 and is one of the great successes of Zimbabwe's Primary Health Care thrust. Studies on coverage show that the percentage of children between 12 and 23 months fully vaccinated in rural Zimbabwe rose from 25 in 1982 to 42 by 1984 and up to between 50 and 80 by 1986.

Urban coverage in 1986 was even higher with surveyed levels of 93 per cent measles coverage in Bulawayo, 80 per cent in Harare and 85 per cent in Chitungwiza. A 1988 survey, however, indicated that coverage had remained the same or changed only slightly in six of the eight rural provinces. In poorer parts of urban areas and in some large-scale farming estates immunization rates are much lower. Vaccination of pregnant women with tetanus toxoid has been introduced since Independence. About 45 per cent of pregnant women received two doses of tetanus toxoid in 1987. Drop-out rates from first to second dose are very high, being around 30 per cent in most provinces and 50 per cent in Bulawayo City. In the October 1988 survey, about 78.9 per cent of pregnant women had TT 1, about 58.8 per cent had TT 2 and about 14.6 per cent had a booster dose of tetanus toxoid.

Although better supervision of vaccination at static facilities will solve problems arising from incorrect administration of vaccines, it is likely that a significant number of children who do not complete their primary courses are from communities or families located in the most inaccessible areas which are also the most marginal in terms of social status. They are also likely to be those most at risk of ill-health and poor nutrition, for whom the morbidity and mortality penalties of non-vaccination are likely to be higher. Ensuring coverage in these groups will require an increase in outreach activities and greater financial allocations to transport, an unlikely prospect given the declining trend in provincial budgets. The availability of road-worthy vehicles and spare parts as well as vaccines, syringes and needles requires foreign exchange and is currently wholly dependent on donor assistance.

Diarrhoeal Disease Control Programme. In February 1982 diarrhoeal disease control was declared a priority by the government. Emphasis has been placed on improved case management, mainly by oral rehydration therapy (ORT), epidemic control, improved nutrition, prolonged breast-feeding and improved environmental hygiene through water supply and sanitation. Although hard data are not available, questionnaire responses and interviews conducted in October–November 1984 suggest that the number of attendances for diarrhoea at health-care facilities has decreased.[9] There has been a significant increase in the percentage of rural mothers who can prepare the correct sugar–salt solution (SSS) for ORT, so that home-based management of the problem is practised increasingly, although with some shortcomings.[10] In a 1988 MCH–EPI survey, 77 per cent of mothers said they gave SSS to their children during their last attack of diarrhoea and 11 per cent had visited a health facility. While 99 per cent said they knew the correct recipe for SSS, in fact only 59 per cent did, the majority having learned it at rural health centres. During a 1991 MCH–EPI survey in Mata-beleland North Province, while 93.5 per cent of mothers had heard of SSS, only 59 per cent knew the correct formula.

National Nutrition Programme. A Department of National Nutrition has been established whose responsibilities include nutrition and health educa-tion, with particular regard to breast-feeding and weaning practices, growth monitoring and nutrition surveillance using child health cards. By June 1984, 80 per cent of children aged one possessed a growth card (as against 71 per cent in 1982) and 83 per cent had been weighed at least twice in the first year of life (58 per cent in 1982).[11] In 1986 the Family Health Project baseline surveys showed that in some areas 98 per cent of under-fives pos-sessed a growth card. This has recently been confirmed in Matabeleland North during the 1991 MCH–FP survey. In a 1988 national survey three-quarters of respondents knew why their children were weighed, although in some provinces up to 40 per cent could not interpret the card.

National Village Health Worker Programme. The National Village Health Worker (VHW) Programme was launched in November 1981 to train multi-purpose basic health workers who were selected and based in the village. Out of a target of 15 000 VHWs, about 7000 had been trained by early 1987. Related to this programme is the Traditional Midwives Pro-gramme (TMP) designed to upgrade the skills of household-level women operatives in identifying at-risk pregnancies, basic midwifery, elementary hygiene and basic child care. By mid-1989 more than 6000 TMPs had re-ceived this upgrading course.

Child Spacing. The Fertility and Child Spacing Association, later re-named the Child Spacing and Family Planning Council, a parastatal institu-tion established in 1981, superceded the voluntary, government-assisted Family Planning Association. Its early emphasis on fertility as well as child spacing has since shifted back towards a concern with population growth, reflected in its most recent new name, the Zimbabwe National Family Plan-ning Council. Largely as a result of its activities, Zimbabwe has the highest rate of contraceptive use in Sub-Saharan Africa, with eight in ten currently-married women reporting having used at least one method of contraception, 68 per cent of these being modern methods.

The Budgetary Implications

All these and other programmes required expansion in government expen-diture. Table 1 shows how the actual expenditure of the Ministry of Health (MOH) changed between 1978 and 1989. At Independence there was an

Table 1. Central Government budget allocation of the Ministry of Health, 1978–79 to 1989–90

	Actual expenditure			Actual growth rates	
	Current prices Z$m	1980 prices Z$m	Budget share %	Current prices %	1980 prices %
1978/79	45.6	57.4		4.8	—
1979/80	53.5	60.7	4.6	17.3	5.7
1980/81	77.4	77.4	5.3	44.7	27.5
1981/82	106.1	113.8	5.6	37.1	47.0
1982/83	123.1	103.4	4.8	16.0	-9.1
1983/84	139.0	117.3	4.8	10.5	13.4
1984/85	156.6	116.2	4.9	12.5	-0.9
1985/86	195.0	128.7	5.3	24.5	10.6
1986/87	239.4	144.6	5.1	22.7	12.4
1987/88	287.3	164.8	5.5	20.0	14.0
1988/89	329.0	172.6	5.3	14.5	4.7
1989/90	352.9	169.4	5.1	7.3	-1.9

Notes: Z$1.6 = US$1 (1985); 1980 prices are calculated using an index of health sector wages.
Sources: 1978–79 to 1983–84: Zimbabwe, Annual Report of the Comptroller and Auditor General, Harare.
    1984–85 to 1986–87: Zimbabwe, Estimates of Expenditure, Harare.

immediate expansion of 44.7 per cent (27.5 per cent in real terms). The Ministry's share of the budget rose to 5.3 per cent, showing that there was also a relative shift in emphasis towards health. This growth continued so that by fiscal year 1981–82, the MOH's actual expenditure had almost doubled in real terms. However, following the downturn in the economy in 1982 and the introduction of stabilization measures in 1983, the real growth has been followed by stable or decreasing levels ever since.

The share of preventive services in the MOH budget has risen from 6.7 per cent in 1980–81 to 14.4 per cent in 1989–90, while that of medical care has fallen from 89.5 to 80.5 per cent. These figures actually understate the shift towards preventive care since some of the costs of such care, especially with respect to immunization, have probably been reduced by the integration of curative and preventive services. This change reflects the impact of the revised philosophy of the MOH after Independence. There has also been a steady rise in the share of the Ministry's budget allocated to salaries and allowances, from 26.8 per cent in 1980–81 to 42.2 per cent in 1989–90. This reflects increasing personnel, rising wages, and the unwillingness of the government to dismiss salaried employees during a period of budget restraint.

The central hospitals' share of the MOH budget has been reduced since Independence. The MOH also assists local authorities, missions and voluntary organizations which provide health care services particularly in outreach programmes such as immunization, diarrhoeal disease control and supplementary feeding. In real terms their grant increased from Z$22.2 million in 1980–81 to Z$35.9 million in 1981–82, and back to Z$24.4 million in 1984–85. This recent fall in real resources constrained their work, especially their ability to perform outreach work during 1984 and 1985.

Resources are also provided to the health sector by foreign donors who play an important part in easing some of the constraints faced by the government. Although the total amount of aid going to the sector has not been large in comparison with the overall MOH budget, it has been significant in relation to the funding allocated to specific projects. In 1983, 18 per cent of the ZEPI budget came from bilateral aid donors.

POPULAR INVOLVEMENT IN THE HEALTH SECTOR

A central feature of the PHC approach is democratization—the process essential to genuine 'community participation'. The health sector policy states: 'This principle of mutual respect and dialogue is at the heart of the new relationship to be created between the health service and the community. Both sides will benefit. The people will feel the health units and activities are "theirs", and will utilize and participate in them as such. The health workers will receive a boost to their morale and motivation; their activities, being responsive to the local situation, will be more effective and efficient in the use of resources.'[8] Popular democratic control is a crucial ingredient for the success of primary health care initiatives and is one— some would say the most important—feature distinguishing PHC from previous approaches.

The State and Popular Organizations

In the case of Zimbabwe, the unfolding relationship before and after political Independence, between the state and institutions of popular organization, is central to understanding the process of popular involvement in all areas of social development including health. It is in situations where the old order and power structures are being contested or have recently been overthrown that comprehensive primary health care has the best chance of succeeding. For it is in such conditions that popular participation in decision-making and collective rather than individual self-reliance grow and flourish.

This situation was most evident in the 'semi-liberated' communal areas, particularly where guerrillas of ZANU (PF), the leading party in the national liberation movement, had been active for a long period. In these areas the party had created popular organizations, initially responsible for supporting the liberation effort but later structured to perform essential social and economic tasks, effectively as an alternative to the Rhodesian State's rudimentary district administration. These organizations were made up of various tiers of people's councils which were set up at village, ward, district and provincial levels. Functions of these various committees differed considerably. Grassroots village committees dealt with the day-to-day problem of feeding and clothing the guerrillas and providing basic services to the community, while those issues involving the outlay of large sums of money would be passed to higher-level committees.

From Direct to Representative Democracy

One of the major gains of this revolutionary experience was the practice of direct democracy where for the first time peasants and workers participated directly in the formulation of policies and their day-to-day implementation and evaluation. Furthermore, the ability of the peasants and workers to control, reject and re-elect representatives became a reality. This was a far cry from their previous experience where they had no vote, and even from the experience of those living in Western democracies where representatives are elected infrequently to parliament or local government bodies without any day-to-day control being exercised over their actions by the electorate. This practice has persisted to some extent in certain parts of the country but is being eroded with the passage of time.

What, then, of developments since the early days of Independence? What is the basic structure of the post-colonial state and what is its relationship to popular organization? Far from being dismantled and supplanted by a decentralized 'workers and peasants' state, a centralized hierarchical structure with permanent institutions, the security forces, civil service, judiciary and health bureaucracy, has *expanded* since Independence. Not only is the standing army much greater in size but the civil service has expanded from under 50 000 to 80 000. It is of course, true that the *racial* character of the state has changed. But has the essential *class* character of the state changed? Perhaps this question is best answered by looking at the relationship between the present-day state and the embryonic 'popular state' previously mentioned.

Between 1980 and 1982 District Councils vested with local administrative development powers were established, replacing the colonial District Commissioners and Chiefs. Although this system of local government is a significant advance over the previous structure with ward representatives elected by popular vote and with greater resources than in the past, it none the less remains an extension of the central state. Full-time local government officials are salaried by and responsible to the Ministry of Local Government and Town Planning. Although councillors are elected every few years, they are neither answerable to their electorate on a day-to-day basis nor subject to recall for unsatisfactory performance. With this extension of the central state to district-level and through the resources available to District Councils, most popular committees, particularly those established more recently, had already become marginalized by 1983. A fragile and evolving system of direct democracy was thus supplanted by representative democracy.

In 1984 the system of local government was further elaborated and extended. As a result of the Prime Minister's directive, decentralized structures were set up 'to facilitate popular participation' in local government. These village development committees (VIDCOs) and ward development committees (WADCOs) were formed 'using popularly-elected local leaders to ensure democratic representation in planning development projects for the people'. However, these structures are less numerous and more geographically removed from the majority of villagers than were the popular committees which were in attendance at the frequent mass meetings held during 1980 and 1981 at village-level.

The extensive human infrastructure created by the liberation effort formed the basis for the early impressive success of two important health sector programmes, the Village Health Worker (VHW) Programme and the Children's Supplementary Feeding Programme (CSFP). However, more recently, bureaucratization and the accompanying popular demobilization have adversely affected these programmes.

The Village Health Worker Programme[12]

Community health worker programmes which are democratically controlled by the poor majority can serve the functions of extending health care to isolated communities and of mobilizing people to transform their living conditions and thus their health. In communities where most people are

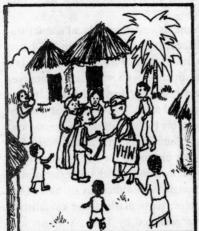 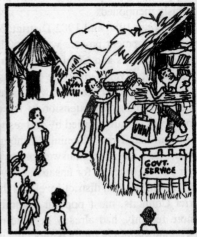

As low-level government employees, VHWs lose their contact and responsiveness to village realities.

poor and often illiterate the tendency is for the better-off and better educated to dominate. This calls into question the very notion of 'community' as a term that suggests a homogeneous, conflict-free group of people. This is almost never the case and certainly not so in rural Zimbabwe where economic stratification exists. Domination by the better-off also has implications for the selection and control of the community health worker.

During the ceasefire in 1980 a health worker at Bondolfi Mission, Masvingo, was approached by the ZANU (PF) District Committee and asked to take on the training of popularly-elected health workers in nutrition, child care, hygiene, sanitation and a little home treatment. The area was well-organized into one political district with 28 branches. Each branch had a popularly-elected committee of 16 members, of whom two were responsible for community health matters. Training commenced for 56 branch health leaders in May 1980. Their six months' part-time training included both theory and practical work, the latter being done after planning with their communities. Due to the project's popularity and increasing community demand, the people decided to have an unpaid village health worker for every one to three villages. As a result, 293 VHWs were selected and trained, 35 from other districts. Selection and control of these workers was at village and branch level with ongoing popular participation. From this project sprang a Development Committee, set up by the people themselves and responsible for coordinating the work done by VHWs in different areas and for organizing other health-related development projects.[13]

In late 1981 the government began its own national programme to train VHWs. These VHWs were to be selected by their own communities in consultation with the District Council. In some areas there really was popular involvement in the selection of these workers. However, in many areas where it was done by the District Council, it was acknowledged that 'there is some nepotism; councillors choose their wives and friends'.[13] The VHWs were paid (Z$33 per month) by District Councils from a grant received from the central government. Inevitably they were responsible to the District Councils rather than to the villagers they served. With widespread rural poverty it would be impossible for many communities to fund their own VHWs.

When the government scheme was set up, ten of the Bondolfi VHWs who were working at the time were taken on and retrained. The government VHWs received a more formal training than the Bondolfi, spending more time in the clinic or hospital. They had to cover a considerably larger area than the Bondolfi women. In effect most of them were full-time workers. By mid-1984 only about 100 VHWs of the original 293 in Bondolfi were functioning. There were a number of reasons for this drop-out, but as one local VHW organizer said: 'When the government scheme started and some were paid Z$33 a month, others stopped working because they were not paid.'[13]

This experience illustrates the general problem that the lack of popular control over VHWs makes them unresponsive to the communities they are to serve. Control at the point of selection, of payment, supervision and performance evaluation are all important, as the Zimbabwean experience demonstrates.

More recently there have been further developments which have virtually eliminated the possibility of popular democratic control over the health sector through the VHW. In early 1988 the VHW scheme was 'handed over' to the Ministry of Community and Cooperative Development and Women's Affairs. VHWs and Home Economics Demonstrators have been combined into a single group of 'village community workers' who, although still notionally part-time, have written conditions of service and are regarded as civil service employees. The nature of the VHW has been qualitatively transformed.

TACKLING THE NUTRITION PROBLEM

The Children's Supplementary Feeding Programme[14]

Soon after Independence a number of nutrition surveys were undertaken in Zimbabwe. In 1980 nutrition surveys by OXFAM in five rural areas identified 30 per cent of children aged 1–5 years as underweight (below the third percentile). Mid-upper arm circumference (MUAC) measurements were below 13.5 cm in 40 per cent and below 12.5 cm in 15 per cent of children. A more extensive survey conducted by the MOH found 61 per cent of children had a MUAC of less than 13.5 cm and 29 per cent had a MUAC of less than 12.5 cm. There was evidence that the prevalence of undernutrition in most areas was inversely related to the availability of food, as revealed by food stocks.

The 1980 food crisis was due partly to an influx of refugees displaced to neighbouring states by the liberation war and partly to the war policies of the former regime whose tactics included destruction of food and agricultural resources. These acute factors aggravated a chronic food problem that was the result of historical inequities in land tenure, in the ownership of the means of agricultural production and in income distribution, to cite only the most important factors.

Recognizing that the impending 1980–81 agricultural season was going to be a crisis period, voluntary agencies and relevant government departments began to discuss a nutrition intervention programme. One hundred and fifty thousand children were estimated to be at risk. Using information gathered in the various surveys it was possible to construct a map of undernutrition which allowed for a more effective selection of areas where the programme should commence.The programme stressed the dual objective of immediate short-term relief and long-term education. It emphasized the importance of using locally-available foods. The supplementary food based on maize meal, beans, groundnuts and oil provided approximately one-half of the daily energy requirements of one- to two-year-olds, and approximately one-third of the daily energy needs of three- to five-year-olds.

The programme was conceived as one of cooperation between the government and non-governmental organizations (NGOs), under the direction of the Ministry of Health. A national working group was set up with representatives from relevant ministries and voluntary organizations and was chaired by a representative of one of the NGOs. Within the provinces, the Provincial Medical Officers of Health set up provincial committees. Local committees included health workers, school teachers, community development workers and women's advisors. Most important of all was the active

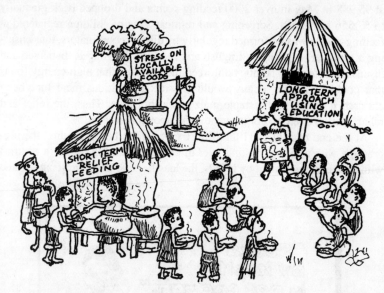

Emergency feeding, with stress on the use of local foods, evolved into a long term nutrition programme.

support of the local communities who were asked to supervise the consumption of food and to teach the importance of energy-rich locally-available foods.

The organization of the programme at district- and village-levels was both complex and unique. The administrative infrastructure developed during the liberation war was utilized to organize the measuring of children, to establish feeding-points close to people's homes and fields and to carry out the cooking and feeding of the supplementary meal for registered children. At village-level, the on-going administration, involving the daily registration of attendance and the preparation and feeding of the meal, was performed by mothers of children enrolled in the programme, who were often organized through the political structure. Children with MUACs measuring less than 13 cm were registered in the programme. The selection of this cut-off point was explained to parents of registered children as well as those whose children were deemed not 'at risk'.

The first feeding-point opened in January 1981 and over the next three months feeding-points were established all over the country. The number of children registered rose from 5824 in January to 56 200 in March. It peaked at 95 988 in May in over 2000 feeding-points and dropped back gradually to 57 556 in August. Screening and re-measuring of children registered at feeding-points was performed regularly by district coordinators, thus ensuring a turnover. A poster in English and the local languages, displayed and discussed at feeding-points, reinforced the message that high-energy foods that could be grown locally would provide a nutritious meal for young children if added to the staple maize meal porridge. Thus, the relief and rehabilitation exercise contained an educational message.

At the end of July 1981 the Ministry of Health began funding the programme with a view to taking over direct responsibility for it. In contrast with earlier management by NGOs, the less-flexible and more-complicated

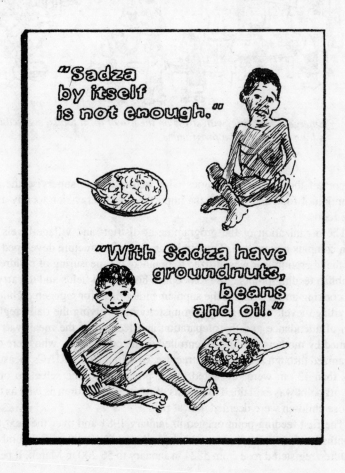

method of government funding led to problems in food purchasing, payment of transport costs and salaries. This resulted in breaks in feeding and near-bankruptcy at provincial level. However, the importance of the programme was recognized and its continuation in critical areas accepted as necessary. It was decided to change the emphasis with less focus on relief, and more on education.

An evaluation of the CSFP was carried out in 1981 in which children in the programme were weighed and compared with children of a similar age range from the same area who had not been registered in the feeding programme. Children in the feeding programme had gained considerable weight. On an average, children attending the programme put on weight at twice the rate of the other children. Children who had attended 30 or more meals gained weight at three times the rate of the better nourished children.[15]

A second part of the 1981 evaluation was concerned with perceptions of the programme among those involved. Most mothers reported improvement in their children's health, and in many areas the educational message had been accepted. Most found the timing of feeding convenient. One-third reported difficulty in participation due to the burden of house-work, agricultural and child-care duties. Perhaps the most striking point that emerged was the geographical variation in food production and usage. While some families were producing considerable amounts of crops, others had very little. Another important finding was a change in intended production patterns: the percentage of interviewees who stated their desire to grow groundnuts in the following agricultural season had risen from 48 to 80 per cent.[15]

The evaluation showed that the feeding programme had achieved much of what it set out to do. Its strength lay in having achieved its aims as a relief programme and having expanded into a programme emphasizing education. It had sustained and built upon grass-roots organization at district- and village-levels. To have local people in control of running a development project is perhaps the best indicator of its successful administration.

Improving Local Food Production

Following the evaluation, some committees approached the organizers of the programme to provide groundnut seed to enable them to grow the crop. Although groundnuts are widely cultivated in Zimbabwe, most of those produced in the peasant areas are sold: economic pressures have turned a nutritious food into a cash crop. Therefore the CSFP Committee drew up a proposal suggesting the development of communal groundnut production plots. If production was collective, it was far less likely that the crop would be sold. This proposal was accepted by the Ministry of Health which made groundnut seed, gypsum and fertilizer available to communities organized to cultivate collectively on a plot that was already or soon would be sited adjacent to a pre-school centre. The harvest from these half-hectare plots was to be gathered and used in the daily meal given to pre-school children attending that centre. Enough of the harvest was to be retained to provide seed for the next year's planting. This scheme was launched in 1981 as a pilot, with a total of over 500 plots country-wide. It was intended that the successful plots would serve as demonstrations for communities not so far involved in this project.

By 1983–84, there were 292 supplementary food production plots in 31 districts. Unfortunately, because of the severe and recurrent drought in Zimbabwe, most of these failed. Due to widespread crop failures, it again became necessary for the government to mount a drought-relief exercise which included a food distribution component. It also proved necessary to maintain and expand the CSFP whose infrastructure was, fortuitously, intact. Over the next few years, the total number of children qualifying for the supplementary feeding increased. During much of 1984 about a quarter of a million children out of approximately 1.4 million 1–5 year-olds were being fed a daily supplementary meal.

Since the end of the drought in 1985 the supplementary food production scheme has diversified. Most plots now produce a mixture of maize and/or beans and/or groundnuts. In most cases these units are situated on land allocated by the District Council to village groups—usually female—who have come together voluntarily to establish a supplementary food production plot. At district and provincial levels Supplementary Food and Nutrition Management Teams have been established. These are chaired by Agritex, the extension arm of the Ministry of Lands, Agriculture and Rural Resettlement, and consist of several government ministries, including Health, and Community Cooperative Development and Women's Affairs.

At present there are two to three thousand supplementary food production plots distributed throughout Zimbabwe's eight provinces. In some districts this scheme has been highly successful, completely covering the young child population in large areas. Perhaps the best example is in the Musami area of Murewa District, some 80 km from Harare. Here there are over 50 food production plots and associated pre-school centres. Maize, groundnuts and beans are produced and in several centres a surplus exists even after the allocation for all pre-school children and retention for seed.

These centres serve not only as activity and day-care centres for all pre-school children but also as outreach points for the health service. When these places are visited each month, immunization, health education and growth monitoring are performed. Those children attending the centre and any children from the 'catchment area' who are too young to be registered for day-care (usually under two-year-olds) are weighed. If growth faltering is detected by serial weighing, the child's parent(s) are counselled. If the child is not already attending the pre-school centre—usually because (s)he is too young—the parent(s) are instructed to bring the child for daily weighing and supervised feeding. Thus, feeding-points have been transformed into comprehensive child care centres and production units. The registers kept at Musami's Mission hospital indicate that the prevalence of young child under-nutrition has declined markedly since the early 1980s and is considerably lower than the country average. Similarly, while an impact evaluation has not been conducted, in Mashonaland West, which has more such units than any other province, the relative reduction of stunting among under-fives was greater from 1985 to 1988 than in any other province.

The Role of Community Involvement

It is instructive to reflect upon the possible reasons for the apparently greater success, particularly in terms of community participation, of the CSFP—especially in its first few years—as compared with the nation VHW programme. The CSFP was launched during 1980 when popular mobilization was both at a high level and widespread, and village community self-organization relatively well-developed. This human infrastructure was consciously utilized and, indeed, formed the organizational base of the CSFP at a time when the old local government institutions had collapsed and the new structure of District Councils, WADCOs and VIDCOs had not yet been formed. Thus, the organizational structure of the CSFP was highly decentralized from the outset, with only a small and very flexible central and provincial administration, unencumbered by the restrictive and complex requirements of government bureaucracy, particularly in respect of financing.

On the other hand, the government VHW programme began slowly in late 1981. From soon after its inception it was administered by the District Councils, frequently with minimal or only episodic involvement of village communities. By the time significant numbers of VHWs had been trained (approximately 500 per district by late 1984), the new local government structures were well established. Direct and on-going involvement of villagers in the management of their communities' affairs had declined since the end of the liberation war. Simultaneously and partly as a reflection of this, local government structures became more centrally accountable, sometimes nepotistic and less responsive to their local communities. Also, the greater technical content of the VHW programme meant that higher-level health workers, often unconvinced of the need for community mobilization, played a much more prominent role in this programme than in the CSFP. This factor may have contributed further to the technocratic and bureaucratic nature of the VHW programme and its undervaluing of community involvement.

Changes in Child Health and Nutrition

The patchy data available indicate that significant progress has been made in addressing Zimbabwe's legacy of ill-health. Most observers agree that there has been a sharp decline in both the infant and child mortality rates since the late 1970s. For example, while the precise levels are not known, a review of existing studies suggests that the IMR currently lies between 60 and 75, having been approximately 100–200 per 1000 in 1980. A study undertaken in 1988 reported that the IMR averaged 52.7 and the U5MR 75.1 between 1983 and 1988. Many observers regard these findings as significantly understating the actual situation, since two other studies in the mid-1980s reported national IMRs of 79 and 73.[16,17] Rural–urban differentials persist, remaining at 2:1 in 1984.

Changes in morbidity are difficult to determine because of problems with comparability of available data for the period under consideration. However, there are indications of a reduction in the incidence of immunizable diseases, although there appears to have been a recent resurgence of tuberculosis in association with the rapid increase in HIV prevalence. Respiratory infections, malaria and diarrhoea continue to be major causes of ill-health although cases of severe dehydration from diarrhoea are reported to be much less frequent than before the implementation of the Diarrhoeal Disease Control Programme. This is evidenced by the decline in diarrhoeal disease deaths both in infancy and young childhood from 10 and 15 per cent respectively of all deaths in those age-groups in 1983, to 8 per cent of infant and 12 per cent of young child deaths in 1987.[18]

Levels of under-nutrition appear to have declined significantly between 1980 and 1983–84 but there is less firm evidence of a decline thereafter. In 1982, a national nutrition survey of under three-year-olds showed 17.7 per cent were under-weight, 35.6 per cent stunted (under-height) and 9.1 per cent wasted (significantly thin). In 1984 another national survey showed 14.5 per cent of one- to five-year-olds to be significantly under-weight. However, due to differing methodologies, these two surveys are not strictly comparable. By 1988 the CSO Demographic Health Survey found national levels of 11.5 per cent under-weight, 29 per cent stunted and 1.3 per cent wasted. While the situation appears to have improved with respect to wasting, levels of stunting remain discrepantly high, particularly given Zimbabwe's aggregate food surplus and her relatively low mortality rates. Once again the comparison with 1982 and 1984 data is made difficult because of differences in anthropometric cut-offs and the different age-groups sampled.

Although these data are sketchy, they suggest a divergence between mortality indicators on the one hand and nutrition indicators on the other. The improvement in the former has probably resulted from the energetic expansion and reorganization of health care described above. The adverse effects of drought, recession and stabilization policies have been partially offset by aid-supported relief feeding programmes and particular health care programmes. However, recession and economic stabilization and adjustment have reduced real incomes for large numbers of rural and urban households since the immediate post-Independence boom. This is reflected in continuing high levels of childhood under-nutrition which has improved only marginally despite the health care drive.

LESSONS FROM ZIMBABWE

The lessons for Zimbabwe are clear. Early post-Independence health policy focused on equity, democratization and the integration of the health sector with other sectors. Its implementation in the context of widespread community self-organization resulted in significant achievements in health care provision and improved health. The revitalization of this policy and encouragement of the social factors facilitating its implementation are, in the current economic situation, not only a moral imperative but an urgent necessity if 'Health for All' is ever to be reached.

Thus, Zimbabwe's experience in the 1980s provides an illuminating case study—almost a 'best case' example—of both the potential of effective health sector interventions and their limitations in the context of a deteriorating economic environment. What are the implications of this for infant and child health during the present international economic recession?

In the now-industrialized countries the large and sustained decline in child mortality was accompanied by reductions in morbidity and malnutrition and largely preceded any effective medical interventions. These advances are generally acknowledged to have been due primarily to improved living conditions. The complex political and economic context of these has been dealt with elsewhere.[19] More recently the decline in mortality, particularly of infants and young children, has been accelerated, especially by the advent of effective chemotherapeutic agents, immunization and advances in newborn care.

Falls in infant and young child mortality in under-developed countries have been largely responsible for the significant increase in life expectancy. This rose by 0.64 years annually between 1950 and 1960, partly as a result of the extension of medical services and partly because of some redistribution of the benefits of the long post-War economic 'boom'. By the mid-1970s the annual increase in life expectancy in underdeveloped countries had slowed to 0.40 years. This reflected the deterioration in living conditions for many as the economic recession spread internationally. During the same period, however, there has been a significant extension of effective and robust child survival technologies, especially immunization and ORT, sometimes even to the most isolated areas of poor countries. This combination of worsening social and economic conditions on the one hand and greater (albeit uneven) accessibility to some child health care technologies on the other has given rise to an unprecedented phenomenon in health: declining infant and child mortality with simultaneous increases in malnutrition, and in many cases, morbidity. The worsening of these latter 'quality of life' indicators among the children of the poor is a probable result of two factors: declining socio-economic conditions with resulting poor diets and deteriorating environmental conditions, and prolonged survival of malnourished children who are more vulnerable to recurrent disease. A mild variant of this situation is being witnessed today in Sri Lanka. Here, although the IMR has continued to decline, the already high rates of malnutrition have increased significantly. Nutritional wasting in children aged 6–60 months rose from 6.1 per cent to 9.4 per cent between 1978 and 1983.[20]

Brazil provides yet another example. During the period of structural adjustment, the IMR in Sao Paulo, the largest city, dropped from 87.1 per 1000 in 1973 to 41.6 in 1983 and the child mortality rate from 3.5 to 1.0. However, stunting and wasting in children aged 6–60 months increased significantly. In the country as a whole, however, IMR increased from 65 to 73 per 1000 as a result of a measles outbreak, as well as an increase in respiratory diseases and malnutrition-related deaths.[20]

It is, however, especially in Africa, particularly sub-Saharan Africa, that increases in infant and child mortality are occurring due to the combined effect of drought and prolonged economic stress and structural adjustment. In Ghana the IMR, which had fallen to about 80 per 1000 in the mid-1970s, was around 100 in 1980 and rose to 110–120 in 1983–84.

These examples are part of a spectrum of situations extending from mild to severe economic recession. In less severe circumstances selected health care interventions can, if widespread enough, continue to reduce infant and young child mortality rates. However, quality of life, as evidenced by morbidity and malnutrition levels remains largely unaffected. In more adverse economic situations, however, the impact of 'selective PHC' on child mortality is likely to be negligible at best, with death merely being postponed. However, such approaches can shift the focus of PHC away from issues of empowerment, social justice and equity, to earlier preoccupations with technologies, a mere palliative amidst deep social ill-health.

References

1. Sanders, D. (1982). Nutrition and the use of food as a weapon in Zimbabwe and Southern Africa. *International Journal of Health Services*. Vol. 12, No. 2, pp. 210–13.
2. Central Statistical Office. (1990). *Zimbabwe Demographic and Health Survey 1989*. Harare.
3. Sanders, D. and Davies, R. (1988). The economy, the health sector and child health in Zimbabwe since Independence. *Social Science and Medicine*. Vol. 27, No. 7, pp. 723–31.
4. Gilmurray, J., Riddell, R. and Sanders, D. (1979). *The Struggle for Health*. Catholic Institute for International Relations, London.
5. Ministry of Health. (1984). *Planning for Equity in Health*. Government of Zimbabwe, Harare.
6. Ministry of Health. (1983). *National Health Manpower Planning and Projections Workshop Report*. Government Printers, Harare.
7. Quoted in Loewenson, R., Sanders, D. and Davies, R. (1989). *Equity in Health in Zimbabwe: a post Independence review*. Study prepared for the Ministry of Health, Harare, p. 7.
8. Campbell, B., du Toit, R. F. and Attwell, C. A. M. (1989). *The Save Study*. University of Zimbabwe, Harare.
9. Loewenson, R. and Sanders, D. (1988). The political economy of health and nutrition. In: *Zimbabwe's Prospects*, (ed. C. Stoneman), Macmillan, London.
10. Cutts, F. (1984). *The use of oral rehydration therapy in health facilities in Zimbabwe*. Save the Children Fund, London School of Hygiene and Tropical Medicine, London.
11. De Zoysa, I. *et al.* (1984). Home-based oral rehydration therapy in rural Zimbabwe. *Transactions of the Royal Society of Tropical Medicine and Hygiene*. Vol. 78, pp. 102–5.
12. Sanders, D. (1992). The State and democratization in PHC: community participation and the village health worker programme in Zimbabwe. In: *The Community Health Worker*, (ed. S. Frankel), Oxford University Press, Oxford, pp. 178–219.

13. Sanders, D. (1984). The State and popular organisation. *Journal of Social Change and Development*. Harare, No. 8, pp. 6–8.
14. Sanders, D. (1991). The children's supplementary feeding programme in Zimbabwe. In: *Diseases of Children in the Subtropics and Tropics,* (eds. P. Stanfield, *et al.*), Edward Arnold, London.
15. Working Group. (1982). *The children's supplementary feeding programme in Zimbabwe*. Report presented to the Ministry of Health, Harare.
16. Zimbabwe National Family Planning Council/Westinghouse Applied Systems Zimbabwe (1985). *Reproductive Health Survey 1984*. Harare.
17. Ministry of Health. (1987). *Primary Health Care Review 1987*. Government Printers, Harare.
18. Government of Zimbabwe and UNICEF. (1991). *Children and Women in Zimbabwe: A Situation Analysis Update, July 1985–July 1990*. Harare, pp. 33–4.
19. Sanders, D. with Carver, R. (1985). *The Struggle for Health: Medicine and the Politics of Underdevelopment*. Macmillan, London.
20. Cornia, G. A., Jolly, R. and Stewart, F. (eds.). (1988). *Adjustment with a Human Face*. Oxford University Press, Oxford, Volumes 1 and 2.
21. Monteiro, C. A., Pino Zuniga, H. P., Benicio, M. H. A. and Victora, C. G. (1989). Better prospects for child survival. *World Health Forum*. Vol. 10, No. 2, pp. 222–7.

CHAPTER 12

Nicaragua: Health under Three Regimes

RICHARD GARFIELD

The author traces developments in health in Nicaragua from the late years of the Somoza regime, through the Sandinista period, to the present Chamorro government. He shows how the swings in policy and practice have reflected political changes and affected people's health status.

Richard M. Garfield, *R.N., Dr.P.H., teaches at Columbia University, New York. He has collaborated with the Ministry of Health in Nicaragua over the past ten years through two regimes and has written two books on Nicaragua's health system.*[1]

INTRODUCTION

Nicaragua is an injured yet hopeful country from which many lessons can be drawn. In its history, disasters have initiated each new epoch. An earthquake in 1931 helped bring the Somoza dictatorship to power. Another in 1972 initiated that government's downfall. A revolutionary war in 1978–79 brought the leftist Sandinista Front (the FSLN) to power, while the Contra war (1983–88), the U.S. economic embargo (1985–90) and a tropical storm in 1988 were its undoing. In 1990 a pro-U.S. coalition headed by Violeta Chamorro came to power in the first peaceful electoral defeat of a socialist government in a developing country. This chapter describes the health care developments which occurred under the Somoza dynasty (1932–79), the Sandinista regime (1979–90), and the Chamorro government (1990 to the present).

Wedged between Honduras in the north and Costa Rica in the south, Nicaragua is the largest of the six countries in the Central American isthmus. Its population of four million is doubling every 20 years (Table 1). The country is dotted with towns, villages and dispersed rural dwellings. More than 5000 communities are located in 135 municipalities. The traditional geo-political division is the department, of which there are 16. To encourage decentralization, the departments were organized into six re-

Table 1. Nicaragua, 1990

Population	4.1 million
Infant mortality rate	62 per 1000 live births
Under-five mortality rate	95 per 1000 population
Crude birth rate	42 per 1000 population
Crude death rate	9 per 1000 population
Population growth rate	3.4 per cent per year
Life expectancy at birth	63 years
Rural population	43 per cent
Total average births per woman	5.8

gions in the Pacific and upland territory and two 'autonomous zones' on the Atlantic coast in 1982.*

The economy of the Pacific region is dominated by plantations of sugarcane, cotton, coffee and bananas. The central highland region is dominated by the cattle industry. The Atlantic region is a centre for small-scale mining, lumbering and fishing. During the 1970s, thousands of small-scale farmers, forced off their land on the coastal plain to make way for export crops, worked as itinerant seasonal labourers on large estates. Wealth and income were highly skewed. The average per capita income of the richest 5 per cent of the population was US $5409. This was 25 times that of the poorest 50 per cent, whose income averaged less than $300 a year in the late 1970s. Annual per capita rural incomes varied from $90 to $225 by region.

By 1979 health status in Nicaragua ranked alongside that of Honduras and Bolivia as the worst in continental Latin America. Average life expectancy at birth was estimated at 53 years. Although infant mortality began to decline rapidly around 1974, in 1979 one of every eight babies still died before reaching one year of age. The main causes were diarrhoeal disease, pneumonia, tetanus, measles and whooping cough. Malnutrition (measured by weight-for-age) affected more than half of all children. Polio epidemics

---

*The Pacific and the upland regions, first colonized by Spain in the early sixteenth century, are ethnically and culturally homogeneous. Almost all the people are Mestizo (of mixed Spanish and indigenous Indian ancestry), Spanish-speaking and Roman Catholic. The Atlantic Coast, a sphere of British influence for more than two centuries, is home to six different ethnic groups. Half the population consists of Spanish-speaking Mestizos who have migrated from the Pacific region. The largest ethnic minority is the Miskito people, descendants of indigenous Indians and Afro-Caribbean slaves. The non-Mestizo minorities belong mainly to Moravian or other Protestant churches.

occurred every few years, leaving hundreds of children permanently disabled.

THE SOMOZA PERIOD, 1932–79

The Somoza family came to power in a U.S.-supported coup in 1932. It was infamous for running the country like a private business, directly controlling about 20 per cent of the land and many major enterprises. Prior to the 1979 revolution that deposed Somoza, Nicaragua's health system was profoundly fragmented. Four separate national institutions and 19 semi-autonomous agencies in the country's 16 states were responsible for health services. Because each institution and agency functioned independently, chaos was the norm, with salaries, record-keeping and working practices differing from one town to the next. Most physicians worked part-time for a public or social security institution but spent most of their time in private practice.

By the 1970s the most powerful health institution was not the Ministry of Health but the National Social Security Institute (INSS), which provided curative health care to salaried employees. With its own hospitals and clinics in the country's two largest cities, Managua and Leon, the INSS controlled half of all health expenditures but provided services to only 8.4 per cent of the population. Health expenditure per person was more than ten times greater for the insured than the uninsured. In 1977 insured patients had more than eight times as many out-patient visits and prescriptions filled relative to the rest of the population.

Although responsible for preventive care throughout the country and curative services in rural areas, the Ministry of Health controlled only 16 per cent of health expenditure, and 75 per cent of this was spent in Managua. The National Guard also ran its own hospitals and clinics, providing high quality care to soldiers and their relatives. Private insurance groups, charitable organizations and local health agencies accounted for most of the remaining health expenditure.

While many of the causes of poor health were to be found in the social conditions of the country, health services themselves also bore much of the blame. The country's health system was uniquely inefficient and inequitable. Paradoxically, and in contrast to what some critics have suggested, a lack of funds was not the main problem. During most of the 1970s the health sector absorbed about 8 per cent of the government's budget (see Fig. 3, p. 282). This was double the average size of health budgets in many developing countries. The public health sector represented 1–2 per cent of the national Gross Domestic Product (GDP), greater than in any other Central American country except Costa Rica.

The system was relatively well-endowed with funds (including foreign aid) as well as doctors and hospital beds. But it was severely imbalanced. There were close to 5000 beds in about 40 hospitals but there were less than 200 health centres in the entire country. Some of these health centres were well-designed and lavishly-equipped but most operated at under 50 per cent of capacity. The system was riddled with corruption and geared almost exclusively to the needs of the affluent.

It was estimated during the 1970s that 90 per cent of Nicaragua's health resources were consumed by a mere 10 per cent of the population. Most of the affluent or medically-insured lived in Managua and Leon. They controlled most of the country's land, commerce and industry. Among these groups, child deaths were about as low and life expectancy almost as high as in the United States.

Only 28 per cent of the Nicaraguan population had effective access to modern health services. Despite the creation of 100 new primary care centres during the 1970s, per capita visits to a physician actually declined. Many people, especially those in rural areas, remained dependent on traditional healers (*curanderos*) and birth attendants (*parteras*) for health advice and treatment.

Many foreign organizations set up hospitals and clinics after President Kennedy set up the Alliance for Progress in the early 1960s. Many donors were religious and/or non-governmental, but the biggest donor was the United States Agency for International Development (USAID). Loans and grants from USAID were used to build rural health centres, set up a mobile rural health programme, train doctors, build hospitals, stimulate community participation and improve sanitation. Despite financial incentives and technical assistance, the anarchic, paternalistic and profit-oriented nature of the Nicaraguan health system defeated USAID's reform efforts. An evaluation in the mid-1970s found:

. . . a combination of poor physical plant, lack of equipment, uncleanliness, and poor quality medical attention. No provisions were made to provide these [health] centres, once built, with adequate personnel, supplies, and management support. . . . The average health centre operated at about 40 per cent capacity in terms of patient visits per medical hour . . .[2]

The major stumbling block to reform was the political and economic system of the country. The evaluation summed up, in a cautious understatement, the effects of the Somoza dictatorship on the health system:

The long history of one-party rule in the country . . . resulted in a centralized decision-making process with limited delegation of responsibility and authority, which often required the President to personally intervene in issues affecting even small amounts of sector resources. Thus the health sector and many health sector personnel lacked the motivation and innovative-experimental approach necessary to make a major impact on the enormous health problems facing the health agencies . . .[2]

Private aid was sometimes more effective. The Council of Evangelical Churches (CEPAD) was set up by Protestant Churches after the 1972 earthquake in order to bypass the government in channelling development assistance to rural areas. CEPAD established and still runs more than 20 clinics in isolated rural communities. Their focus on home gardens, latrines, water systems, breast-feeding and health education has been exemplary.

THE END OF A REGIME

The Sandinista party, organized in the early 1960s, aimed to lead the people in a Cuban-style uprising to effect land reform and bring health and other social benefits to the poor. By the late 1970s, Nicaraguan society grew increasingly polarized. U.S.-funded community health initiatives were begun to train birth attendants, improve rural sanitation and promote community involvement. Such reforms, however, threatened to undermine the Somoza system of control and to bypass powerful leaders. Rural programmes were subverted to help defend the dictatorship against growing support among peasants for the Sandinistas. Indeed, as Somoza's political position weakened relative to the growing revolutionary movement, so did his restraint. Union leaders were jailed, murdered or simply 'disappeared'. Many health workers, especially nurses, left the country because of political harassment or lockouts. Finally the National Guard turned its fury on the hospitals themselves. During the last months of the revolutionary war in 1978–79 four of the country's public hospitals were destroyed and five others were damaged in air or artillery attacks by the Somoza government.

Meanwhile, growing numbers of doctors, nurses and medical students abandoned hospitals, private practices and universities to join the revolutionaries. Clandestine networks were established to move injured or sick guerrillas out of the country for treatment. Doctors and nurses (including some from Germany, Costa Rica, Honduras and Mexico) also trained medical orderlies who were attached to Sandinista combat units. In towns where the National Guard lost control, the Sandinistas established clandestine hospitals where doctors operated on the war-wounded. Many health workers lived a dual life—an official one working in a government hospital or clinic and a secret one treating FSLN guerrillas and their families. It was a perilous existence. Dr Fernando Silva worked with the FSLN in Managua:

We would collect needles, syringes, penicillin, gauze and other medical supplies to send to the countryside and the fighters. I remember the day when the Medical Director came to the Social Security clinic where I was working. He said he was convinced I was working for those sons-of-bitches the Sandinistas. This shook me because my white jacket was bulging with a pistol. I was in the habit of travelling armed because I was treating guerrillas. 'After you finish with these patients, come to my office so that we can talk,' he said. I did not know what to do. I needed to get rid of the gun. I was trembling in fear that I would be shot because of the gun. There was a man nearby, holding a baby in his arms covered by a blanket. He touched me. 'Don't worry', he said. He took the gun and put it under the blanket. I was saved from certain death. That night they attacked my house, but I had already fled.

In neighbourhoods supporting the Sandinistas, food, water and other basic supplies ran out as the government attempted to starve the people into submission. A branch of the FSLN responded by organizing Civil Defense Committees which acted as provisional local governments, storing and distributing food, water and essential commodities such as kerosene and cooking oil. The Committees also constructed street barricades, deployed lookouts and messengers to support the guerrilla fighters, coordinated health volunteers, trained orderlies to treat the sick and wounded, and organized the burial of the dead and the disposal of household refuse.

In effect, Somoza and the National Guard forced the Sandinistas to create a new health system in 'liberated' communities, staffed entirely with volunteers. By July 1979 when more than four decades of Somoza rule finally came to an end, the Sandinistas had established a make-shift system with widespread community involvement in health care.

THE SANDINISTA PERIOD, 1979–90

Health was a high priority on the Sandinista political agenda. This agenda proposed to empower people to identify their health needs, organize them to realize their health goals and involve them in the institutions and programmes that developed.

Within the Ministry of Health (MINSA), Sandinista leaders with strong trade-union links argued that the health system should be oriented to the organized work force, private medicine should be prohibited and all health professionals should be employed by the state. On the other hand, revolutionaries who had fought in the mountains, believed that the peasantry was the heart of the revolution. They argued that government should give top priority to those in rural areas. Some wanted to follow China's example and down-play the roles of urban hospitals and fully-trained doctors.

More moderate Sandinistas sought to legitimize the new regime by favouring the middle-class and technical experts, such as doctors. They favoured a pluralistic approach to preserve private practice and respond to the interests of the urban middle-class. New public health programmes staffed by auxiliary nurses and volunteers could be developed for the poor and rural populations, but doctor-based hospital care and imported pharmaceuticals were their ultimate objective. After all, weren't these the goals of most doctors who took part in the revolution?

All three groups were represented in the political coalition which brought the Sandinistas to political power, and all three took part in the compromises needed to establish a national health policy at the end of 1979. MINSA's main focus became urban and rural labourers, small-scale farmers, and women and children. These were the groups which had been most disenfranchised under the Somoza regime.

While initially preserving the private medical sector, MINSA planned to orient the entire system, including doctors and hospitals, towards rural areas and urban slums. Revolutionary rhetoric emphasized preventive health care, health education and community participation. The primary health care strategy, with its focus on equity and community participation, seemed to fit well with the Sandinistas' political values and health objectives.

Towards Primary Health Care

The practical implications of planning and implementing PHC throughout the country presented enormous obstacles. The health policies of the new government contained the seeds of conflict. On the one hand the government proclaimed the need for low-cost, community-based, preventive health services. On the other, it also promised wide access to curative care in modern hospitals. This well-intentioned commitment to sophisticated medical care was inconsistent with the primary health care approach; it was also medically unnecessary and financially overwhelming.

Responding to popular demands for change, the revolutionary government brought about two sudden changes in urban health services. Medicines were distributed without charge and the social security facilities were opened to the entire public. These early reforms were to shape the direction of primary health services throughout the decade.

, In the towns and cities demand for free health care at clinics created early morning lines that snaked down the street in the hot sun as far as the eye could see. Hospitals were also deluged with patients. Alta Hooker worked as a nurse in the regional hospital of the Atlantic Coast town of Puerto Cabezas:

> Before the revolution we never filled the 27 beds in the hospital. About two months after the war of liberation . . . the people were really starting to come in. It became impossible to work—you'd nearly walk on the patients lying on stretchers or on the ground between beds. The Ministry of Health told us that we'd have to be patient, that it was the same everywhere and we'd just have to wait our turn. We increased the number of beds from 27 to 69 in that first year and in 1985 we got a new wing with 22 more beds.

Almost everyone agreed that massive expansion in primary care centres, hospitals and doctors was needed to achieve equity. By 1982 more than 300 new health posts were built (Fig. 1). Only about half of these new facilities were constructed by the government. The remainder were built by communities themselves. In many places existing buildings were converted into health centres or posts. In the town of El Cua a notorious prison was converted into a health centre with beds. In many small towns the elegant homes of Somoza supporters who had fled the country in 1979 were turned into spacious health centres. In Waslala the first revolutionary health service was staffed by a physician captured from Somoza's retreating army. He was convinced to work for the Sandinistas on the promise that following a

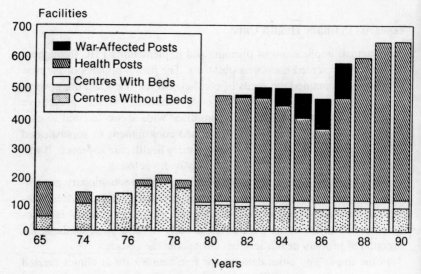

Fig. 1. Primary health care facilities, 1965–90.

year of public service he would be exempted from prosecution. One of Managua's better-designed health centres was once a brothel owned by one of Somoza's colonels. When the revolutionary government proposed turning it into a prison, community groups persuaded the government that the building, with its rows of small cubicles, would be put to better use for medical consultations.

Curative Facilities

In 1980 Managua had a doctor for every 1000 people while in some remote regions there was a doctor for every 10 000 residents. The disparity in nursing coverage was also huge. The best-endowed region had one graduate nurse for 3000 residents, while the worst region had one nurse for every 20 000 people. As large numbers of health workers were trained and assigned to facilities in rural areas, geographic inequalities decreased dramatically. By 1983 the best and worst health regions had only a two-fold difference in coverage with nurses and doctors.

The growth in use of basic curative care was most dramatic. Provided in part by 700 foreign doctors, half Cuban, a quarter sent by other sympathetic governments and the rest ideologic volunteers from North and Latin America, medical care reached many previously-unserved communities. In 1971, 12 per cent of the country's doctors, 11 per cent of the nurses and 9 per cent of the auxiliary nurses worked in primary care. By 1981, as a result of the large influx of health workers into rural areas, 36 per cent of the doctors, 30 per cent of the nurses and 30 per cent of the auxiliaries—including almost all new graduates—worked in primary care. Public health programmes for rural areas, maternal and child health and occupational medicine expanded enormously. Outpatient care and prescriptions—the curative services most neglected for the general population prior to 1979—showed the most dramatic increases. From 1977 to 1983 hospitalizations and surgical procedures rose more than 50 per cent, out-patient medical visits tripled (Fig. 2, p. 276), and the number of vaccinations increased more than four-fold.

By 1982 at least 70 per cent of the population received some medical care from trained staff, a dramatic increase over the 28 per cent getting modern health care at the end of the Somoza era. The number of visits per capita to a doctor more than doubled. Northern Zelayau zone on the Atlantic Coast had the highest rate of doctor visits, with more than three consultations per capita each year. None the less, towns and cities were still better served than most rural areas. In 1982 residents of Managua averaged 55 per cent more medical consultations than people in the rest of the country.

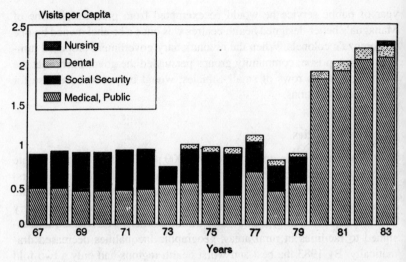

Fig. 2. Medical, nursing and dental visits, 1967–83.

Community Participation

In many remote parts of the country the first health workers to arrive were young volunteers (*brigadistas*) with only two weeks training in health care. Beginning eight months after the Sandinistas came to power, the National Literacy Campaign recruited close to 100 000 volunteers—mostly high-school and university students—to teach basic literacy skills, to 400 000 adults between March and September of 1980. The newly-formed Ministry of Health trained 15 000 of these literacy *brigadistas* in first aid, sanitation, and malaria and diarrhoea control at the newly-formed Polytechnic Institute in Managua. Apart from teaching literacy skills, these young men and women also worked as rural health aides, collected information on local herbal medicines and folk healing practices, and helped to construct health posts.

In 1980 the government established People's Health Councils from the neighbourhood committees set-up during the revolutionary war to 'mould the aspirations of the people into concrete programmes' and 'channelize the activities and concerns of the people in a coordinated manner'. The Councils took responsibility for organizing Peoples' Health Days; campaigns to combat particular health problems. For example, in 1980 an estimated 30 000 volunteers took part in a series of Health Days focusing on polio and measles immunization, dengue (eliminating peri-domestic mosquito-breeding sites) and environmental sanitation (largely community clean-up and trash disposal). On each occasion volunteers attended weekend training sessions and made door-to-door visits to explain the purpose of the forthcoming Health Day. For the immunization campaigns the volunteers also carried out a census of infants and children who required vaccination in their neighbourhood. Each campaign was followed by regional 'Analysis and Summary' meetings involving doctors, nurses and health volunteers.

In 1981 the Councils again mounted four campaigns: vaccinations against polio and measles, a further effort to clean garbage and environmental waste, an anti-dengue mosquito-breeding site campaign and—most ambitious of all—an anti-malaria campaign involving about 200 000 voluntary workers. In a single nation-wide effort, all persons above the age of one year were administered three daily doses of primaquine-chloroquine—a total of 15 million pills given to over 80 per cent of the population. The malaria incidence rate plummeted and was maintained at a low level by the health services for more than a year thereafter. Within MINSA, the department dealing with campaigns, the Division for Education and Popular Communication for Health (DECOPS), became so large and active that other, more conservative offices were alarmed. It was even feared that DECOPS might take over the Division of Preventive Medicine.

Both conservatives and radicals were concerned about the meteoric growth in health campaign activities. Conservatives lacked trust in the *brigadista* programme because it threatened to replace professional medical care which was the heart of the health system. On the other hand, radicals were concerned that the volunteers might weaken the push to re-orient physicians toward the poor majority. The 'appropriate technology' of volunteers and preventive campaigns might therefore free doctors from the pressure of public service to continue 'business as usual' with their urban, middle-class clientele.

In 1981 the membership of Health Councils was broadened to include health professionals, mostly doctors—a decision that many later felt discouraged autonomous community initiative. Religious missionary Celine Woznica lived in the township of Ciudad Sandino at that time:

> The over-riding problem with the People's Health Councils is the dominance of the Ministry of Health. This stands in the way of broad and effective community participation.[6]

Financial conflicts between government and community groups were common. For example, in 1981 the health committee in Ciudad Sandino decided to collect one Cordoba (worth about as much as a bus ride) as a 'voluntary contribution' from patients waiting to see a physician. The purpose of these collections was to buy medical equipment, construct benches and chairs and support community health activities. Because the policy of the government was to provide health care without charge, the Committee obtained special permission from the Ministry of Health for these collections. By 1983 such collections had become common in many parts of the country, providing the communities with a small but useful discretionary fund for initiating their own health activities. However, in 1984, the regional MINSA office ordered the Committees to stop collecting money from patients. With national elections scheduled for November of that year, the official policy of free health care assumed greater political importance, over-riding the issue of local autonomy. The Committee in Ciudad Sandino did not challenge the directive even though it meant the loss of its only regular income, and with it the power to initiate health projects. Left out of the decision-making process, the Committee slipped into a more passive role. The attendance of *brigadistas* at health committee meetings fell and more dropped out of community health activities. Similar discouragement occurred when MINSA clinics recalled the weighing scales which were being used by health volunteers for well-baby check-ups and food supplement distribution in the community. The constant see-saw between centralized socialist policies and decentralized community control and initiative, between professional health care pushed more into the periphery and paramedical and volunteer services arising among community groups made the development of health care erratic.

The Effects of the Contras

Paradoxically the Contra war in 1982–88 led to some positive changes in the health system. Among these were more efficient use of resources, better organization, the setting of clear priorities and increased administrative decentralization.[7] According to former Sandinista Health Minister Dora Maria Tellez: 'The tighter things are, the better we have to organize things so as to obtain maximum usage of our resources.' While concentrating formerly-scattered, rural communities into new settlements quickly led to localized epidemics, it also made it much easier for health workers to reach families with preventive and curative services.

A two-tiered system of care emerged with the Contra war. The rural system was run by *brigadistas* at the primary level; the urban system was led by surgeons and other specialists needed for war-related pathologies.

However, as the curative hospital system was being strengthened in cities, health resources were being stretched to breaking-point.

Between 1982 and 1988, 128 of the country's 600 health facilities were closed, damaged or destroyed. The losses included one hospital, seven health centres and 115 posts in six regions of the country. Close to 10 per cent of the country's inhabitants and at least a quarter of those living in war zones—about 300 000 people—lost access to health services because of the war (personal communication). Nearly one in every ten hospital admissions between 1983 and 1986 was for war-related injuries.[8]

Many hospitals had running water only part of the day, electricity failed during surgery and back-up lights broke down. On three separate occasions in a single year, a surgeon in Esteli was left in the dark with a patient's abdomen wide open during a gastro-intestinal operation. Whenever the electricity failed or respirators in an intensive care unit broke down, a nurse had to maintain the oxygenation of the patient by hand for up to 24 hours.

Approximately 0.2 per cent of the Nicaraguan population, some 6000 people, has some kind of physical disability. About half of them were disabled in the Contra war. Treatment and rehabilitation for these people became a heavy burden on the country's already over-stretched medical and social welfare services.

To make matters worse many people continued to use hospitals as primary health centres. Doctors contributed to this. Accelerated training of new doctors led many to treat their health posts mainly as referral pathways to the health centres and hospitals. As a result increased funds for hospitals were used only to keep up with increased demand for services.

Social security clinics and hospitals, restricted to insured workers during the Somoza era, had been opened to the public. But developments in primary care created massive demands on the hospital sector. Since health posts were staffed by graduate physicians, people began to look to hospitals for care. Self-referral and physician-referral to out- and in-patient facilities in hospitals became common even for simple problems. It became clear that even local physicians, trained in First World type medicine, were unable to function effectively in a poorly-supplied health system which had to respond to Third World health problems. Ironically, as the primary care system developed, hospitals took on increasing importance as the backbone of the health system. Many urban workers agitated to re-establish restricted access to social security facilities. The regime's commitment to equity made it impossible to accommodate this desire.

By contrast, the revolution's most successful health programmes—malaria control, polio and measles immunization and promotion of oral rehydration therapy—used low-cost health technologies and involved tens of thousands of non-professional health workers. Nicaragua became the first Central American country after Costa Rica to report no new polio cases. Epidemics of measles and whooping cough, so common in the past, were not seen. Oral rehydration centres popularized the concept of early and aggressive treatment of diarrhoea to prevent dehydration. The number of diarrhoea cases presenting at hospitals or registered as deaths was cut nearly in half.

The financial crisis which developed through the mid-1980s on account of war, economic embargoes, and economic decline had a profound effect on the concept of good health care. In 1980 leaders believed that high-tech doctor-provided care would be made available gradually to the whole population. By 1988 MINSA openly embraced the concept of low-cost health care by the people. Then Minister Tellez, addressing the need for latrines, said:

Any kind of latrine is better than defaecating in the open air. If we don't have the resources to make latrines with good seats, even just a simple hole in the ground will suffice. We have to be ready to meet our needs with whatever minimal resources are available, and not wait for better conditions.

Despite limitations, rural health care throughout the 1980s remained a clear example of the commitment and effectiveness of government-led services. The proportion of personnel dedicated to primary care remained high and the involvement of the community significant. This was not the 'selective' strategy advocated by some experts for primary care in poor countries. The 'selective' model usually involves a package of services provided in a uniform manner by national-level administrators. By contrast the Nicaraguan approach evolved from local needs and interests. It is administered regionally or sub-regionally via 'territorial health systems' and municipal government offices. It depends on decisions and resources which are generated in part from local offices of government ministries and community organizations. This approach resembles the 'comprehensive' primary health care approach intended to provide a full array of services. But due to limited resources it focuses on a few activities selected on the basis of dialogue and epidemiological analysis in individual communities. The Nicaraguan system thus appears to be a unique hybrid: a selective primary health programme within technologic and resource limitations and comprehensive primary health care in its social and political dynamics.

Drug Policies

More than any other act, the 1981 decree that all drugs dispensed in public hospitals and health centres would be free convinced people that the health services were indeed theirs. With the advent of this policy, everyone wanted to fill their medicine chests. Doctors often responded by providing unnecessary injections and drugs for ailments that required little or no medication. The financial implications of the policy soon forced the government to retreat from this promise.

In March 1982 the Ministry of Health imposed a 'registration' fee for prescriptions, though drugs themselves were still free. In 1986 a more radical shift occurred: a charge was levied on prescription medicines. However, not all drugs were charged for and most were heavily subsidized. Those needed in special programmes, such as tuberculosis, venereal disease control and immunization were still free, as were drugs for hospital in-patients.

In 1987 direct subsidies were slashed. Except for drugs used in several special disease control programmes the prices of essential drugs at government health facilities and private pharmacies were similar. However, essential drugs still received an indirect subsidy through a favourable foreign exchange pricing policy. Private pharmacies continued to sell more non-essential, 'popular' drugs which provided them with the bulk of their profits.

The policy took another spin when a single rate of foreign exchange was established in the national monetary reform of February 1988. Meant as an emergency measure to combat inflation and to improve the business environment, it also eliminated the indirect subsidy for medicines. The effect was a five-fold increase in the price paid by the consumer. The public's reaction was immediate. 'There is a drastic reduction in demand', said Byron Ramirez of the Ministry of Internal Commerce. 'If someone needs ten pills, at best he will only be able to buy five now.'[3] Medicine sales fell so drastically that prices had to be cut by 35 to 50 per cent to avoid letting the products become outdated prior to sale.

Despite the elimination of subsidized prices, Nicaraguans often still consumed medicines which were ineffective or harmful. Sixty per cent of all imported medicines are antibiotics; enough are consumed to provide each person with five full courses of treatment in a year—more than is used in Europe or the U.S. But people often take antibiotics for only one or two days at a time making each dose ineffective and promoting resistant bacterial strains. With the recent elimination of pharmaceutical subsidies, the tendency to take less than a full course of treatment is even greater.

The misuse of modern medicines was a common feature of the Somoza era when most people lacked effective access to doctors and hospitals. It grew worse in the resource-poor Sandinista era when populist health policies eroded the formerly-overwhelming authority of physicians.

Investments in Health

With the revolution, health investments rose rapidly. By 1981 the health sector represented 13 per cent of the government's budget and 4.7 per cent of GDP. Despite rising inflation the value of public funds invested in health rose far more rapidly. Furthermore, MINSA accounted for only about 40 per cent of all health-related expenses in the country. Private physicians and dentists, private medicine purchases and health investments by other ministries together surpassed MINSA expenditures (Table 2). Total health spending constituted 10 to 15 per cent of GDP during the mid-1980s (Fig. 3).

After 1984 further increases in the number of Cordobas devoted to the health system were eaten up by inflation. In 1986 MINSA had only slightly more inflation-adjusted Cordobas to spend than it did in 1980. Compared to other Central American countries where economic problems have been less severe the Nicaraguan health sector has none the less fared very well.

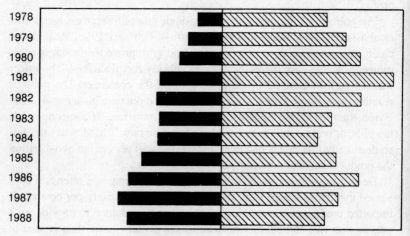

Fig. 3. Ministry of Health expenditure as per cent of GDP and of total government budget.

Table 2. Estimated expenditures for health in Nicaragua, 1986[13]

Source	Billions of Cordobas
Government	
Ministry of Health	23.8
Water and Waste	2.4
Armed Forces	2.0
Social Welfare	0.5
University Health Training	0.5
Total government	29.2
Private individual payments	
Private physicians	14.1
Private dental care	1.8
Water supply payments	5.3
Private pharmaceuticals	3.4
Charges for public pharmaceuticals	0.4
Private hospitals	1.2
Lab tests and eye glasses	0.5
Folk practitioners	0.5
Total private	27.2
Charities and health industries	
Red Cross	1.4
PROVADENIC	0.3
Popular organizations	0.2
Health industries	0.6
Total charity and industries	2.5
Estimated Total Health Expenditure	58.9

THE CHAMORRO PERIOD, 1990 TO THE PRESENT

The election of Violeta Chamorro in 1990 was a blow to rural health. Cuba withdrew most of its 100 physicians who were staffing rural primary care centres, pharmaceutical supply from Eastern Europe deteriorated, and Nicaraguan administration of rural health programmes weakened. As a result many health posts and some health centres were forced to close. While MINSA was committed to maintaining these facilities, it had not found a way to ensure the staffing and medicines. Furthermore, with new, conservative doctors installed as regional health authorities, interest grew in hospital and specialty care and rural care was no longer the priority for resource allocation.

In a situation reminiscent of the time when the Sandinista government was new, mobile medical services were promised to areas lacking in doctors. In some towns private doctors helped to fill the vacancies created by withdrawn Cuban specialists at health centres. Health campaigns fared badly. Without cooperation from other ministries and lacking political links (unlike the Sandinista neighbourhood groups), MINSA's health campaigns reached only about half as many people in 1991 as compared to those in previous years. While routine health services were able to fill some of the demand for immunization, a large outbreak of measles occurred in early 1991, perhaps sparked by lower coverage service, but also reflecting reduced immunization activity in the late Sandinista years. In some areas community health committees and *brigadistas* associated with right-wing parties were formed. Such efforts were short-lived; they could not make up for a breakdown in the already extensive national primary care system.

The greatest fear was of radical privatization. Former Health Minister Tellez viewed this philosophy as 'the right to health for the rich. The poor, the workers, can have as much health as they can buy.'[9] But contrary to accusations from the Left, the new Health Minister Salmeron had no intention to privatize. Rampant inflation and fixed budgetary allotments as a result of new decentralization policies led health centres and posts to run out of supplies quickly. Hospital directors spoke of shortages worse than any they had seen in years. Some health centres were able to purchase only a quarter of the medicines they had received just months before. Yet the consumption of medicine and visits to doctors declined only slightly. More people simply had to purchase medicines in the open market after getting a prescription through MINSA services. In this way privatization crept uncontrollably into the health system.

To make matters worse, the new health leaders drawn from the ranks of urban private doctors lacked the experience needed to face such a crisis. Some in positions of authority worked only half a day, devoting the rest of their time to private practice.

The loss of careful administrative control further exacerbated the trend towards privatization. Earlier, limits had been imposed on the number of pills an individual could receive through the public health system. When this regulation was abolished in 1990 a small number of people purchased large amounts. Similarly, vaccines for health campaigns fell short as they were distributed indiscriminately without regard to previous vaccinations. Some hospitals began to charge for X-rays and some oral rehydration centres even started to charge for packets of rehydration salts. The use of these services began to decline. Small and large-scale robberies of pharmaceuticals, last seen in 1985, reappeared.

This deterioration was the product of the polarization and poverty which beset the country in 1990. The Minister of Health and most of his new assistants worked hard to hold the system together. Some of the former Sandinista leaders continued to work for MINSA, others did so indirectly via Pan American Health Organization (PAHO) and UNICEF, and still other Sandinistas who had not been in MINSA were appointed to Vice-Ministerial posts. The new leaders obtained funding for health programmes from a meeting of government-related donors in Europe in the summer of 1990. These programmes—the campaign to defend the lives of children, water and sanitation systems and care for the disabled, among others—were nearly identical to programmes promoted by the former administration. A five-year health plan developed by late 1990 similarly took its priorities and programmes mainly from the health plan for 1988–91 developed under the Sandinista administration.

Aid to the Health Sector

Following the Chamorro election the U.S. economic blockade ended and new moneys started to flow. USAID spent about $14 million for health-related services for Contras returning from Honduras, provided over $4 million directly to MINSA for emergency pharmaceutical purchases and several million more for health through U.S. organizations such as Project HOPE. European governments pledged even more in a $70 million package to be administered by the World Bank and InterAmerican Development Bank. These funds would nearly double the effective budget of MINSA, but were not made available until loans in arrears were re-negotiated. As a result, MINSA, like the rest of Nicaragua, was still starved for development funds a year after Chamorro took over.

In fact foreign moneys still supported most of the health system. Primary care most likely would have proceeded differently in the 1980s if foreign support had not subsidized inefficient pharmaceutical, food supplementation and health personnel policies. Even the Sandinistas favoured the politically vocal urban populations for the sake of domestic peace. The Eastern Block had provided the second largest pool of international resources for health prior to 1990, exceeded only by UN agencies. This supported inefficient practices and doctor-centred curative service. Suddenly this source disappeared. At the same time, declining financial support from pro-Sandinista solidarity groups was disbursed directly to community groups and non-governmental organizations, by-passing MINSA. The new Ministry faced worse financial pressures than its predecessor.

Western European governments and the US nominally supported the government which their war had brought into power and partially made up for lost sources of funds and materials. However, with attention turned to Eastern Europe and the Persian Gulf by 1991, these funds fell far short of needs.

Politics

In 1990 the situation grew confusing as both the Sandinistas and the Chamorro coalition split over various health policies. On the Left, some kept to the policy of 'governing from below' by refusing to work with or support the government, encouraging alternative institutions and strikes. Others pursued critical support for the government in what became known as *concertacion*, or harmonization. The *concertacion* faction gained steam with the reappointment of Sandinista leader Humberto Ortega as Minister of Defence, and MINSA became a test-case for the policy of working together for common goals despite political differences.

Chamorro centrists, led by Minister Salmeron, supported policies favourable to doctors and the private sector but defended the need for a public health system that responded to the needs of the poor majority. Radical rightists were determined to undo everything the Sandinistas had created and were intent on destroying the public health system. They saw the policies of Dr Salmeron and President Chamorro as virtual treason to their cause. The situation led the Minister to cry that he was 'caught between two groups of bandits'.

The attack on health from the Right came primarily from other government ministries. The new Minister of Social Welfare touched the most vulnerable nerve by stating publicly that social security funds should be withheld from MINSA in order to build a 120-bed social security hospital. The Minister of Health sounded a bit like a Sandinista in his defence of public care:

If you want to invest $100 million in a private hospital with 100 beds and modern, scientific technology, welcome . . . But please get it out of your head that there might be any government resources to finance private investments in medicine.

From the Left, the health workers' union, FETSALUD, took on renewed importance in 1990 not seen since the anti-Somoza strikes of the 1970s. It participated in two general strikes in 1990 and helped organize a doctor's

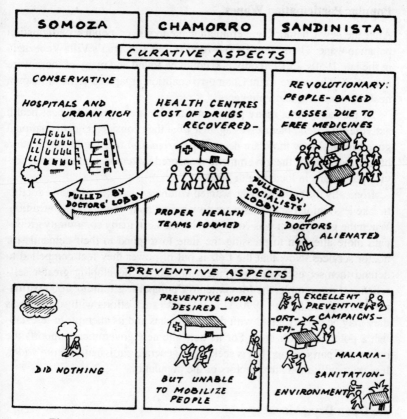

The varied effects of Nicaragua's political systems on health care.

strike in early 1991. In the first strike, most of the government was shut down amidst demands for wage adjustments, worker participation and an end to arbitrary firing. Salmeron testified that the demands were just but depended on resources and on policies which could be made only by the President. MINSA was one of two government ministries to remain partially open during the strike.

The second strike was more extensive and militant. All ministries were closed and health workers took over several clinics. One clinic in a rightist Managua neighbourhood suffered an armed attacked by 60 government supporters and ex-Contras to dislodge what was considered a Left stronghold.

Popular Participation Wanes

After the new Chamorro government came to power, popular participation began to wane. There were 1200 *brigadistas* in Managua's Villa Venezuela in the late 1980s. In 1990 only 800 could be found and many of these were not active. The centre–right Chamorro coalition organized some of its own health committees and volunteers.

At the same time, many poor communities are organizing local health activities to defend themselves against what they consider a hostile national government. Many more are demanding *brigadista* training in anticipation of a withdrawal of the government-sponsored system stationing social service physicians in local health posts.

Ironically the populists who wanted volunteers to take more (and doctors to take less) initiative in health are now seeing their dream come to fruition. When the government was controlled by the Left, many community groups paid more attention to pressing the state to respond to their demands for doctor services. Now that the Left is out of power they feel compelled to defend themselves from government neglect by developing greater self-reliance. For example, the Movimiento Comunal was training 7000 permanent *brigadistas* by late 1990. USAID views such efforts with suspicion as they may be closely allied with the Sandinistas and its attempts to re-establish a political power-base. For its part, the new government supports the concept of participation but is seeking to generate participation from wider, less politically-motivated sectors of the population.

An Open Drug Market

Nicaragua's drug policy got caught up in the wave of privatization sweeping the country and Eastern Europe in 1990. Even orders which were already paid for were not shipped as newly-privatized firms in Eastern Europe refused to honour commercial commitments made when they were still state-run companies. As a result, remaining subsidies and free medicine programmes disappeared in Nicaragua. Medicines went to market value just as hyper-inflation returned to destroy the buying power of salaries.

In addition, tight central controls imposed by MINSA on distributing medicines were lost. In their place health units were to order medicines of choice through fixed budget allocations. Lacking careful norms and supervision and under new leadership, pharmaceutical distribution deteriorated. Several devaluations reduced the power of health units to buy imported supplies. Health centres and hospitals complained of shortages worse than any they had experienced under the Sandinistas, and many health posts reported no medicine deliveries at all for months. Minister of Health Salmeron reiterated MINSA's policy of free medicines for high-priority groups and asked for public assistance in policing the pharmacies. However, in the environment of radical privatization, this became increasingly difficult. State pharmacies were privatized *de facto*, while 80 new, profit-oriented pharmaceutical importing firms sprang up in addition to the 380 existing previously. Free or subsidized medicines became a thing of the past except for vaccines and tuberculosis drugs which were guaranteed by UNICEF and the International Union for the Prevention of Respiratory Diseases, respectively.

International Assistance

Both Left and Right groups had important foreign supporters. The University and community groups continued to receive assistance from many small solidarity organizations in the U.S. and Europe. Aid which formerly had been provided to MINSA was shifted rapidly to non-governmental organizations in what must be the first international campaign to privatize leftist assistance for health! This was justified with the statement that 'progressive leadership . . . has come only from the Sandinistas or its supporters'.[11] The coordinating committee of the U.S. health solidarity network even adopted a policy that no member group could solicit or accept funding from USAID.[10]

The Cuban government had reacted to the Chamorro election by immediately withdrawing most of its health and other technical staff. Although they had good reason to be concerned for their physical safety, some Cuban doctors were soon sent back to Nicaragua. Fidel Castro suggested that more doctors could be sent if the government was willing to pay. Minister Salmeron looked upon this offer favourably as Cuba charged only about 20 per cent as much as the German and Soviet governments for physicians. By August 1990 there were again 113 Cuban doctors while there had been 175 at the beginning of the year.

The most active foreign supporters of the Right were those groups which had formerly assisted the Contras in Honduras. The biggest of these is the Miami Medical Team, a group of anti-Castro Cuban exile doctors deeply committed to the Contra cause. They had flown in regularly from Miami during the war to provide surgery at Contra bases. The Miami Medical Team Director, Dr Alzucaray, flew into Managua following the election and proclaimed: 'Today Managua, tomorrow Havana'. Other supporters included religious and/or political groups considered rightist and engaged in health work, including the Dooley Foundation, Freedom Medicine and the Pan-American Development Foundation. One ministerial aid commented, 'Frankly, I don't have much use for either the solidarity or the rightist groups. Both arrogantly assume they know all the answers and can tell us what to do.'

Many of Nicaragua's new leaders are highly motivated and concerned professionals. But in the absence of a government policy and public commitment to health for all, programmes will continue to drift, often at the whim of private concerns and the profit motive.

LESSONS FOR OTHER COUNTRIES

Like Socialist revolutions in other countries, the Sandinistas in Nicaragua developed health services in two stages. The first was a rapid expansion of curative medical care in response to pre-revolutionary goals and plans. The second was a re-formulation of health plans to fit the revolutionary economic, political and social environment. Some countries did this amidst conditions of extreme scarcity, such as the USSR during the New Economic Plan in the 1920s. Others, such as Cuba which began its community medicine programme in 1976, did it in relative affluence. Nicaragua re-formulated its health system between 1983 and 1986 in response to scarcity and war, without nationalization or affluence. The major successes of this reorientation provide important lessons for other countries attempting to do more for health with less money.

— Decentralization of budgeting and priority-setting. This led to more community involvement, improved ability to mobilize local volunteers and finance, and better responses to the felt needs of residents. User fees, even at a low $0.05, gave local committees the means to take action in response to local needs. Even international finance often went directly to small towns through independent fund-raising, sister-city arrangements and solidarity peoples' movements. Local resources made participation meaningful.
— The modification of developed-country technologies to developing-country conditions. Appropriate technologies included oral rehydration centres, a midwifery training programme and herbal medicine development. All of these used modern information and research methods to guide the development or implementation of simplified, inexpensive interventions useful both in poor urban and rural communities.
— Encouragement and coordination of volunteer efforts including one-day

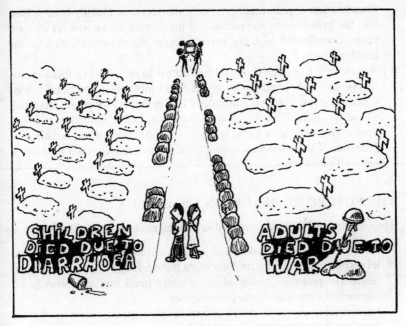

Needless deaths—a national tragedy.

health campaigns, mothers' clubs, *brigadistas* and the involvement of mass organizations in health promotion. The ability to sustain large-scale mobilization throughout their decade in power reflects the ability of these programmes to motivate the population. Although it was assumed that mobilization was equivalent to empowerment it is not possible to quantify the impact of health education and popular campaigns during the 1980s. There is no doubt that the mass campaigns against malaria and vaccine-preventable diseases gave a huge boost to efforts to control these serious health threats. They also succeeded in involving large num bers of people in health activities. Local areas used the approach for specific problems such as TB case-finding in the North, recruitment of village workers along the Atlantic coast, occupational health and protection from pesticides in the Pacific agricultural areas.

— Careful utilization of both large-scale and small-scale international support for personnel, training and treatment. Relatively large funds were available but charges of waste, corruption and inefficiency were seldom heard. Decentralized funding led to both participation and accountability.

— Coordination of public and private health services. Initially seen as hostile, the government accommodated the private sector and, in its later years, coordinated with the private sector via decentralization of the health system.

— A slow shift from universal and free access to services to a focus on the groups and individuals most in need and most likely to benefit from public services. This was particularly true in the field of pharmaceuticals where the initial free provision of drugs was later confined to essential drugs, and still later to only those essential for public health programmes. This meant that very limited resources were used in increasingly efficient ways.

THE FUTURE OF HEALTH IN NICARAGUA

The election of Chamorro changed several aspects of the health system:

— International assistance declined in 1990 and then grew by late 1991 to levels never seen during the Sandinista period. Large inter-governmental funding is promised to the Ministry while small private resources are channelled more directly to communities.

— Intersectoral coordination disappeared, leaving all responsibility for health to the private sector and MINSA.

— Attention to primary care declined as interest shifted back to doctors and hospitals.

— The private sector grew while the system of public care declined.

— Community participation shifted towards defending the poor from government neglect rather than collaborating with the public health system.

To manage and mobilize resources, socialist governments in developing countries, including China and Cuba, nationalized their economies. By the 1980s this model had lost much of its appeal, having led to the development of a privileged bureaucratic elite and condemning each country to isolation from potential markets, sources of capital and modern technology. Thus revolutions following the Vietnam War looked for models which might generate less social dislocation and more rapid economic growth. Nicaragua and Zimbabwe were prime experiments of a more moderate road to socialism (see also the chapter by Sanders in this book). The strategy paid off for both countries, albeit in limited ways. Providing loans and credits to the private sector in Nicaragua stimulated the economy in the early 1980s and may have reduced or delayed hostile acts, including possible direct U.S. military intervention. It permitted the simultaneous growth of Socialist government health initiatives, populist health promotion policies and a thriving private sector in health. One drawback was that this moderate, mixed public–private road toward socialism in health led to a more capital-intensive, doctor-based health system than might otherwise have occurred. Thus, when the Chamorro coalition won, conditions were ripe for a return to the exploitation and neglect that had accompanied the earlier capitalist medical model.

The Sandinista political agenda preceded by a decade the primary health strategy which was elaborated at Alma Ata in 1978. It evolved sometimes in unexpected ways. Sandinista plans were often modified under pressure from doctors, community groups or other ministries. Ironically it is only under the Chamorro government that community groups are independently defining and meeting their health needs. Faced with the collapse of socialist political commitment, local social cohesion is at last taking responsibility for the health needs of the community, rather than waiting for government action. Earlier, political expectations had encouraged unrealistic demands and diminished local initiative.

Strong input from doctors was an enduring element of the Sandinista political programme. The input can be seen as limiting primary care development because training and services retained a curative, resource-intensive orientation. More might have been achieved if the Sandinistas had, instead, adopted a more aggressive approach to primary care. This could have worked in either of two ways. The entire health system could have been nationalized, requiring all doctors to pursue the priorities of the public system of care. Radicals argued for such a Cuban-style approach, while moderate leftists feared alienating doctors and other middle-class groups. Since these were the terms of the debate, a second option was not considered. The hospitals could have been left in the hands of conservative doctors, but without public subsidies. MINSA then could have concentrated on primary care using newly-trained paramedicals and doctors committed exclusively to public service. Freed from the administrative, financial and political burdens of running a system full of unsympathetic doctors, the Left could have achieved more in primary care and community participation.

It is worrisome to see the public system shrink under today's overwhelming financial, organizational and ideological burdens. Yet many of the innovations of the 1980s, including the demand for equity, preventive health campaigns, basic medicines and simplified technologies and community involvement, have remained enduring elements of the system. It will be instructive to see how politicians from the Left, labour unions, community groups and public health workers can work together to limit the extent of privatization. Decentralization was developed in the 1980s to empower communities. It could also be used to oppress them by freeing government of the responsibility to organize and provide care.

Economic recessions in the 1980s and early 1990s, together with the collapse of state socialism in Eastern Europe, have unleashed a wave of privatization and shrinking governmental social welfare spending in much of the developing world. Although many groups defend the importance of government in the provision of social services, the health sector in many countries has been affected by this trend.

Even as MINSA tries to avoid privatization, this is happening through reduced employment in the public health sector, the closing of primary care sites, requirements that services to the poor become self-supporting, and the relaxation of administrative mechanisms which earlier limited the role of hospital-based curative care in the nation's health system. Some of these changes express the political perspectives of the Chamorro government. Others were responses to the shortage of resources available to the health system due to decreased voluntarism, loss of intersectoral coordination and diversion of 'solidarity' donations.

Most of the health innovations of the Sandinistas appear equally relevant under the current, more conservative regime. Some of them, like the experiments at decentralization and cost-recovery, can dangerously facilitate the decline of public responsibility for care.

Large-scale international assistance will be required for an extended period of time to rebuild the country. While such assistance appears to be increasingly available, it is also necessary for donors to engage in a dialogue with national leaders to help ensure that these funds efficiently reach those in greatest need.

Health for all in Nicaragua will require an end to atrophy in the public system of care, increasing resources devoted to prevention and basic care, extensive education among doctors and patients on the rational use of pharmaceuticals, renewed cooperation among government ministries, and increasing attention to nursing and paramedicals. The issues are not Left or Right, black or white—they relate to the compromises necessary to develop a financially-viable, technically-sound and socially-equitable form of health promotion and medical care for all. Struggles over these issues most likely will define the nature of primary health care in Nicaragua and many other countries through the decade ahead.

References

1. Garfield, R. M., Williams, G. (1992). *Health care in Nicaragua: primary care under changing regimes.* Oxford University Press, New York.

2. USAID. (1976). *Health sector assessment for Nicaragua*. USAID Mission, Managua.
3. Kuhl, C. A. (1980). Report on the health situation in Nicaragua to the 33rd World Health Assembly. MINSA, Managua.
4. Garfield, R. M. and Vermund, S. H. (1983). Changes in malaria incidence after a mass drug administration in Nicarauga. *Lancet*, Vol. 2, pp. 500–3.
5. Garfield, R. M. and Vermund, S. H. (1986). Health education and community participation in mass drug administration for malaria in Nicaragua. *Social Science and Medicine*, Vol. 22, No. 8, pp. 869–77.
6. Woznica, C. (1987). Community participation in health as an empowering process: A case study from Nicaragua. Ph.D. dissertation, University of Illinois, Chicago, p. 258.
7. Braveman, P. and Siegel, D. (1987). Nicaragua: A health system developing under conditions of war. *International Journal of Health Services*, Vol. 17, pp. 169–78.
8. Garfield, R. M. (1985). Health and the war against Nicaragua, 1981–1984. *Journal of Public Health Policy*, Vol. 6, No. 1, pp. 116–31.
9. Garfield, R. M., Frieden, T. and Vermund, S. H. (1987). Health related outcomes of war in Nicaragua. *American Journal of Public Health*, Vol. 77, No. 5, pp. 615–18.
10. Lomba, M. (1990). Privatizar la salud seria asestar estocada al pueblo. *Barricada*, July 4, p. 1.
11. National Central American Health Rights Network. (1990). Report of the post-election delegation to Nicaragua. NCAHRN, New York.
12. National Assembly. (1990). Debate over the Agency for International Development. *Links*, Vol. 7, No. 2, p. 22.
13. Roemer, M. I. (1986). The health system of Nicaragua under fire. Los Angeles, CA. Mimeo.

CHAPTER 13

The Dynamics of China's Health Care Model

SUSAN RIFKIN

The author examines the relevance of China's revolutionary approach to universal health care during the recent rapid economic and social change in the country. Several of the features of China's much-heralded model have been jeopardized and the future remains unclear.

Susan B. Rifkin, Ph.D., was the first Coordinator of the Asian Community Health Action Network, ACHAN, in Hong Kong. She has been a lecturer at the Liverpool School of Tropical Medicine, U.K., and is presently lecturer at the Institute for Tropical Hygiene in Heidelberg, Germany.

INTRODUCTION

China is the world's most populous country. With its limited resources, its attempts to adapt the advances of modern science and technology to benefit its massive population are legendary. This quest began in the late nineteenth century with the disintegration of Chinese imperial rule and continues today under a strong, centralized government. Its search for answers to problems of development has inspired individuals and countries throughout the world.

One of the areas in which the attempts have had considerable success is in the area of public health. Known in the past as 'the sick man of Asia', modern China's health achievements are ones which many countries, particularly those with large populations and scarce resources, seek to copy. Combining the past with the present, ideological political commitment with pragmatic solutions, and health care with socio-economic development, the Chinese health care model became the inspiration for the WHO–UNICEF policy of Primary Health Care. Here we describe that model and the experience of its application in a very large and diverse country. In conclusion, we look at lessons and the challenges that remain as the year 2000 approaches.

THE BEGINNINGS

The history of modern China is the history of revolutionary struggle in which the collapse of a feudal empire was followed by a long period of civil war. The country finally emerged as a strong centralized Communist state in 1949. The leadership that achieved this unity had confronted very difficult problems including a long trek over a large part of the country, pursued by both the Japanese and internal political opponents. The lessons learned during the hardships of this period became the underpinnings of the new government when it emerged victorious in 1949.

The leadership of the new nation, the Peoples' Republic of China, built its government on the principle of equity. This was a radical change from the previous period when scarce resources were squandered on a small minority by those who had armies and power. From the early days of the new government, social policy became a focus to ensure the millions and mainly poor, rural Chinese rapidly became beneficiaries of the new political order. In 1950 a national conference established the four principles on which the Chinese health care system was based. These principles were:

— *Health must serve the common people*. This laid emphasis on the health needs of the rural masses rather than the urban elites who commanded resources prior to the Communist period.
— *Place prevention first*. This demanded that emphasis be placed on a strong preventive network rather than on large curative institutions.
— *Unite traditional with modern medicine*. This called for all available health resources to be integrated and used for the great task of health improvement.
— *Integrate health campaigns with other mass campaigns*. This sought to mobilize people to understand the new orientation of the government and to undertake public health activities in which everyone participated, such as street-sweeping, killing flies, building and using latrines, and adopting family planning.

BUILDING THE CHINESE MODEL

On the basis of these four principles China created a model for health care which differed radically from those existing in other countries. Several features of the model became the principles of Primary Health Care and the framework for the global strategy towards Health for All by the Year 2000.

The first feature and principle of PHC was that of equity. The Chinese model rested upon the belief that the greatest resource of a nation was its

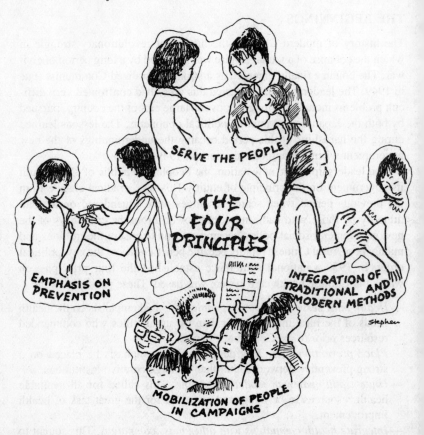

people. For the nation to expand and develop, the needs of the people must be met. Echoing the analysis of the Swedish economist Gunnar Myrdal that health and education were 'investments in man', the Chinese leadership committed time and resources to develop a system where most people had some access to health care. The principle of equity was confirmed by the revolutionary restructuring of the Chinese state. It has been pursued over the past 40 years by both the Communist Party and the government of the Peoples' Republic of China but not without major problems and setbacks.

The second feature of the model was the priority accorded to prevention. Confronted with massive disease and health problems, the government chose to attack these difficulties at the point of prevention rather than cure. With this strategy China did not build large urban hospitals or invest in expensive, advanced technology. Rather, the government put maximum ef-

Table 1. Incidence per 100 000 population of four infectious diseases
in 1959 and 1986

	Diphtheria	Pertussis	Measles	Poliomyelitis
1959	22.4	240	1432	2.60
1986	0.07	7.97	18.9	0.17

fort into measures to reduce loads on the existing institutions. As a result rapid gains were made in reducing and controlling communicable diseases which accounted for the majority of deaths and morbidity in the pre-Communist period (Table 1).

The third feature of the Chinese model was its emphasis on participation. Participation by all members of the Chinese state in the political process was a foundation of the new government. Participation was not by choice but by obligation. Mobilized for 're-education', for mass campaigns which included health campaigns, and for support of external and internal government policies, people participated to ensure support to the government's radical approaches to create a post-feudal China. However, participation enabled the majority of people, who had never had access to health care let alone have any say about how it should be delivered, to be involved in decisions which affected their daily lives.

A fourth feature was an emphasis on appropriate technology. In searching for modernization, the Chinese government did not allocate massive resources to build a modern industrial base but rather, it used its massive labour power to search for alternative strategies. Many, like the backyard furnaces during the Great Leap Forward, were doomed to fail. However, others, like the use of acupuncture as an anaesthetic and for the treatment of chronic inflammation, provided China with appropriate and acceptable techniques to stretch scarce resources to cover many more people.

Another feature of the model which influenced PHC was its intersectoral approach to solving health problems and providing health care. Health in the Chinese Communist view was not the responsibility of a single sector in a modern state. Good health could only be the result of improved food supplies, better education and an improved national income. It was a state responsibility to ensure that its people could both contribute to the modernization of China and reap the benefits of that modernization by being sound in both mind and body. Interpreting health as a key part of socio-economic development meant that health professionals were necessary but not sufficient to ensure health improvements. Even the technical features of health care became the responsibility of local people through the deployment of the barefoot doctors. This holistic approach was one of the most important in pursuing the new health strategy.

Of all features of the model, however, the one which most definitely ensured its development and expansion could be called the 'political will' of the Chinese government. The leadership was committed to a restructuring of the State as well as of the health care system. Health policy implementation was ensured by the state's new infrastructure supported by that of the Communist Party. Without a strong centralized state and the support of the political leadership the Chinese health care system would not have been possible.

PUTTING THE MODEL INTO PRACTICE

To put these principles into practice, the government undertook a number of important steps. The first was to create a health service infrastructure which reflected the stated priorities. The health care system, like the administrative system, was decentralized, based on units responsible for agricultural production in the rural areas where 80 per cent of the people lived. The production team comprising 200 to 700 people was the smallest unit. Several teams made up a brigade. The commune of 10 000 to 60 000 was the largest rural grouping with five to ten forming a county or *Xian*, the lowest level of civil government. Health units were established to correspond with each of these units thus re-enforcing the political and managerial infrastructure and interlinking accountability of officials from the lowest local unit to the national level. Urban health infrastructures were slightly different but nonetheless decentralized. In addition, to ensure preventive activities, anti-epidemic stations were established. These local units became responsible for the reporting of communicable diseases and for carrying out public health and sanitation work in their regions. They were the basis of the earliest rural health infrastructure and for the heavy emphasis on preventive measures.

A second important step was the development of health and medical manpower. In 1944, for a population of about 500 million people, there were 12 000 Western-style doctors in China, 60 per cent of whom were qualified. Even with the expanded number of doctors (estimated to be 70 per 100 000 in 1986), the supply was rather limited. As a result, much of China's health care relied on the training and deployment of various categories of other medical auxiliaries. Table 2 lists some of the most important and gives a description of their education and tasks.

Table 2. Selected health care workers—education and role

Position	Education	Typical role
Non-salaried workers		
Barefoot Doctor	Highly variable, primary education (or more) plus 3- to 6-month special course, plus continuing education	Service to field production teams and brigade health station
Rural Doctor	Upgraded barefoot doctor	Posted in brigade health station
Middle-level salaried staff		
Assistant Doctors (of Western and Chinese Medicine)	Specialized senior secondary school	Play assisting role in city hospitals, roles of greater leadership in commune health centres
Nurses	Specialized senior secondary school	Support role in hospitals
Senior salaried staff		
Western Doctor	Varied over time; currently 5 to 8 years post-secondary	County general hospitals; urban and enterprise hospitals
Doctor of Chinese Medicine	Currently 5 years post-secondary	County and district general hospitals; hospitals of Chinese medicine
Public Health Doctor	Same as Western doctor, except for less clinical training and more public health	Staff and manage county and provincial anti-epidemic stations

Note: There are many more types of personnel in each of the categories listed, and there is an additional category of primary-level salaried staff. Most workers are, however, of one of the types listed here.

By far the most famous category of health personnel identified with the Chinese health care model was the barefoot doctor. Although dating from the 'Great Leap Forward' in 1958, the barefoot doctor was trained and promoted widely in the 1960s as part of the Cultural Revolution. As a working member of the Chinese brigade in the commune, the barefoot doctor was trained for three months on an average, and then returned to his production unit both to contribute to the labour force and to serve as a front-line health worker. Paid usually by 'work points', the salary basis of the production unit, he/she was responsible to the production unit and not to the commune medical personnel. The tasks of these part-time health workers included promotion of preventive activities and local health campaigns, health education, advice on family planning, treating simple diseases and referring more complicated ones, as well as collecting and reporting health-related information. The creation of this type of health worker was to enable China's great rural population to gain access to health care through a rapid and radical change in the health delivery system.

Incorporation of traditional medicine was also an important feature of health care in China. In the early period the 500 000 traditional doctors were recognized as key resources to fulfil health care objectives and were given recognition for their contribution toward this goal. Subsequently, training institutions were established and Western-trained doctors were given opportunities to study traditional practices. An academy of traditional medicine was established. This decision not only increased the available manpower and resources for medicines substantially, but also gave the patient a choice of treatments.

Another important strategy was the mobilization of the people to take part in health campaigns. Linked directly with the creation of mechanisms to ensure the active participation of the masses in the new political order, these campaigns covered activities from individual home cleanliness to the eradication of major communicable diseases. Two of the most famous campaigns focused on venereal disease and schistosomiasis. During the former, people with the disease were identified, treated, their contacts followed up and prostitutes, the main carriers, were trained for more constructive employment. During the drives against schistosomiasis millions of peasants engaged in campaigns to bury the disease-carrying snail which lived along the banks of water channels, at the same time improving irrigation for the rice fields.

Financing the new health care system did not depend on massive injections of cash or on massive allocations of foreign aid. Rather, it depended on mobilizing existing resources and building a financing system based on the local production units. The Central Ministry provided funds for the central hospitals and training institutions and for the health insurance of State employees. However, rural health units, the more numerous health care structures, were paid for by the local production units. In fact, this meant that the more wealthy units provided a better service. However, altogether, the system provided far superior care for most people than was ever possible during the earlier period.

THE MODEL'S PERFORMANCE OVER TIME

In pursuing the four health care principles, the Chinese government has had to respond to three major influences over the past 40 years: political change, changing public demands and expectations, and rising population. These influences, which have also affected other developing countries, have modified the health care model, brought new challenges and raised a series of issues for the achievement of health for all. They suggest lessons which might be useful to other countries.

The first influence was rapid political change. In the Peoples' Republic of China it meant several marked upheavals throughout the country. Although no lasting threat has come so far to the Communist leadership, political changes paralyzed that leadership for long periods of time and created major problems in the pursuit of national policies. Table 3 gives a chronology of the major domestic upheavals and the corresponding important changes in health care delivery.

Political instability resulted in constant revision of health activities to reflect the current Party line. In periods of intense political activity, the continuity of health care delivery was often broken. During these periods the health infrastructure suffered from either excessive attention or neglect. A good example is the Cultural Revolution when urban doctors were sent to the countryside to staff anti-epidemic stations. Preventive networks broke as a result of massive defections of these doctors to commune hospitals where they could use their training. In many areas diseases like malaria and schistosomiasis increased rapidly. More recently, modernization efforts have resulted in a shift away from fully state-supported health care to free market, private sector services.

In addition, political changes in China have affected the training and deployment of all levels of health personnel. In the 1950s and 1960s highly-trained medical professionals were squandered on menial health tasks in order to improve attitudes to and understanding of State goals. Also, millions of people were called upon to perform medical treatment tasks without adequate training or supervision. In the 1980s the return to professionalism and upgrading of health care quality has resulted in the expanded production of fully-qualified medical personnel. One result could be the overproduction of doctors and the undercutting of training of health auxiliaries who provide health care to millions of poor rural Chinese. Such policy shifts put great pressure on both the training and planning establishments as well as on the personnel themselves.

The second major influence on the Chinese health care model has been

Table 3. Chronology of major political changes in the People' Republic of China

	Political changes	Health care development
1949	Establishment of the Peoples' Republic of China under the Chinese Communist Party after the defeat of both the Japanese and the civil war opponents of Kuomingtong.	Health care restructured based on decentralized agricultural units.
1958	'The Great Leap Forward' supported a massive thrust for industrialization and intensified collectivization by promoting small-scale industries at the very local level and demanding that technical experts be under supervision of Party people.	Beginning of use of local people for health care delivery.
1966	'The Great Cultural Revolution' launched, promoting Party loyalties above expertise, ending with a fight for control between the moderates and the revolutionaries.	Urban doctors sent to the countryside and millions of peasants trained to do front-line health care.
1969	Fall of 'The Gang of Four', the four people who (after the death in 1976 of Mao Zedong, the man who led the Peoples' Republic since its creation) pursued a fundamentalist approach to revolution, resulting in a continual struggle with more moderate groups. 'Household responsibility system' established.	Free markets and private health care encouraged. One Child Family Policy promoted. Promotion of preventive measures and rise of paid curative medicine.
1989	Tien An Men Massacre in which the emerging moderate leadership used the military to end protests to its rule, thus causing condemnation by the international world and another split between the hardline and moderate groups within the leadership.	Implications still unclear

the rising and increasingly immediate expectations of millions of Chinese people for material improvements after years of sacrifice and promises of improvement. The moderates who emerged in 1979 under the Chairmanship of Deng Xiaoping confronted these concerns and reorganized the economic system by replacing the collective production units with a 'household responsibility system'. Essentially this meant that each household was responsible for their own earnings and expenditure.

This decision had major consequences throughout the country. In the health field it resulted in a shift from state responsibility for health and medical care to individual responsibility. It meant that in the future people would pay for their health care and providers would charge fees for their services.

Reflecting rising expectations, people in villages began to forsake the rural health units and seek treatment at a higher level. Farmers began to travel to urban hospitals and surveys showed that nearly 20 per cent of villagers in some areas preferred treatment in the county hospitals or the township health centres to local health care.

Corresponding to this shift was the decrease in support for the cooperative medical systems and the barefoot doctor. It was estimated that in 1975, 84.5 per cent of the rural Chinese population was covered by the cooperative medical system. By 1985, this coverage had fallen to 39.9 per cent. A survey undertaken by Zhu and his colleagues in four rural counties suggested that health status deteriorated because there was no money available for barefoot doctors to update skills or buy better or even standard equipment. While the new policy allowed barefoot doctors to seek higher qualifications and to charge fees, the low fees and lack of State recognition and support for such amenities as examination rooms began to take its toll. The barefoot doctors were now spending more time in farming and less on health work.

CRITICAL QUESTIONS

The developments occurring as a result of political changes and rising expectations raise a series of critical questions directed at the Chinese health care model. The most obvious is: What will happen to equity if consumer choice and not the State directs the supply of health care? Evidence suggests that even under State support there were large differences in the availability of resources between production units. Differences are now apparent even among people living in the same geographic area. Who will pay? Will the poor be left out?

Another question concerns the role of the barefoot doctors. Although the government continues to promote these rural auxiliaries as the backbone of rural health care, it has not committed resources or framed clear policies of support. As a result, there is uncertainty about their future, and local people see little reason to use their services. Linked directly with the question of poor utilization is the lack of incentive for village people to work in the

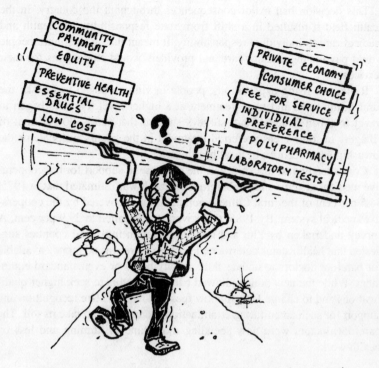

Health in China faces a critical balance between private curative services and more equitable essential primary health care.

delivery of first-line health care. Both monetary compensation and social prestige have declined markedly.

What is the implication of this new direction for preventive work? Preventive activities are not only one of the principles of Chinese health care but also a prime factor in the rapid improvement of health status. Now there is evidence of neglect. Immunization rates fell in the early 1980s but were dramatically raised to the highest in the world by 1990 through a concerted national campaign. Sanitation and environmental conditions have deteriorated visibly. This deterioration may in part reflect the lack of perceived need for preventive services and work. In China, as in other places, people will pay for curative care but prevention is neither promoted nor valued under present conditions.

Finally, there is the question of community support—financial and motivational—for the health care system. The experience of allowing people to take decisions collectively about events which affected their daily lives was a critical part of the formation of the new China. With continuing emphasis on curative care and private service provision it is possible that health care will be an activity only of professionals, and services bought only by those who have money. It will no longer remain an important glue which binds the State and people comprising the Chinese nation.

THE EFFECTS OF POPULATION GROWTH

The third influence which has radically affected the Chinese approach to health is population growth. China's population has nearly doubled since the 1950s and has resulted in great pressure on resources. One major consequence of this growth is the development of a structured birth control policy designed, on paper at least, to reduce both the birth rate and the absolute numbers of people. The early Chinese Communist leadership was ambivalent about family planning. On the one hand it recognized and promoted a modernization approach which relied on labour-intensive inputs. On the other it saw the threat of this rising population to the inputs. It was not until the 1970s that official policies of population control were introduced. By 1979 these policies had been tightened to promote and enforce the 'one-child family'.

The one-child-family policy was based on a system of incentives and punishments. Those families which complied had access to substantial benefits including pay bonuses, extended maternity leave, schooling and job placement for the child. Families which refused to conform were in danger of being asked to pay for all benefits received and to pay penalties. In their most extreme forms, the punishments led to forced abortions and sterilizations.

The implementation of this policy appears to be uneven across the nation. For example, evidence suggests that it was enforced better in urban than rural areas in part because of the stronger and more concentrated structures in China's cities. Evidence also suggests that policies were pursued with different degrees of vigour within China's rural areas. In some areas officials rigorously enforced the one-child policy while in others officials were lax, not imposing fines and inflating statistics to show success.

Lack of data as well as good methodological analysis of existing data makes it extremely hard to analyse the effects of these policies both on demographic patterns and on changes in human behaviour. While it is clear

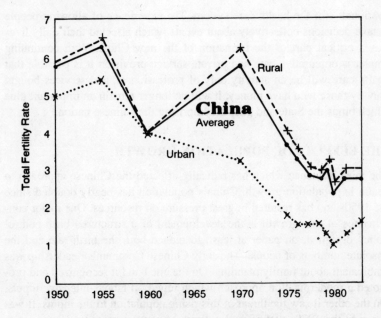

Fig. 1. Total fertility rate in China—rural and urban areas, 1950–82.

there has been a radical change in fertility in the last 20 years (Fig. 1) it is hard to attribute this change only to alternation in birth control policy.

Available data suggests that there have been fluctuations in the vigour with which the one-child policy has been pursued over time as well. For example as late as 1986, approximately one-half of births were of second or higher birth order. In addition it is not at all clear that the policy has in fact changed people's attitudes and beliefs concerning the desirability of children. Sons are still preferred to daughters and thus families will risk breaking the rules if the first born is a girl. Rural people who have actually lived through radical swings in other policies cannot be blamed for thinking that this one too will change. Then, traditional beliefs about large families could well escalate China's population growth again.

The pressure of millions of Chinese on resources has had major implications for the Chinese health care model. It utilized scarce resources for the development of a birth control programme which was vertical rather than integrated. Support for broader activities such as vaccination in the health care of mothers and children diminished as efforts focused singularly on the one-child family. Thus the contention of a holistic Chinese health care system must be questioned. But can China afford single-problem health programmes?

In addition population expansion calls for the government to make choices in resource allocation. For example, the choice between rural and urban health care acquires new relevance as the urban population exhibits the disease patterns of industrialized populations rather than of rural Chinese people. There is a choice of technologies to develop, and questions arise on whether to stress prevention and how to support mass mobilization and community participation. Ultimately the government will focus on the choices that will ensure continued political support from a rapidly changing, growing and urbanizing population.

LEARNING FROM CHINA

Some of the most important questions regarding the Chinese health care model are not particular to China. They are equally pressing in other countries, especially those with low incomes, large populations and demands for modernization. The Chinese responses to these questions, therefore, have relevance to other countries. As the year 2000 approaches, a few lessons are of use both to China and to other nations.

One major lesson is that it is possible to rapidly transform the patterns of health of a poor, populous nation in a radical way. It is arguable that a revolution is a pre-condition for such change. Certainly a committed political leadership capable of motivating and mobilizing the population is.

The choices made by the Chinese leadership enabled radical transformation. The choices which the leadership continues to make will determine whether the benefits of earlier decisions can be maintained. The most important choice which determined the nature and development of other decisions was the choice to pursue equity. To give all citizens an opportunity for good health was critical to achieving such positive results. Today the leadership faces challenges to that decision through a changed economic structure. Evidence already suggests that if equity is not rigorously pursued in the future, large gaps will appear among different groups of people and those whose access to resources is not ensured by the State will suffer.

The choice of equity determined the shape of the health care system. By giving state support to decentralized health delivery, China established a resilient health care system. Flexible enough to integrate change but strong enough to deflect major shifts in direction, the decentralized infrastructure is both enduring and pervasive. It has survived the political stresses and strains of time. Another lesson, therefore, is that the creation and especially the support and maintenance of a strong decentralized health care delivery infrastructure is a key factor in improving health and health care for large numbers of poor people.

Strong infrastructure has enabled preventive activities to function well. These activities were a major contribution to China's health improvements particularly in the early years of the new government. However, in the light of recent changes, a corollary might be added—that preventive work is necessary but not sufficient to ensure the support of people. Curative activities make major contributions to health and also provide motivation for most people to use health care services. The tension between preventive work, usually state-supported, and consumer demands for curative care

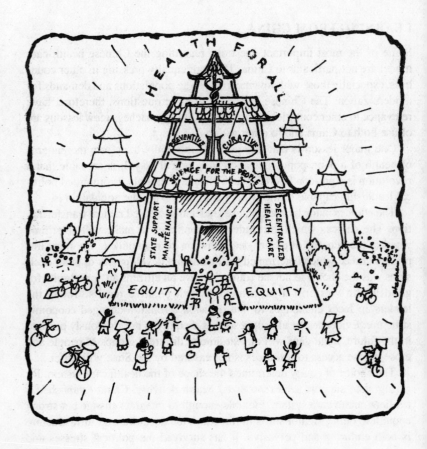

plagues modern health systems throughout the world. It is reflected in decisions about resource allocation. Although these decisions take into account scientific and technical outcomes, in the end they reflect the political and social priorities of the state.

In conclusion, the Chinese experience shows us the political nature of health. It is perhaps this lesson which will be most remembered. Throughout history, whenever the political dimensions of science and its technological applications have not been recognized, it has remained of benefit largely to its discoverers and developers. Only in its political guise has it enabled improvements to the great majority who, most often, lack opportunity, resources and hope.

CHAPTER 14

Transitions in Health Care in China

CARL TAYLOR

The author examines current trends in health service delivery in China and finds that compromises with the basic principles have made China's health system successful and worth emulating.

Carl Taylor, *M.D., Dr.P.H., was founding director of the Department of International Health at Johns Hopkins University, Baltimore, USA, following over a decade of public health work in India. He was Representative of UNICEF in China from 1984 to 1986. He is a regular consultant to public health programmes throughout the developing world.*

INTRODUCTION

In the past decade rapid economic transitions in China have jeopardized the health services that were an important model for the 1978 World Conference on Primary Health Care at Alma Ata, USSR.[1] A shift away from a centrally-controlled economy towards private enterprise, especially at the rural commune, reduced community-based financial support for programmes in health, education and welfare, which had been among the main achievements of the period from 1950 to 1980. During the following ten years, village people discovered that they would no longer automatically be provided the complete health care that they had taken for granted. The resulting process of adjustment demonstrates the importance of giving priority to equity in health care during periods of rapid economic transformation.

EXPERIENCE BEFORE THE ECONOMIC REFORMS

Before 1949, health conditions in China were among the worst in the world. At the time of liberation, ideological commitment to equity in a classless society permeated all decisions. The Russian model of centralized health care was not feasible because China's war-devastated economy could not

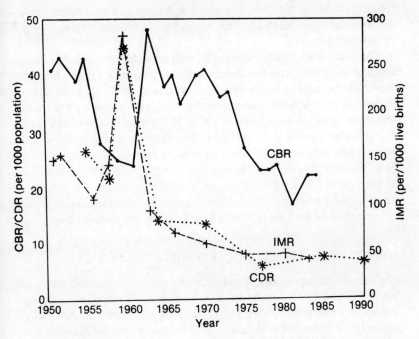

Fig. 1. Mortality and fertility declines in China, 1950–90.

finance free care for one-quarter of the world's people. Local control and funding of health care was established under the commune system in the 1950s and 1960s.[2] By 1980 China had lowered mortality rates, especially child mortality, almost to the levels of developed countries even though the country's per capita income was less than US $100 per year. Figure 1 shows the decline in mortality and fertility since liberation. By the 1970s China was saving the lives of over a million children a year who would have died in other countries at equivalent levels of economic development.[3]

A great deal of progress occurred in social and economic spheres but many feel that the most important reason for China's mortality decline was the rapid extension of community-based health services. Communes supported their own cost-effective services through health cooperatives. Equity at the local level was almost complete. One of the most perceptive observers of China's health transition was Dr Ma Haide (George Hatem—an American who became a Chinese citizen). He was the architect of the national campaigns that eradicated venereal diseases and controlled leprosy.

He gave credit for the overall mortality reduction to the 'constant day-to-day availability of health care that works year-in and year-out as provided by barefoot doctors'.[4]

The Chinese experience shows that with equitable distribution even the simplest and lowest-cost health measures can have great impact. It is more important that care at community level be readily available to all with no barriers of cost or social constraints than that it be of the highest quality. Infant mortality fell from levels of 100 to 200 in most counties but it tended to plateau at more than 50 per 1000 live births in poor provinces in the western half of the country, and at 20 to 50 in more affluent counties in the East. The four provinces and autonomous regions in the extreme West have 11 per cent of China's population and an IMR of over 70. The differential distribution of infant mortality ranges from under 20 in the ten best provinces and cities of the East to over 100 in Xinjiang and Xizang (Tibet).[5]

EXPERIENCE AFTER THE ECONOMIC REFORMS

The massive disruption of cultural traditions and social structure during the late 1960s and 1970s was followed by a rejection of many of the changes that had been imposed. When Deng Xiao Ping terminated the political excesses of the Cultural Revolution in 1978 there was great relief and enthusiasm among the people. Particular resentment had focused on local party cadres who had become increasingly authoritarian and overt in appropriating benefits for themselves. Centralized production policies had resulted in massive ecological devastation and deforestation. Change was especially rapid and drastic among the 80 per cent of the population who lived in rural areas. The commune structure was dissolved and China returned to the previous three-tier organizational structure under the County (Xian). Townships (Xiang) replaced communes and natural villages replaced production brigades and production teams. However, some good social innovations were also lost along with the oppressive political controls.

In Sichuan, a province which has 100 million people, making it the equivalent of the eighth largest country in the world, an experiment developed which rapidly spread to the rest of the country. It was observed that agricultural production on family plots of land was double that on communal land. As a trial, in a portion of the province all the land was given back to family control under a contract with the local government. The family had to sell to the government the amount that would have been grown under previous patterns of production, but they could now sell in the free market anything more that they could raise. The experiment proved so successful that the next year it was extended to the whole province, and then by 1982, the 'contract responsibility system' was extended to the rest of the country.[6] Agricultural production nearly doubled after 1982. In the early 1980s there was more per capita money available in 'better-off' villages than in most cities; new homes were built and many small industries started.

By the late 1980s this rural economic boom had lost its early momentum which had been based mainly on the fact that people worked harder for their own economic benefit than for the common good. They had returned to traditional but inefficient agricultural practices such as ploughing with buffaloes rather than tractors and harvesting by hand.[7] A need to rationalize traditional practices with the mechanization of agriculture and to farm units larger than the small family plots has become evident. Contracts have been extended to periods of 15 years or more to encourage investment and ecological protection.

China's economic reforms were at first widely applauded in Western countries because it was assumed that the Chinese would also liberalize politically. However when China's leaders reimposed strict political control after the 1989 uprising at Tienanmen Square, the pace of economic modernization slowed. A wide range of unanticipated social as well as political adjustments had to be made. Both families and local governments were concerned mainly about economic growth which caused considerable slippage in attention to social benefits.

THE EFFECTS ON HEALTH CARE

Especially pervasive in its social impact was the loss of most community-based activities for children when economic decision-making was taken away from communes and returned to families.[8] Private enterprise and the shift away from work-points for remuneration of health workers weakened the financial base for equity in health care.[9] Barefoot doctors were upgraded into a smaller number of village doctors. Instead of about two million part-time barefoot doctors there are now about 1.2 million village doctors, most of whom work nearly full-time (Table 1).[10] About half have passed examinations to acquire new credentials after a variable period of up to two years of hospital training.

Government workers are still covered by health insurance and each industry has to provide health care for its workers. There were large variations in health expenditures, with urban health care costing three times more than rural in 1981 (33 yuan vs. 10 yuan per capita). State expenditures were about nine times more in urban than rural areas (26 yuan vs. 3 yuan). By

Table 1. Number of Barefoot Doctors and Birth Attendants in China, 1970–86[10]

	Barefoot Doctors	Village Doctors (Total certified)*	Health Assistants	Birth Attendants
1970	1 218 266			
1975	1 559 214			615 184
1980	1 463 406			634 858
1984		1 396 452 (117 236)	2 006 560	584 565
1985		1 293 094 (341 972)		513 977
1986		1 279 935 (341 783)		507 538

*Figures in parentheses indicate the number of village doctors who have been certified by passing credentialling examinations. The others continue to practise without certification.

contrast private expenditure in rural areas was almost double that in urban areas (5 yuans vs. 3 yuan). Most of the people in rural areas were left with greatly-reduced health coverage.[10] Decentralized decision-making has resulted in great variability in local financing. A few of the more affluent counties have maintained their health cooperatives with each family paying a premium, or county funds from local economic enterprises are used to support health services and schools. However, most counties decided against funding health services by any collective system. A general feeling developed that if private enterprise under the contract responsibility system is good for farm families, then this privilege should be available also to local health workers. Most village doctors support themselves by fee-for-service private practice. In better-off areas village doctors are doing very well financially, often earning more than party cadres or assistant professors in local medical schools.[8]

One negative aspect of this shift has been that curative care has crowded out the earlier emphasis on prevention.[11] People everywhere are usually willing to pay for treatment of acute illness. Long educational effort is needed, however, for people to understand the importance of paying adequately for preventive services. Because village doctors have discovered the money to be made by dispensing medicines, a serious emerging problem is overmedication with expensive and toxic drugs. The commonest cause of deafness in children, for instance, is overuse of antibiotics.[12]

Local health officials have found that they can no longer tell people what to do and expect universal compliance. For instance a county in Sichuan received national recognition in the late 1970s because they had achieved over 95 per cent installation of sanitary, home biogas units which digested faeces to produce methane gas for cooking. After decision-making was returned to families, they also went back to the traditional practice of using fresh excreta as fertilizer on fields because there was more of it than could be digested in a biogas unit. People have to be educated to understand practices they had complied with earlier simply because they were ordered to.

Of great concern to the government, which still gives priority to equity because of ideological convictions, is the slippage in health care coverage of those in greatest need. As people have to pay even for preventive services, the poor obviously have less access to care than the rich. The costs of illness care for one individual can be devastating for the economic future of a family. Detailed data are not yet available but there is a trend towards stratification in care. Newly affluent families go to hospitals in towns and cities or to private practitioners. Ordinary people increasingly bypass their village doctors and go to township hospitals. Village doctors respond to the competition by doing whatever people ask, and by giving the costliest medicines used by hospital doctors. Polypharmacy is frequent—a single prescription may contain as many as six to eight drugs for a minor complaint. The poorest people are having increasing difficulty paying even for the care provided by local village doctors.

This trend is not yet firmly established, largely because there is still a strong residuum of community concern and action. The old barefoot doctor spirit still causes village doctors to care for neighbours in greatest need. When communities turned health posts over to village doctors, often in group practice, part of the deal was that they would continue to provide preventive services at low cost as a community service. This was sometimes explicitly stated as being in exchange for the privilege of practising. In some villages community committees still function to promote action for social services. However when people are asked to participate in mass activities such as the old patriotic health campaigns, their response often is 'pay me'. As a result there are reports of a recrudescence of previously controlled infections such as schistosomiasis.[5]

According to UN estimates, the IMR has not declined much since the 1982 census—39 per 1000 births dropping to 31 (Fig. 1).[12] A recent na-

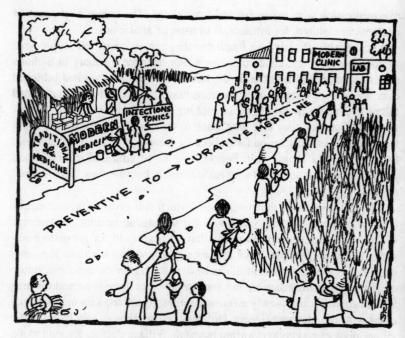

People travel further to modern curative facilities, bypassing local health posts which emphasize preventive services and traditional remedies.

tional maternal mortality survey gave a rate of 95 per 100 000 in contrast with earlier estimates which were about half that figure.[13,5] Neonatal tetanus rates are more than eight times higher than previous estimates.[14] In both instances it is not clear whether this is because of earlier under-reporting or due to a decline in the quality of services. As an increasing number of pregnancies and births are not reported because they are beyond birth quotas, the impact of these babies on fertility and mortality rates is unknown. These births and the increasing size of the floating population are jeopardizing even well-organized national programmes such as EPI which depend upon registration and follow-up by a responsible provider. Despite China's high immunization coverage there have been outbreaks of poliomyelitis presumably due to non-immunization of these children.

Personal conversations with party cadres at county level indicate a consensus that health services are less systematic and complete than ten years ago. In one small study there was almost an inverse relationship between the amount of time spent on preventive MCH services and the total income of the village doctor.[15] As long as income depends mostly on how much medicine is dispensed, the neglect of preventive services seems inevitable. This means that the deterioration of these services will continue and may not be limited to poor areas.

CURRENT EFFORTS

The Ministry of Public Health is aware of these problems and is attempting to re-establish cooperative arrangements for preventive services adapted to 'present realities'. Increasing public education in prevention, stimulated by the great concern to do everything possible for a family's one child, is leading to improvements, especially in the more affluent areas. However in poor areas, community resources are insufficient to pay for preventive services. General budget cuts make it difficult for health services to assume these costs. Under the economic reforms each institution and government unit is expected to earn sufficient income to cover costs. Visits to rural areas show that MCH stations and centres are shifting their effort from the earlier preventive focus to opening wards and clinics to care for paying patients. They purchase expensive equipment, such as beta ultrasound units to monitor pregnancies, allowing them to charge high examination fees rather than continuing to focus on supervising home-based MCH services. Anti-epidemic station staff feel the pressure to sell laboratory services to earn money. An important factor pushing up overall health care prices is the rapid escalation of costs in urban areas.

Considerable experimentation is going on to discover Chinese solutions to problems of local financing. An innovative approach was developed as part of the national expanded immunization programme. In 1988 China successfully met the goal of 85 per cent immunization coverage in every province.[5,16] About five years earlier when the programme started it had been decided that families should pay village doctors for each immunization. A fee of 10 fen (3 cents) was suggested but each county was to adjust the amount to local conditions. A year later I participated in a review which showed that in counties where village doctors were being paid 30 to 40 fen, coverage was 95 per cent or more. In poor counties where people could pay only 5 fen, coverage was only 45 per cent. Then one county tried a contract system which proved very popular and quickly spread to much of the country. A family paid a single fee ranging from two to seven yuan (50 cents to $2) for the entire series of immunizations for a baby. This proved attractive because the contract specified that if the child got any of the six diseases, all health care for the illness would be free and the family would also receive an indemnity of about 100 yuan ($30). By 1989, 68 per cent of counties had adopted this system, but only about 20 per cent of all young children were covered by these counties.

A more general approach to promoting equity which is being tried and implemented gradually is the provision of subsidies for poor areas. This approach attempts to correct inequalities in regional health care distribution. For instance the only part of China where health and education are completely free is in the Tibet Autonomous Region.[5] Per capita government expenditures on health are about three times more in Tibet than in the rest of the country. In other poor areas there are partial subsidies depending on economic level, but the money is given in a block grant and local officials often use it for other local priorities.

Inequalities in local distribution of services are more difficult to correct than inter-regional disparities. For these local inequalities a system of financing health care should be designed that will reach the poorest people in each community. Studies are being made of alternative forms of insurance. For instance the contract system developed for EPI is being expanded in some areas to cover all care from pregnancy through the first year of a child's life.

An intensive effort was made in the MCH Model Counties Project supported by UNICEF to test local ways of financing preventive services under the guidance of the provincial MCH bureau.[10] This project started in the early 1980s in ten counties spread over the country, each county associated with the local school of public health and medicine. The project was expanded progressively to 35, 95 and then 300 counties. Systematic action-research was used to find innovative means of providing comprehensive child health care adapted to each region of the country. Major changes included the training of village doctors to use specific priority interventions decided on locally in order to maintain a better balance between preventive and curative work. This applies especially to high-risk monitoring of pregnancy and child growth and surveillance to provide early treatment for the main causes of mortality and morbidity, such as pneumonia and diarrhoea in children. There is also a deliberate process of introducing better management with emphasis on supervision to improve the quality of care.

The MCH Model Counties Project now covers over 120 million people. The commitment of the government to equity is shown by the fact that the present phase of expansion is to the poorest 300 of China's 2271 counties.[5] This expansion is also supported by UNFPA in order to test ways of integrating family planning with maternal and child health care in an educational approach, as part of the move away from implementation of the strictly vertical family planning programme developed during the Cultural Revolution. Similar large efforts in primary health care are being supported by WHO, the World Bank and the Central Government's own resources.

PROSPECTS FOR THE FUTURE

With the pragmatic flexibility that has characterized China's development in recent years there is no doubt that much will be learned in the present transitions about how primary health care can be provided in a rapidly changing economy. It is probable that the patterns of health care being developed now will be more relevant to conditions in other developing countries than was the earlier much-publicized commune system. Visitors to China before the economic reforms would eloquently express their admiration but then shake their heads and say that their people would never tolerate so much regimentation. With what is essentially a mixed economy China is now having to develop new methods of coping with local financing. The extreme decentralization has created a massive natural experiment in which local administrators have been told to develop their own solutions. By observing the evolving patterns much can be learned about alternative approaches and principles in local financing of health care. Among the many questions that still remain to be answered, the following three seem especially important.

First, how can decentralization provide for local adaptation while still maintaining minimum standards for the whole country? The present pattern of health planning is that central authorities set national norms and guidelines. Local authorities then have to evolve solutions based on what works best under their conditions but they are held accountable for results. There is a great deal of interest in seeing what other counties are doing, leading to informal sharing of experiences. This can be systematized by comparative research and evaluation mechanisms such as have been developed in the MCH Model Counties programme.

Second, how can an appropriate balance be maintained between the trend toward increasing professionalization of services and the great strengths of past patterns of community participation? The trend in recent years has been strongly toward specialization and elitism in open disagreement with Maoist principles of deprofessionalization. Health officials have long been embarrassed by the international attention given to the notion that Chinese health workers were going around barefoot. These officials recognized the generally low level of knowledge and skills of workers and have endeavoured to upgrade them into competent medical professionals. Great effort is being devoted to improving training to re-establish the credibility of the qualified physician. The greatest weakness of current training is that it is didactic and dogmatic with massive memorization in the Confucian tradition but with little opportunity for learning systematic problem-solving. This traditional authoritarian teaching has an unfortunate tendency to denigrate rather than empower the capacity of communities and families to solve their own problems and, therefore, it encourages dependency on the health system.

The third question and the greatest cause for concern is how to correct the emerging inequalities in the distribution of services. A concern for social justice has been recognized to be an essential principle of primary health care as enunciated in the slogan 'Health for All by the Year 2000'. The only way that population-based indicators of health can be improved is by taking services to the people among whom health problems are concentrated, the poor and neglected. Equity was the characteristic of China's health care that used to be most distinctive in comparison with Western countries. Commune health services provided egalitarian care. Now that the financial base for earlier uniform coverage has been largely lost, there are two activities that seem necessary. Systematic surveillance for equity will help the community to become aware of where and what their health problems are and then help them to identify how these problems can be corrected. This requires that professional assistance be deliberately designed to strengthen community capacity rather than to weaken it. The second need is frank recognition that care for the poor will have to be subsidised. This should be done regionally to correct disparities resulting from differences in the relative affluence of various areas. It also needs to be done locally to make basic services available for those in greatest need in each community. China has the capacity to resolve these basic dilemmas. Other countries have much to learn from its experience.

References

1. WHO/UNICEF. (1978). Report of the International Conference on Primary Health Care, Alma Ata, USSR.
2. Sidel, R. and Sidel, V. (1983). *The health of China*. Beacon Press, Boston, 1982. *Health care and traditional medicine in China, 1800–1982*. Routledge and Kegan Paul, London.
3. Grant, J. P. (1991). *The State of the World's Children Report, 1991*. Oxford University Press, New York.

4. Burchett, W. and Alley, R. (1976). *China: The quality of life*. Penguin Books, Great Britain.
5. UNICEF. (1989). Children and women of China: A UNICEF situation analysis. Beijing.
6. Schell, O. (1985). *To get rich is glorious—China in the 1980s*. Mentor-Pantheon, New York.
7. Feinberg, R. E. *et al*. (1990). *Economic reforms in three giants: U.S. Foreign policy and the USSR, China and India*. Transaction Books, New Brunswick, USA.
8. Hinton, W. (1990). *The great reversal: The privatization of China, 1978–1989*. Monthly Review Press, New York.
9. Kan, X. G. (1990). Village health workers in China: Reappraising the current situation. *Health Policy and Planning*, Vol. 5, pp. 40–8.
10. Taylor, C. E., Parker, R. L. and Jarrett, S. (1988). The evolving Chinese rural health care system. *Research in Human Capital Development*, Vol. 5, pp. 219–36.
11. Taylor, C. E., Parker, R. L. and Zeng, D. L. (1991). Public health policies and strategies in China. *Oxford Textbook of Public Health*. Oxford University Press, Oxford.
12. Sheng, J. H., Shao, X. L. and Wu, X. Y. (1985). One hundred seventy five cases of deafness caused by gentamycin. *Chine ENT Medical Journal*, Vol. 20, No. 2, p. 135.
13. UNICEF. (1991). *The State of the World's Children, 1991*. Oxford University Press, Oxford.
14. Bannister, J. (1987). *China's changing population*. Stanford University Press, Stanford.
15. Lin Liang Ming. (1989). Analysis of retrospective sample survey of children's death in 9 provinces in 1986. Paper for the Seminar on Children's Survey in China, Beijing.
16. Study of MCH services and financing of these services. Shanghai Medical University, 1990 (unpublished report).
17. Cao, Q., *et al*. (1985). Immunizing the children of China. *Assignment Children*, UNICEF, Vol. 69, No. 72, pp. 347–68.

CHAPTER 15

Primary Health Care in Vietnam

JAMES ALLMAN

The author contrasts the health care systems of North and South Vietnam which have encountered increasing difficulty in meeting the health needs of the population as financial constraints have worsened progressively over the past 15 years. Privatization has not removed the need for improved public health services.

James Allman, Ph.D., has worked on health and population projects in the Middle East, Africa and the Caribbean, most recently serving as consultant to the World Bank, UNFPA and several NGOs in Vietnam. He has taught and conducted research at Columbia University, Harvard University and the American University, Beirut. He is currently Senior Lecturer in Demography at the Sorbonne, Paris, and Visiting Professor of Population Studies at the National Economics University of Hanoi.

INTRODUCTION

Vietnam's approach to health for the people was viewed positively in the late 1970s and early 1980s by international observers.[1,2] During its heroic 30-year struggle for independence beginning in 1945, Vietnam developed a system of health care that focused on providing low-cost, basic coverage for all, using local resources including traditional medicine and considerable mobilization and education of community members through mass organizations. The first World Health Organization Representative in Hanoi saw Vietnam as a model of what the primary health care (PHC) approach could achieve in meeting the basic health care needs of underdeveloped countries. He even claimed that 'the whole of Vietnam can be considered as one well-designed (PHC) project'.[3]

More sober and realistic views of the health care system and the health needs of the population in Vietnam began to emerge in the mid-1980s as UNICEF and WHO began to work with the Ministry of Health on programmes of expanded immunization, control of diarrhoeal diseases, and maternal and child health.[4,5] UNFPA support for population programmes,

Swedish bilateral aid and the work of a few non-governmental organizations (NGOs) similarly indicated many difficult and pressing problems. The past few years have seen numerous evaluation studies which, when taken together, allow an appreciation of the significant progress and accomplishments of Vietnamese primary health care efforts. On the other hand, they also point to the many remaining needs and challenges that face the country as it attempts to improve its socio-economic conditions and provide health for all.

This chapter assesses the health care situation in Vietnam based on recent reports and on field visits by the author during 1989–92. It looks first at Vietnam's exceptional and undeniable accomplishments in moving towards Health for All. It then examines the limits of the revolutionary government's efforts. Finally it considers the major socio-economic and political changes in Vietnam during the past few years and their implications for primary health care.

ACHIEVEMENTS OF VIETNAM'S REVOLUTION IN HEALTH

Vietnam's per capita income was only around US $200 in 1991 and has been at this low level for over a decade.[6,7] Health and population statistics have been very scarce and it is therefore difficult to discuss trends. Fortunately, recent data collection efforts—notably the 1989 Census and Census Sample and the 1988 Demographic and Health Survey—have received considerable technical and financial support and are of good quality. The infant mortality rate is relatively low—around 50 per 1000 live births. Other demographic indicators (Table 1) show that Vietnam is clearly in the midst

Table 1. Estimated vital statistics and development indicators, Vietnam, 1989

Population	64.4 million
Infant mortality rate	50 per 1000 live births
Crude birth rate	31–32 per 1000 population
Crude death rate	7–8 per 1000 population
Life expectancy at birth	63 years
Contraceptive prevalence rate (modern methods)	38 per 100 married women aged 15–49 years
Literacy	88 per 100 persons over 10 years of age
Per capita GNP	US $200

Source: Vietnam Population Census, 1989

of demographic transition. Life expectancy is estimated at 63 years. The fertility rate has declined from over 6 in the early 1970s to around 4 in 1988–89.

What are the main features of Vietnam's development and health system that have contributed to the vital revolution indicated by these demographic data? They include government policies and programmes, health infrastructure and manpower, community participation, women's status, water and sanitation, and international cooperation in Vietnam.

VIETNAM'S POLICIES AND PROGRAMMES

Vietnam has followed socialist policies, stressing equity in all aspects of economic and social life and human development through education, health system improvements and mobilizing people through mass organizations. These measures have raised levels of literacy dramatically and greatly improved the coverage of the health care system. Economic policies and programmes included agrarian reform through land distribution and cooperatization and setting up state industries and bureaucracies. The government attempted to control the economy closely but, as in other socialist economies, the results were far below expectation. The economy has remained stagnant and the population very poor. Since the sixth Party Congress in December 1986, liberalization policies are giving people more freedom. Vietnam is entering world markets through joint ventures, increases in exports, and a renewal of trade with many countries of the world. The economy is now starting to take off and there have been major improvements in agricultural production and food availability. The private sector currently accounts for more than half of GNP and is growing rapidly.[8]

North Vietnam's efforts to improve the health of its people through socialist mobilization, campaigns to attack major health problems, a stress on preventive services at the commune level and training of numerous health workers, among other strategies, were effective during the 1960s and 1970s. As shown in Table 2, both death and birth rates declined significantly between 1960 and 1975.

The situation in South Vietnam was quite different. While there were a small number of well-trained health workers catering to the well-to-do and the army in urban areas, rural areas of the South were neglected. The health situation worsened considerably during the 1965–75 period due to massive bombing, defoliation and the ravages of war.

With unification after the American departure in April 1975, the socialist

Table 2. Estimates of vital rates (per 1000 population) in North, South and
Unified Vietnam, 1960, 1975 and 1989[27,30]

| | North Vietnam | | South Vietnam | | Unified Vietnam | |
	1960	1975	1957–67	1968–74	1976–80	1989
Birth rate	46	31	42	42	39.5	31–32
Death rate	12	5.5	12	14	8–9	7–8
Rate of natural increase	34	25.8	30	28	32	22–24

government made major efforts to improve the situation in the South by
sending health professionals from North to South, training staff and building new health facilities. There was expansion of health services in the
South and stress on education. These factors and the end of armed conflict
led to declines in death and birth rates.

In the North, during 1975–85, the health system apparently regressed.
While accurate data is difficult to come by, many knowledgeable people
would agree with David Marr, a distinguished historian of contemporary
Vietnam, that 'the DRV medical system of the 1950s and 1960s was far
better integrated, and probably more effective than the system today, which
sees a small number of research and teaching hospitals trying to maintain
international standards, while province and district hospitals struggle with
cases referred to them from below, and thousands of village clinics are
unable to deal with routine disorders for lack of basic supplies'.[9]

I asked a senior official of the Ministry of Health whether he agreed with
this analysis. He said he did. Why the change? 'In the past, people believed
in the government. Since 1975 this is much less so.' He agreed that the
health situation in the south improved after unification due to education,
training of more health workers and strengthening of the health institutions
serving rural people. But in recent years the south of the country has been
improving more rapidly than the north, both in regard to its economy and
health care system. 'There remains in the south of the country a spirit of
initiative which allows people to make decisions and develop creative approaches to solving problems. Doctors are much less under the thumb of
central authority and can decide what to do themselves. The private sector
is booming.'

Despite recent progress, Vietnam is still unable to feed its population
adequately. A summary of food and nutrition studies noted that the Vietnamese were getting only 1950 calories per day on an average compared to

the required 2300 calories. In the countryside, 40 per cent of the population have low calorie meals (17 per cent with less than 1500 calories and 23 per cent with 1500–1800). Only 17 per cent of the population can afford 2400 calories a day.[10] The Vietnamese diet is highly imbalanced, with people eating about 450 grams a day of rice on an average compared with less than 370 grams of starchy foods on average for the world.[11]

The threat of famine during natural calamities continues in Vietnam. When typhoons and other natural disasters occur the people of the north and those living in coastal areas are threatened with starvation, as they were in 1988.[12] Transport and organizational skills are inadequate to move the surplus from the Mekong Delta to areas experiencing shortfalls.

HEALTH POLICIES

The Ministry of Health is the major and, until recently, practically the exclusive health care provider. There is an extensive traditional medicine sector, well-integrated into the national health system.[1,13,14] Many facilities including commune health stations have trained traditional health workers. There is extensive use of locally-produced herbal medicines. There are specialized traditional medicine hospitals in the major cities. Since 1989 the Ministry of Health has encouraged the development of the private sector. Recent health policy documents provide for payment for services, designed to generate income to pay staff and run facilities better. The integration of traditional medicine and new approaches to health manpower education and retraining are also advocated.

Six priority national health programmes have been identified: (1) consolidating health services at village, ward and district levels to implement the ten elements of primary health care; (2) population and family planning within the context of maternal and child health; (3) expanding services for diagnosis and treatment; (4) malaria control; (5) the Expanded Programme of Immunization; (6) essential drugs and supplies. In addition, there are three other important programmes to control diarrhoeal diseases, malnutrition and acute respiratory infection. Except for the unrealistic goal of reducing the population growth rate to 1.7 per cent by 1990—Census data suggest it was over 2.1 per cent in 1989[15]—quantitative goals are not set.

HEALTH INFRASTRUCTURE

Vietnam has developed an extensive network of health facilities reaching into all areas of the country. The lowest rung in the health system is the

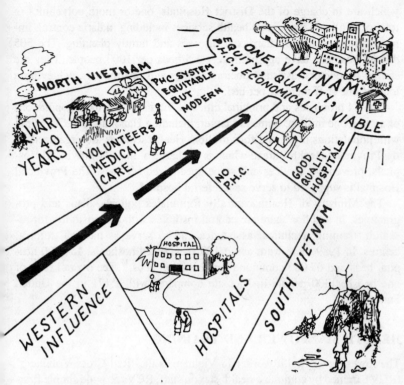

The challenge to Vietnam is to integrate the best elements of the contrasting health systems found previously in the North and South.

commune health station which serves a population of between 2000 and 20 000. The 9383 health stations are supposed to provide the usual broad range of primary health care services including health education, maternal and child health and family planning, immunization, hygiene and sanitation, prevention of locally endemic diseases, drug supply, curative services and referral. These health stations should be staffed by an assistant doctor, a nurse and a midwife and sometimes a pharmacist and specialist in traditional medicine. The size of the population served, the resources available and support from community leaders all influence the staff size. Generally there is an attempt to have one health worker to serve 1000 people.

The next level is the district with an average population of around 150 000. Health services are organized by the 449 District Health Bureaus which are in charge of the District Hospitals, one or more polyclinics (a total of 676), and preventive health services including malaria control, immunization, control of diarrhoeal diseases and family planning. The 505 district hospitals have approximately 1.5 beds per 1000 people. They are staffed by doctors, assistant doctors, nurses and pharmacists, achieving a total of one staff member per bed.[16]

The 44 provinces and principal cities of Vietnam each have populations of around one million. Some are larger, including Hanoi and Ho Chi Minh, with populations of around four million. Health services are organized by the Provincial Health Bureau which is in charge of the 174 Provincial Hospitals, preventive services and some specialized services. The Provincial Hospital is supposed to serve as a referral hospital.

The Ministry of Health centrally formulates policies, plans and programmes. In addition there are central institutes with responsibility for research, training, technical assistance and to serve as national referral centres. In 1989 there were about 100 specialized hospitals, 154 000 hospital beds and 67 000 commune health station beds.[17] The overall ratio of one bed per 300 people in Vietnam compares with 1:171 in the United States.

HEALTH MANPOWER AND TRAINING

The lowest-level health worker in Vietnam is the 'Red Cross Volunteer' (RCV), trained by commune health station staff. RCVs provide simple first-aid treatment and family planning advice on a part-time basis. There is no national data on their numbers or activities.

The next level includes assistant nurses, midwives, pharmacists and technicians, trained for three to nine months at the district. There is no data concerning their numbers and activities either. Some cadres such as the brigade nurses, attached to cooperatives and other state work units, virtually disappeared as the liberalization of the past years reduced funds to pay them.

Secondary level health workers including nurses, midwives, pharmacists, assistant doctors and various types of technicians who are trained for two-and-a-half to three years at provincial secondary medical schools. These workers staff the commune health stations, district and provincial hospitals.

Doctors and pharmacists are trained for six years at a university faculty of medicine or pharmacy. There is also a new course at university level for nurses, midwives and laboratory technicians. Graduates of this level work almost exclusively in hospitals. Postgraduate specialization is also available, generally requiring five years of experience.

Medical schools were established in Hanoi in 1902* and in Saigon in 1947. The number of Vietnamese physicians practising in the country increased from 95 in 1920 to 200 in 1937 and 310 in 1953. Ten years after the division of Vietnam in 1954, an American study found 6000 physicians in the north and only about 750 Vietnamese physicians in the south, mostly practising in Saigon.[18] Another report noted that South Vietnam had 'one of the most severe doctor shortages in Southeast Asia. Of approximately 800 practising physicians, some 500 serve in the army and another 150 are in private practice in Saigon. Thus about 150 doctors, or one for about every 100 000 persons are available for the rest of the country.'[19] The US. presence in the south of Vietnam had led to the establishment of Saigon Medical School which provided high-quality clinical training. However, not much was done for training in community health. Health personnel remained concentrated in the cities; the rural areas were virtually ignored.[20]

Since unification in 1975, efforts at training health manpower and staffing a broad system of health institutions have been remarkable. Currently, there are a medical–pharmaceutical university, seven medical faculties, two public health colleges and a college of pharmacy. Approximately 2000 physicians and 330 pharmacists graduate annually. Table 3 shows the availability of medical manpower in Vietnam in 1989. Looking only at physicians, Vietnam's ratio of 2.7 doctors per 10 000 population is considerably better than that of Sri Lanka (1.2), Thailand (1.6), Philippines (1.5), but below India's 3.9. In general, 'in comparison with other countries of similar or slightly greater GNP, Vietnam has a larger number of all categories of health personnel'.[16]

ACCESS TO HEALTH CARE

Official data suggest good access to health care in Vietnam. This is clear if we look at such factors as the health worker: population ratio, the distribution of health facilities, urban and rural differentials in access, policies and practices concerning payment for services, and selected indices of use of services such as immunization among one-year-olds and use of contraceptive methods. However, this access is not uniform: De Vylder and Fforde estimate that 'while virtually the entire urban population has access to

*The Hanoi school was founded by Paul Documer with Dr Yersin as Director. The latter, a disciple of Pasteur, had founded the Institute of Bacteriology at Nha Trang in 1895.

Table 3. Estimates of medical manpower available in Vietnam in 1989

Category	Numbers	Per 10 000 population
Physicians	23 800	2.7
Assistant physicians	46 400	13.8
Midwives	14 000	4.6
Nurses	84 300	7.6

Source: Ministry of Health, Health Statistics Data, 1990

health services, only some 90 per cent of the population of rural provinces in the Red River Delta and 40 per cent in the Mekong Delta are covered by functioning health centres'.[6]

In the past, health services were provided free so cost was not a barrier to their use. The situation changed in 1989 with efforts by the government to recover costs. Today there are fourteen categories of people (including war veterans, government workers, workers in state firms and cooperatives, and members of ethnic minorities) who do not have to pay for health services. It has been difficult to recover costs of drugs in community pharmacies which are attempting to be self-sufficient. The recent introduction of fees for services and drugs apparently already has reduced the number of patients using government facilities, even the better ones.[21]

During a 1991 survey in the north in which the Ministry of Health looked at private as well as public health providers, I visited commune health centres, polyclinics and private doctors. Typically a commune health centre with five or six health workers would see five to six patients a day, a good polyclinic with a staff of 17 would see about 40 patients, while private doctors were each seeing 20 or more patients. Surely, this tells much about the perceived value of services.

Data on immunization coverage suggest that most of the population is being reached with some preventive interventions. With strong support from UNICEF and WHO the number of communes participating in the EPI programme increased from 74 per cent in 1987 to 91 per cent in 1989. On the basis of special studies WHO reported that 70 per cent of children under one year were fully immunized as of December 1989,[22] and the government reported the following coverage rates among infants at the end of 1990—90 per cent for BCG, and 87 per cent for DPT3, Polio3 and measles.

Recent data on contraceptive use also indicates that modern methods are reaching women in all parts of the country. Of married women in the reproductive age, 54 per cent were using some contraceptive method in 1988. Twenty-nine per cent in urban areas and 34 per cent in rural areas reported using IUDs, 8 per cent used the rhythm method, and just over 2 per cent were sterilized. However, other modern contraceptive methods are in short supply and by 1990 over one million women were terminating pregnancies by abortion in a year. Unmet demand for family planning services appears to be high.

OTHER SOCIAL ACHIEVEMENTS

Community Mobilization and Participation

Mass organizations such as the Vietnamese Women's Union, the Youth Union, Farmer's Union and the Red Cross are found in each commune and at every higher level in Vietnam's social organization. They have been mobilized for health education, environmental sanitation activities and, most recently, for EPI. The Women's Union has been particularly active in the family planning programme as well as in maternal and child health activities.

The Vietnamese Army has also played an important role in providing a large part of the population with basic health information and encouraging improvements in hygiene and sanitation. Between 1945 and 1975 the majority of able-bodied men in the North and the guerrillas in the South spent time in the military, providing a captive audience for health education. Health practices taught and enforced in the army have been carried home to become a part of cultural practice.

Women's Education

Women participate extensively in economic activities in Vietnam. Their rights and status have received particular attention from the government. One important indication of progress to date is their access to education. The 1989 Census found that over 84 per cent of women over age ten were able to read. This may be a critical factor in improving children's health as educated mothers appear to have better knowledge of effective ways to prevent, recognize and treat their children's health problems. They also have greater access to and are more receptive to modern health information.

Water and Sanitation

For the past 35 years the government has been conducting mass campaigns to encourage people to improve the environment and to promote the construction and use of wells, rainwater tanks, bathrooms and latrines. In 1955 less than one per cent of families had a well or sufficient rainwater storage facilities. By 1985 the Ministry of Health estimated that 39 per cent had such facilities. However, only 40 per cent of these facilities met the Ministry's standards in terms of quality. Similarly, in spite of incentives such as cement to construct latrines, currently only 10 per cent of the rural population have latrines of an approved type which are also hygienic and well-maintained. The Ministry of Health estimates that about 90 per cent of the population is infested with one or more types of intestinal worms—100 per cent in the North, 60–70 per cent in the central provinces and about 40 per cent in the South. According to a UNICEF report, 'the high prevalence of intestinal parasites in the North is directly connected to the traditional habit of using excreta as fertilizer'.[22] The double-vaulted latrine, promoted by the Ministry of Health as an effective way of using excreta and widely heralded in the West as a public health breakthrough, has not proved practical. The composted waste is neither safe nor convenient for farm use, and most people have reverted to direct application of human waste to gardens and fields.

Although there has been progress in recent years in improving water and sanitation, UNICEF concludes that 'major extension of coverage will require considerable external support' and that currently 'problems related to lack of safe water and adequate environmental sanitation have a very severe impact upon the health of the population in Vietnam, particularly the most vulnerable groups'.[22]

INTERNATIONAL COOPERATION FOR HEALTH

WHO, UNICEF, the World Food Programme and the UN Population Fund have had active programmes for over a decade. In addition to providing needed supplies and materials, particularly prized by the government, the programmes have also been a source of support for considerable in-country training, some training and study abroad, and have encouraged the introduction of new ideas and thinking about health and related problems. With the exception of the Swedish aid programme which has provided about $10 million in assistance for health, initially for hospitals but increasingly for primary health care, there has been little bilateral aid. International non-governmental organizations have been involved in small projects and the government has allowed a few to establish offices in Hanoi after 1988 and to send their staff into rural areas to support and monitor projects.

THE LIMITS OF PROGRESS

There is a consensus that the quality of health care in Vietnam is currently low and deteriorating. The improvement of health services has been hampered by economic stagnation, difficult climatic conditions, pervasive poverty and the continuing growth of the rural population.

The lack of economic development in Vietnam—per capita GNP has hovered around $200 for the last 15 years—has meant that the central government has had very few resources to support health efforts in the communes, districts and provinces. As Woodside has noted with regard to education: 'The economic anaemia of the Vietnamese state prolonged the existence of notable and historical regional differences in the acquisition of effective schools. . . . There was . . . no real agricultural surplus with which a centralized authority could finance comprehensive educational modernization.'[23] A similar situation exists in health.

The funds available for health services are relatively low—less than 4 per cent of the national budget and around $2 per capita per year. Low salaries paid to health workers oblige them to have other jobs to make ends meet. Since most of the health budget goes to salaries, drugs and supplies are not available in sufficient quantities. The physical structures are generally in very poor shape and maintenance is neglected.

The Ministry of Health is struggling increasingly to maintain services with very limited funds. A recent UNDP–Ministry of Planning report estimated that 'the government health budget can meet no more than 40 per cent of the minimum requirement which is needed to maintain the current level of services; health workers are usually only paid about 50 per cent of their salaries'.[24]

However, getting more money from the central government to the local areas should not be considered the main solution to the paucity of funds in communes and districts. Attention to creating local financing through generating local demand for services is critical. As de Vylder and Fforde note, 'continued support for the unreformed . . . model of centralized control and high-tech medical facilities will only inhibit this process'.[6]

The determination of the government to improve the country's economy is leading to a stress on privatization and decentralization. This may mean a reduction in support for public services and the expansion of private medical care.

Some observers argue that health workers are active in EPI and family planning because of the considerable support from UNICEF, UNFPA, WHO and other international groups. They wonder how sustainable these programmes are if support were to diminish. The donors have promoted a series of vertical programmes that operate independently of each other. Little attention has been focused on community support and participation or on the integration of services. The economics of health has been virtually ignored, and social science research on public health problems in Vietnam is just beginning. Health care administration and management courses are very recent in Vietnam.

The data on the quantity of hospitals, health institutions and beds, while impressive, is misleading. For example, there are stated to be over 9000 commune health stations, one for each commune in the country. However, when one goes into the field it is apparent that some stations are simply the homes of health workers, are housed with the People's Committee, or are in inadequate buildings. Further, since allocation of funds is related to the number of beds the institution has, beds are kept on the books even when they are rarely, if ever, used. Underutilization of health facilities is a very serious problem.

Similarly, data on health workers presents an overly optimistic picture. It is clear that in rural areas health workers generally have to farm, raise animals and do many other things to make a living, leaving little time to deliver health services.[26,27]

Although the EPI programme is seen by UNICEF and the government as a great success, a review by Schofield noted that 'no reliable epidemiological system for managerially useful reporting on the six EPI diseases yet exists in Vietnam'.[28] He further found that 'generally, within the health services, the Evaluation Team found the concepts of analytical epidemiology to be absent. This is not surprising,' he felt, since 'this science has been growing up only since the middle of this century . . .' when the Vietnamese 'professional public health cadres were working in isolation from the growth centres of epidemiology in the world'.

The lack of managerially useful data to monitor and evaluate programmes and health status is a general problem in Vietnam. Health statistics are very weak. International experts have serious reservations concerning accuracy. There have been numerous studies and surveys but, as Abbatt notes, 'these are very hard to consolidate into a comparative survey as they have been carried out in different ways and in different parts of the country'.[16]

However, we can be confident that there is indeed a vital revolution taking place in Vietnam, not by looking at health statistics but rather because of recent demographic data produced by the 1989 Census and special surveys such as the 1988 Demographic and Health Survey.[15]

The concept of primary health care which has evolved among public health professionals since Alma Ata is not widespread in Vietnam. Health workers often believe the term used for primary health care (in Vietnamese '*cham soc suc khoe ban dau*') refers to first care, the first medical actions taken to deal with health problems. There is often a lack of understanding of the importance of active community participation and of the need for intersectoral economic development activities to provide resources for better living and health.

Many observers believe that primary health care in Vietnam is at a turning point. 'The quality of the work must now replace quantity of output as the main objective of public health policy, of management, of training, of technical supervision and of the reporting systems in the health services.' The problems in the EPI programme, and in most others, are not due only to economic underdevelopment but also 'to the lack of public health management training and experience which is evident throughout the health services'.[28]

SIGNS OF CHANGE, HOPE FOR THE FUTURE

Several lessons emerge from Vietnam's attempts to provide health for all. Socialist policies created stagnation and a low standard of living for decades in the North, and for all of Vietnam between 1975 and 1986. This seriously limited government investment in health as well as education. Attempts to redress the situation have led to considerable economic growth since 1988–89, especially in the South, but the social sectors are now in crisis. Structural adjustment is causing hardship to the poor. It remains to be seen how basic services will be provided to all in need. At the same time the stress on universal basic education, leading to high levels of female literacy, has probably been a major factor in reducing mortality and fertility to relatively low levels in this predominantly rural population and economically backward economy.

Since 1986 the Vietnamese government has sought to improve prospects for economic development with its renovation policy ('*doi moi*'). Recent developments suggest that this policy is paying off. In 1989 Vietnam became the world's third largest rice exporter. Production and exports of rice increased more in 1990 in spite of problems in securing enough fertilizer due to decline in imports from the erstwhile USSR. Food consumption has also improved greatly within the country. Business is beginning to boom and Vietnam is entering world markets through joint ventures, increases in exports and a renewal of trade with many countries of the world. The private sector currently accounts for about 65 per cent of GNP and is growing rapidly.

Short-run economic prospects in Vietnam are fraught with difficulties as Vietnam weans itself from Soviet and Eastern European aid, estimated at almost $5 billion per year. Party leaders see hard times ahead but appear determined to liberalize the economy, encourage individual initiative and actively seek cooperation with new economic partners.

It is encouraging that the government is beginning to support NGO efforts in PHC. Several NGOs are bringing in new ideas, particularly focusing on community participation, income generation and multisectoral

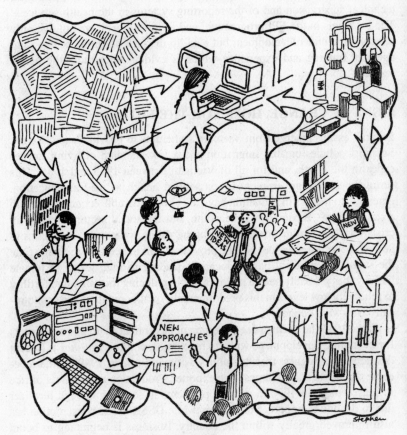

Increased contact with the outside world is rapidly bringing needed change to the health care system.

activities, and are setting up pilot and demonstration projects. Some relatively inexpensive, useful activities such as translating '*Where There is No Doctor*' and '*Helping Health Workers Learn*' into Vietnamese, holding workshops and seminars, and providing training for key people can contribute to opening new directions in PHC in Vietnam as they have in other countries.

There is a growing awareness of the need for greater community participation in PHC, especially in the area of payment for services and local, commune support of health workers. Some health institutions are thriving in the new system. They have managed to make user-fees available to pay reasonable salaries to staff, buy drugs and basic supplies and maintain physical facilities. Abbatt is correct in noting that a major challenge for the health system in Vietnam 'is to find ways in which the charges levied for services and drugs (especially at commune level) can be used to increase the motivation of staff and the quantities of available drugs. If this challenge is met, then there is great potential for existing health care staff (supported by retraining programmes) to raise standards of health care delivery'.[16]

However, community participation 'implies not just the mobilization of the community's resources but a process through which people gain greater control over the social, political, economic and environmental factors affecting their health'.[29] Much more remains to be done in this area in the future in Vietnam. Vietnamese organizations involved in health and population information, communication and education still use the word 'propaganda' ('*tuyen truyen*') to explain how educators, health workers and mass organizations are supposed to transfer ideas and information to the people. It is a top-down approach intended to encourage people to go along with the decisions taken at the top.

Fortunately, however, the Ministry of Health and other groups concerned with health are beginning to be exposed to new ideas and approaches to information, education and communications as well as in the areas of management, supervision and training. Concepts such as 'sustainability' of PHC activities and community financing of essential drugs, which are part of the Bamako Initiative, are being applied and tested. The new health manpower plan focuses on strengthening the commune level and avoiding an overproduction of doctors.

Increased contact with the outside will bring in new ideas and approaches which should favour the expansion of the primary health care movement. Although technical assistance and learning from the experience of other developing countries could remedy many weaknesses in public health in Vietnam, as they have with the collection of demographic data, collaboration with outsiders is still difficult. There is an elaborate system of travel permits and the foreign community, particularly in the north, is relatively isolated and cannot easily mix with the Vietnamese. The situation has been improving in recent years and the strong Vietnamese interest in learning from others so that they can improve their country is starting to break barriers.

Vietnam's past history of determination, persistence and courage in the face of seemingly overwhelming obstacles suggests that the next decade will see the country advance rapidly in providing its people with better socio-economic conditions. Hopefully, Vietnam will continue to view health as the right of every individual, 'an essential precondition to successful PHC' and surely a major reason why Vietnam has accomplished so much thus far with such limited resources.

References

1. McMichael, J. (ed). (1976). *Health in the Third World, Studies from Vietnam.* Nottingham.
2. Ladinsky, J., Levine, R. E. (1985). The organization of health services in Vietnam. *Journal of Public Health Policy.* June, pp. 255–68.
3. Djukanovic, V., Hetzel, B. A. (eds). (1978). The Democratic Republic of North Vietnam. In: *Basic Health Care in Developing Countries, An epidemiological perspective.* Oxford University Press, Oxford, pp. 102–17.
4. Vogel, U. (1987). The whole of Vietnam can be considered as one well-designed project—Some reflections on primary health care experience in Vietnam, 1945–1985. Dissertation for the M.Sc. (Economics) in Tropical Epidemiology and Health Planning, University College of Swansea, University of Wales.
5. Quinn-Judge, S. (1986). Shortages confront Vietnam's health care. *Indochina Issues.* No. 65, April.
6. De Vylder, S., Fforde, A. (1988). *Vietnam, an economy in transition.* Swedish International Development Authority, June.
7. *Vietnam, stabilization and structural reforms.* (1990). World Bank, Washington, D.C.
8. Heibert, M. (1990). Vietnam regains role as major rice exporter. *Far Eastern Economic Review.* 10 May, pp 32–4.
9. Marr, D. G. (1987). Tertiary education, research, and the information sciences in Vietnam. In: *Vietnam, dilemmas of Socialist Development,* (eds. D. G. Marr and C. White), Cornell University, Southeast Asia Program, Ithaca, New York.
10. Vietnam News Agency, 16 September 1990, p. 1.
11. Brun, T. A. (1989). *Agriculture and food production sector review—Vietnam, food consumption and national status.* State Planning Committee/Food and Agriculture Organization of the United Nations, Rome, July.
12. Crossette, B. (1987). Vietnam tells of wide malnutrition. *New York Times*, 14 May, p. 41.

13. Marr, D. G. (1987). Vietnam's attitudes regarding illness and healing. In: *Death and Disease in Southeast Asia*, (ed. N. G. Owen), Oxford University Press, Singapore, pp. 162–86.
14. Ladinsky, J., Volk, N. D., Robinson, M. (1987). The influence of traditional medicine in shaping medical care practices in Vietnam today. *Social Science and Medicine*. Vol. 25, No. 10, pp. 1105–10.
15. 'Sample Results'. (1990). *Vietnam Population Census, 1989*. Central Census Steering Committee, Hanoi.
16. Abbatt, F. (1990). *An analysis of health and health manpower, Vietnam, 1989*. Sweden–Vietnam Primary Health Project report, Hanoi, February.
17. *Vietnam demographic and health survey, 1988*. (1990). National Committee for Population and Family Planning, Hanoi, November.
18. *Democratic Republic of Vietnam, North Vietnam* and *The Republic of Vietnam, South Vietnam*. (1966). Health Data Publications, October and January. Walter Reed Army Institute of Research. Walter Reed Army Medical Center, Washington, D.C.
19. Smith, H. H. *et al.* (1967). *Area handbook for South Vietnam*. U.S. Government Printing Office, Washington.
20. Ruhe, C. H. W., Hover, N. W., Singer, I. (1988). *An Experiment in International Medical Education*. American Medical Association.
21. Wahlquist, E. (1989). *Organization and management of primary health care in two districts in Quang Ninh*. Sweden–Vietnam Primary Health Project report, Hanoi, December.
22. *The Situation of Children and Women*. (1990). Hanoi, UNICEF.
23. Woodside, A. (1984). The triumphs and failures of mass education in Vietnam. *Pacific Affairs, 1983–1984*. Vol. 56; pp. 401–27.
24. *Report on the economy of Vietnam*. (1990). United Nations Development Programme, Hanoi and Socialist Republic of Vietnam, State Planning Committee, January.
25. *Studies on social aspects of community health*. (1990). Center of Human Resources for Health, Ministry of Health, Hanoi.
26. Allman, J., Nguyen Thi, Phuong Mai. (1990). *Primary health care needs in PhuLuong district, Bac Thai Province, Vietnam*. CIDSE, Hanoi.
27. Allman, J., Vu Qui Nhan, Nguyen Minh Thang, Pham Bich San, Vu Duy Man. (1991). Fertility and family planning in the Socialist Republic of Vietnam. *Studies in Family Planning*.
28. Schofield, F. C. (1989). *Report on an EPI field visit to Sr. Viet Nam*. UNICEF, Vietnam.
29. Morley, D., Rohde, J. E., Williams, G. (eds). (1983). *Practising Health for All*. Oxford University Press, London.
30. Jones, G. W. (1982). Population trends and policies in Vietnam. *Population and Development Review*. December, Vol. 8, No. 4, pp. 783–810.

CHAPTER 16

Health for Too Many: India's Experiments with Truth

MEERA CHATTERJEE

The author describes developments in health care in India during the 1980s and identifies approaches which prevail at the beginning of the 1990s. These are likely to determine India's health paths in the near future, raising serious questions about the likelihood of Health for All being achievable in India's current economic and socio-political environment.

Meera Chatterjee, Ph.D., a health scientist and planner, has worked and written extensively on Indian health policy and has been involved in the design as well as evaluation of and research for health, nutrition and family planning programmes. She has lived in New Delhi since 1978 after completing her doctorate at Massachusetts Institute of Technology (M.I.T.) (1976) and post-doctoral training at the Harvard Medical School and M.I.T. in the USA.

AN UNCERTAIN BEGINNING

In India, the 1980s began amid disquiet. The Janata Party Government, a socialist government of the people, was in a shambles and even Indira Gandhi's detractors predicted that she would return to power in the nation-wide elections scheduled for January 1980. She did, occasioning considerable speculation on the policies her Congress-I Government would follow. The fate of the Janata Party's leaders and the policies which they had barely put in place over 1977–79 also hung in the balance. Mrs Gandhi had been Prime Minister from 1966 to 1977. During the declared state of Emergency from 1975 to 1977, her son Sanjay Gandhi, young and impatient, had personally spearheaded a massive campaign to control population growth. Unfortunately, this had unleashed excesses such as forcible sterilization on men—young and old alike, within a general atmosphere of muscle power in northern India. Tragically, a sizeable segment of India's intelligentsia supported this approach which included punitive action against persons with dissident views. Would the Congress Party continue such policies or had Mrs Gandhi's brief period out of power (1977–80) changed its approach?

India's economy was also in an unsettled state at the beginning of that decade. One of the century's worst droughts had occurred in 1977–78. Food prices had risen sharply, the government's buffer stock of grain was depleted, and the meagre resources of the poor were severely strained. There had been many deaths from food and water shortages. The Janata Party Government had somehow staved off a calamity—largely, it was believed, because the nation was so relieved by the restoration of democratic freedom after the Emergency that even the spectre of death did not deter the people. However, during its brief rule the Janata Party had pursued several populist policies which had strained the government exchequer, and little sympathy remained for 'socialism' within India's restless private sector or the international aid community.

The situation in the health sector around 1980 mirrored this political and economic uncertainty. Within the previous five years the public health system had carried out first the hardline policies of one government and then the vague, community-oriented approaches of another. Under the Congress Party family planning had become the be-all and end-all of the health system, while under the Janata Party the term 'family planning' became strictly taboo and was substituted by the more inclusive 'family welfare'. Under the latter government India had signed the Alma Ata Declaration in 1978 and began its own exercise to translate that commitment into a programme for the country. J. P. Naik, a committed intellectual and follower of Mahatma Gandhi, was the moving spirit behind a committee set up to frame India's approach to Health for All. In August 1980 this committee* produced a report which advocated 'radical change' in the path which India had been following to health.[1] However, as the Congress-I had returned to form the Government that January, the fate of this document was unclear, and with it the fate of millions of unhealthy people in India.

Treading a New Path to Health

The Government of India (GOI) responded to the Health for All movement by formulating a National Health Policy in 1982, the first such statement of intent since India's Independence in 1947.[2] This resembled, in spirit and

---

*Known as the ICSSR–ICMR Committee as it was set up jointly by the Indian Council of Social Science Research and the Indian Council of Medical Research.

substance, the report of the Bhore Committee of 1946 which had prepared the ground for the development of India's multi-tiered public health system.[3] Although the Bhore report, three decades earlier, had enunciated many of the same principles as the Alma Ata Declaration, by the late 1970s many in India's public health community recognized that the country's health planning had gone awry. It had emphasized curative, high-technology medicine and urban hospitals, and pursued 'elitist' health manpower policies which undermined the possibility of widely-available basic health care. The National Health Policy hoped to correct this by steering the country towards the 'universal provision of comprehensive primary health care services'. It broadly envisaged that this would require reorganization of the health infrastructure, major modifications in the existing system of medical education and paramedical training, and integration of health plans with those of health-related sectors, such as water supply and food production, as well as with socio-economic development processes.

The Policy gave pride of place to the community health worker and expanded eloquently on community participation in health care. It paid tribute to the voluntary health sector on account of several successful projects, calling for it to play a major role in the future development of India's health. It also squarely recognized the importance of social and economic development to health, giving responsibility for health improvement to several sectors of development. These amounted to clear promises to reach out to those who had remained beyond the pale of formal health services, to improve living conditions which affected health, and to give people control over health care. Through these and other mechanisms India aimed to reduce its prevailing high mortality, morbidity and fertility rates.

HEALTH DEVELOPMENTS DURING THE 1980s

As the 1980s advanced, India made slow but perceptible progress towards better health, judging by its overall demographic and health indicators (Table 1). General mortality fell by 20 per cent as did the more intractable infant mortality, with a four-year increase in life expectancy. Even fertility declined by ten per cent. But the decade clearly exposed the differentials that exist among the country's states and between its rural and urban areas, females and males, children and adults, rich and poor. Far from bringing about Health for All, health policies clearly benefited some more than others.

During the decade, the path to health deviated considerably from that mapped out by the 1982 Policy. On the one hand, some developments in the

Table 1. Demographic and health indicators in India during the 1980s

	1980	1983	1986	1989*
Crude death rate				
Rural	13.7	13.1	12.2	11.1
Urban	7.9	7.9	7.6	7.1
Combined	12.6	11.9	11.1	10.2
Infant mortality rate				
Rural	124	114	105	98
Urban	65	66	62	58
Combined	114	105	96	91
Life expectancy at birth		81–86(P)	86–91(P)	
Males	54.1	55.6	58.1	
Females	54.7	56.4	59.1	
Persons	54.4	56.0	58.6	
Crude birth rate				
Rural	35.1	35.3	34.2	32.0
Urban	27.8	28.3	27.1	25.0
Combined	33.7	33.7	32.6	30.5

*–Provisional; (P)–Projected on the basis of 1980 value

health sector—a few unanticipated—contributed to improvements in health. These included: expansion of the rural health infrastructure, the Universal Immunization Programme (UIP), and the Integrated Child Development Services Scheme. On the other hand, several developments have made the achievement of Health for All a more distant dream. Prominent among these is the virtual demise of the Community Health Workers' Scheme, and with it almost all hope of community-controlled health care. Very slow progress in raising living standards and continuing lack of education for vast numbers of people have stymied the contribution of the social and economic development vector to health. Despite economic growth, over 40 per cent of the population lives in poverty; and despite substantial increases in food production, there was slight improvement in the nutrition of the poor, half of whose children suffer from moderate or severe malnourishment.

Towards the end of the 1980s, economic pressures led to stringent government health budgets which took their toll of state-supported health care. Alongside, the private health sector burgeoned and health policy-makers and planners began to pay it increasing attention. Economic liberalization is expected to fuel further growth in the drugs and medical technology sector, bringing urgency to the need for quality and price controls to protect the health of all. Most certainly, economic policies will determine what India will provide by way of health care in the 1990s. While the ups-and-downs of the past decade may be ascribed to the ideological confusions that prevailed in politics, economics and the health sector, current directions in health care clearly do not favour those who are most in need.

Development of Rural Health Infrastructure

The 1980s saw considerable 'construction activity' geared toward expansion of the governmental health infrastructure in rural areas where 75 per cent of India's population lives. India's multi-tiered health system is one of the best-developed in the industrializing world. At its base, catering to approximately 5000 people in four or five villages, is the Sub-Health Centre. This facility is staffed by a pair of male and female Multi-Purpose Workers who are expected to provide basic health care, maternal and child health services including family planning, and undertake simple sanitation and health education tasks. Until 1985, 20 to 25 of these sub-centres were supported and supervised by a Primary Health Centre (PHC). In addition to supervising the community health outreach work, the PHC offered general medical and simple surgical services provided by two or three doctors and eight to twelve paramedical staff, including registered nurses, lady health visitors, a pharmacist, a health educator, and a laboratory technician. These PHCs had ten in-patient beds and catered to about 100 000 people.

In 1985 the pattern of health infrastructure was modified, and the latter part of the decade was devoted to establishing the new structure. A PHC with one Medical Officer and one Community Health Officer (both doctors) and seven paramedical staff was allotted to every 30 000 people and designated to supervise six sub-centres. A new, higher-order facility was introduced to serve every 100 000 people—a Community Health Centre (CHC) with four medical officers providing specialist medical, paediatric, obstetric and surgical services, seven nurse-midwives and other paramedical staff, 30 beds and complete diagnostic laboratory and pharmacy facilities. Thus, the rural health system is now a four-tiered one: sub-centres, Primary Health Centres, Community Health Centres and, at the apex, *Taluka* and District hospitals. The former serve about half a million people and the latter about 2 million on an average, providing full-fledged medical and surgical services. At the district level there is also a large health administration responsible for communicable disease control programmes and family planning in addition to medical services. In addition to filling in this structure, the health system has felt compelled to keep pace with the development of other infrastructure in India, such as roads and communications, increasingly entering remote areas, acquiring the latest technology, replenishing growing inventories of 'hardware'—buildings, vehicles and equipment, and expanding health manpower cadres.

In 1980 there were 5484 Primary Health Centres and 47 112 sub-centres in the country. By 1991 these numbers had grown to 22 065 and 130 983, respectively, and 1932 Community Health Centres had been established. In addition, there were about 1500 *Taluka* hospitals and 460 District hospitals. In fact, the 'targets' set for infrastructure for the year 2000 were achieved by 1990, except for a number of CHCs which remain to be established in the decade ahead. These targets were intended to keep the public health service system abreast of population size. However, the revision of norms and underestimation of the rate of population growth have meant that the system has been running, simply to stay in place!

Indeed, the health system's focus on meeting numerical targets for health facilities has been at the expense of attention to their quality. In some in-

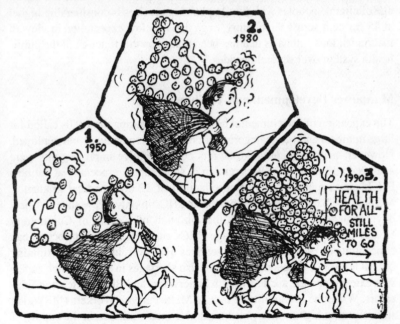

As health planning in India is based on population norms, the burden of increasing numbers makes reaching health for all difficult.

stances, health centres exist only 'on paper'. For example, PHCs have been considered 'established' when buildings are requisitioned, or 'upgraded' to CHCs simply when staff positions are created, rather than when the staff are in place. In fact, deficiencies in the quantity and quality of staff are widespread. Workers are often not competent or willing to perform necessary tasks, and their attitudes to people (particularly the poor) are manifest in rude behaviour or neglect. The state of equipment and availability of supplies are usually poor; essential drugs are grossly inadequate at all levels. The health centres are consequently inefficient and underutilized as they inspire little confidence in people. At the same time, outreach services from PHCs and sub-centres have been inadequate on account of poor management and inattention to 'software' such as training and communications. As a result, the primary health centre system provides less than eight per cent of the medical care sought by rural households, and public hospitals a further 18 per cent. The remainder is acquired from various private practitioners (see below). About 13 per cent of pregnant women in rural areas register for ante-natal care at public facilities, and only eight to ten per cent of deliveries are attended by trained government personnel. While the coverage of eligible couples with family planning services is considerably higher at 45 per cent across the country, even this is below expectation in view of the tremendous emphasis that has been placed on this function of the public health system over several decades.

Manpower Development and Training

The expansion of governmental health facilities during the 1980s called for large numbers and new categories of personnel to be trained and deployed. However, neither quantitative targets nor qualitative improvements were achieved adequately. Doctors remain in short supply especially at the new PHCs, despite India's annual production of 12 000 medical graduates. Medical specialists have been posted at CHCs in only a few states. A new development in the 1980s was the initiation of a cadre of Community Health Officers (CHOs) to manage PHCs and CHCs, so that doctors can concentrate on providing medical services. However, in most states training of CHOs has not yet begun. There are also shortages in cadres which supervise extension work, such as Health Supervisors and Block Extension Educators. While the availability of female Multi-Purpose Workers (MPWs) at sub-centres is higher, there is considerable local variation in the supply of these important front-line workers. For the most part, male MPWs are not functioning as the government's intentions to retrain workers from the earlier vertical programmes into a single, integrated cadre have been stymied by administrative bottlenecks and legal proceedings. Thus, ensuring adequate staff and their actual presence at health centres is a major immediate task to improve the quality of care in the rural health system. Greater attention has also to be paid to developing the 'health team' and its managers, and to instituting procedures to enable them to implement comprehensive primary health care.

The re-orientation of medical and paramedical personnel to community health needs has long been considered important in bringing about the universalization of primary health care. The National Health Policy of 1982 envisaged a thorough overhaul of medical education and training systems to accommodate health priorities. Instead, the 1980s were characterized by marginal tinkering in the area of manpower reorientation: brief 'refresher' courses were given to large numbers of health workers and administrators, leaving really substantive modifications to be made in the decade ahead.

The Heart of the System

In essence, while India built a vast network of health centres and hospitals between the 1950s and 1980s and provided this infrastructural 'skeleton' with the 'muscle' of some 22 500 doctors and almost 300 000 paramedics, this large body has lacked in 'head' and 'heart'. The inadequacy of know-how and appropriate skills and the want of a 'service motivation'—empathy for the sick, the needy and the isolated—became painfully apparent in the 1980s. Many and varied attempts were made during the decade to improve management, including training several cadres and reviewing and reformulating job descriptions and work routines. Greater sensitivity was sought to be introduced into health care through motivational training of workers and managers. At the same time, strategies were employed to make the system resilient to the idiosyncrasies of workers, including management information systems and 'information, education and communications' (IEC). It was believed that creating demand for services through IEC would force greater accountability on workers and managers, and thereby increase their effectiveness. However, the same workers who were responsible for service delivery were put in charge of IEC programmes and, in the absence of inherent motivation and communication skills, they gave IEC little priority. Consequently, there is continued lack of understanding of and demand for preventive health care, even for clinical services such as antenatal care or aseptic delivery. Low levels of prevention have, in turn, resulted in a growing need for curative services. But the public health sys-

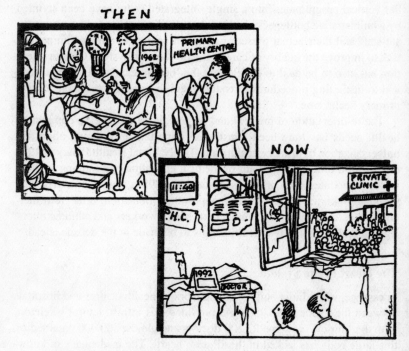

*Rapid expansion of public health infrastructure has led to poor
quality services and, in turn, to increasing use of private providers.*

tem is increasingly unable to provide what is demanded, even though most
of its resources are spent on curative care and little on prevention! There
has been no abatement in this vicious cycle, which remains a major con-
straint to India's hopes for Health for All.

The continued inadequacy of 'head' and 'heart' can be attributed to several factors. First, the health system is gigantic—for all workers to have
their skills meaningfully upgraded, their managerial abilities honed, and
their teamwork abilities developed requires an enormous number of training days for each cadre, far too many for health administrations to handle.
District Health Officers have been heard to lament that if they actually
carried out the amount of training advocated for key district health staff
(numbering more than 2000), they would be doing little else! They are
constrained also by a paucity of good training institutions and trainers. By
the 1980s, many institutions which had been established in the 1950s and
1960s were becoming obsolete. They were unable to cope with the health

system's expansion and had difficulty in introducing new methods and innovative thinking. Financial resources to establish new institutions were limited and the appropriate human resources not readily available to the government sector.

Growing needs have meant that increasing numbers of non-governmental institutions have become involved in training for health. Their quality has been variable, a second reason for a decline in the managerial capabilities of the public health system. The need for quality control and coordination has led increasingly to standardized approaches and bureaucratization, a third major reason for the lack of thoughtful management and commitment in the system. Workers at all levels complain of excessive paper work—recording, reporting and monitoring requirements are heavy, norms and procedures to be followed are laid out in great detail, decisions are inevitably passed upward to be taken at higher levels—some even to 'the highest level', an Indian euphemism for the Prime Minister's Office. Thus, bureaucratization has also meant excessively centralized control. Part and parcel of such control are the nature and direction of resource flows—almost all meaningful primary health initiatives are funded from the top, with money passing down from Centre to State, district, block and, eventually, village.

Indeed, the single vital effort to make the health system perform during the 1980s was the Universal Immunization Programme which was centrally-controlled and managed. Through this programme, attempts were made to develop health management capacity at short order, to instil a sense of purpose in workers who had become demoralized after the debacle of the family planning programme during the Emergency, to overcome the inertia that had set into service delivery after family planning was downplayed, and to bring some accountability into the organization. Another programme which became a counter to the ills of the health system, built on a parallel structure, was the Integrated Child Development Services Scheme. This too had highly-specified norms and was controlled by the Central bureaucracy, but expanded rapidly throughout the country in the 1980s. While both these programmes have been successful in some ways, they have revealed some additional obstacles to reaching Health for All.

The Universal Immunization Programme

The Universal Immunization Programme (UIP) was launched in 1985 with the objective of immunizing 85 per cent of infants and 100 per cent of pregnant women by 1990. The programme was directed by a National

Technology Mission, a high-level Central committee established by the then Prime Minister Rajiv Gandhi which included bureaucrats and technocrats. It was managed by specially-appointed immunization officers at the state and district levels but used existing workers to deliver services. It planned to cover India's 400-plus districts in a phased manner, which it did by 1989. An extensive cold chain was installed from the points of vaccine manufacture or import to the level of sub-health centres. Indigenous capacity to manufacture all but polio vaccines was enhanced. Trained managers and management mechanisms were put into place to ensure coverage and accountability. The logistics of delivering vaccines, equipment and supplies to the village-level were streamlined. Workers were retrained in immunization techniques. Individual immunization cards were distributed to mothers to record antigens received by their children, and remind them to return for follow up doses. Public education messages on radio and television, tinplate posters hung in village day-care centres, health centres and even post offices, and slogans painted on walls were used to increase public awareness and demand. Almost for the first time on a nationwide basis, nongovernmental organizations such as the Rotary and Lions' Clubs and private medical practitioners affiliated to the Indian Medical Association were drawn into a public health campaign. Indeed, the programme demonstrated what the health system in India is capable of performing under the force of central authority and direction and with adequate managerial input and support. Although official claims of 80 per cent coverage by the target date of 1990 are believed to be somewhat inflated, perhaps 70 per cent of target children were immunized (with 90 per cent contacted for at least one dose) in the first five years of the programme throughout this vast and diverse country, despite its widespread poverty and illiteracy.

While UIP demonstrated that health services can be provided in remote villages, overcoming physical constraints and traditional resistances, it revealed the unevenness in the health services of India's many states almost more than any programme had demonstrated previously. Diverse levels of commitment were reflected, for example, in the speed with or extent to which the basic strategies of UIP were implemented. Differences in performance among states and even smaller units such as districts or blocks are a hallmark of Indian development. They are a positive sign, on the one hand, of decentralized functioning (even of a scheme as centrally-controlled as UIP!), but also unfortunately a symptom of the low priority accorded to health by public administration, and to preventive health measures within health organizations. This low priority has in fact been responsible for the vast differentials that are seen across the country in health, as indicated by

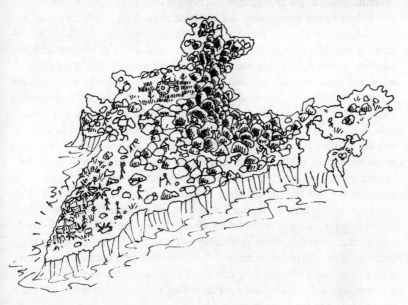

The difficulty of improving health increases from south to north in India.

infant survival or fertility levels. In UIP, the worst performance occurred in states with the worst health situations and, thereby, greatest preventive health needs! As the Central Government hands management of the immunization programme over to the states not only are differences in quality likely to become more apparent, but overall performance may well decline.

There is considerable concern in the public health community regarding the sustainability of UIP. To date, it has been a centrally-sponsored scheme, with start-up funds provided by UNICEF and other international donors. Working conditions in rural areas make maintenance and replacement of equipment difficult—in the past, the health system has suffered severe setbacks in programmes because inputs (such as vehicles which are so critical for the immunization programme) have not been maintained. Perhaps more troubling are manpower concerns—training and motivating workers to deliver immunization services effectively requires continuous effort, particularly as camp approaches must give way to routine identification and immunization of pregnant women and infants.

Currently, attempts are being made to piggy-back other services onto immunization, as the programme has been severely criticized by sections of the Indian health community for its verticality. The 'Child Survival and Safe Motherhood' programme which will be implemented in all 500 districts in the country over 1991–95 includes immunization, oral rehydration, vitamin A prophylaxis, Acute Respiratory Infection (ARI) control, antenatal and intra-partum care, and birth control. The rationale that a system capable of delivering immunization can and must be utilized to provide a range of MCH services is sound. But critics allege that this is 'old wine in new bottles' as the mandate to improve maternal and child health has existed over the past four decades. MCH services are not as easily delivered or monitored as immunization and in the not-too-distant past were subverted by the pressure on workers to meet family planning targets. The potential for this to happen again is evident in the experience of UIP in some districts where immunization and family planning officers clashed, competing for the same staff and resources. Even at the PHC and sub-centre levels, staff found it more profitable to carry out family planning tasks because of the financial incentives built into that programme. Thus, it remains to be seen whether UIP can be re-integrated effectively with MCH services, ensuring quality care and reaching those most in need. This is a major challenge for India in the 1990s.

Integrated Child Development Services

In fact, a programme which combined child health and maternal care, the Integrated Child Development Services (ICDS) Scheme, was a significant effort of the 1980s. It proved only too clearly how worthy the concept of integration is, but how difficult it is to achieve. ICDS consists of a 'package' of supplementary nutrition, immunization, health check-ups, referral, nutrition and health education, and pre-school education. The concept of integrating nutrition, health and child development services emerged from the disappointing experience of nutrition supplementation programmes in the 1950s and 1960s when it was realized that a broader response was required to the widespread problem of undernutrition in children, including a range of health activities. At the same time, the links between undernutrition and poor school performance led to the belief that providing pre-school education could redress the problem of low enrolment of poor children into the formal school system and the learning difficulties they face.

Because of its conceptual origins and intentions, the scheme is managed by the Department of Women and Child Development and involves the Department of Health only in the provision of primary child and maternal .

health services. At the beginning of the 1980s it had completed a five-year pilot phase. By 1985 it expanded to 1000 development blocks; and by 1991 to almost 2600, encompassing some 230 000 villages and 227 urban areas, and a total population of over 230 million in the country.* It targets nutritional supplements at 17.1 million pre-school children and 2.8 million mothers, making it the largest supplementary feeding programme in the world. Indeed, a remarkable achievement of ICDS has been its 'staying power'— the government's commitment to expand it during a time when political ups-and-downs negatively affected almost all other health programmes. A leading reason for this is that the programme is preferentially located in backward areas and focused on very disadvantaged groups, India's 'untouchable' castes and indigenous tribal people. Administrators have adhered to the principle of feeding all children 'below the poverty line' in these needy areas, in order to promote social equity. This strategy of 'universal feeding' has come under fire from those who are conscious of its high cost (about US $4.5 per beneficiary per year) and lower effectiveness than 'selective' feeding (which is practised, for example, in the Tamil Nadu Integrated Nutrition Programme described by Jayshree Balachander in this book). Indeed, alleged low cost-effectiveness may limit the programme's expansion in the future.

ICDS is designed as a community-based programme. A local woman who has received three months' training is the mainstay in each village (or cluster of 200 urban homes). At the *anganwadi*, a centre based in a village home, she prepares and distributes the food supplement daily, providing each child with 300 kcal and pregnant/lactating women and severely malnourished children with 500 kcals. The '*Anganwadi* Worker' (AWW) also conducts nonformal pre-school activities and nutrition and health education for mothers. Health services are provided by the female Multi-Purpose Worker who visits periodically from the nearby health sub-centre. The AWW is supported by an ICDS Supervisor, a woman graduate who oversees 17–25 *anganwadis*. In a block there are up to 100 *anganwadis*, managed by a Child Development Project Officer, who liaises with the Primary Health Centre Medical Officer to ensure the provision of health care within the programme.

However, the links between ICDS and health personnel have been weak, with the result that health care at *anganwadis* has remained sporadic. Until the advent of UIP, the MPWs largely ignored the ICDS *anganwadis*. Sub-

---

* A rural block currently has an average population of 110 000–120 000, while tribal blocks are considerably smaller, 35 000–50 000.

sequently, many MPWs understood the advantages of having a local person list and gather children and mothers for immunization, and utilized them to increase immunization coverage. High coverage with immunization occurred most often where an active *Anganwadi* Worker, resident in her own community, was involved in the organization of immunization sessions each month. But immunization performance in ICDS areas has still fallen short of the full coverage which the programme's registration system could support. Despite the side benefit of increased contact between MPWs, AWWs and the youngest children in their communities, most MPWs have yet to provide other health inputs in a systematic manner, or undertake health check-ups regularly, or establish a working referral system in *anganwadi* villages.

In the absence of regular visits by the MPW, most communities do not perceive ICDS as a health programme. The AWW is not considered a basic health worker as it is known that she has not been trained to provide health care. Thus, while the programme intends to give children a headstart by providing ante-natal care and nutrition to their mothers, and offering safe, clean deliveries, it has been poor in reaching mothers and has not generated demand for these services. Ante-natal registration by the AWW alone is of little use as she is not trained to provide pre-natal or safe delivery services herself.

Instead, communities view ICDS as a pre-school and/or feeding scheme. Where *Anganwadi* Workers are available regularly, mothers have come to appreciate the day-care provided by the *anganwadi*. Where food distribution is reliable, poor families attach value to the supplements as these allow reallocation of meagre food resources available within the household. Most *anganwadis* are attended by pre-school children who are old enough to walk the distance from their homes, sometimes with older children who carry their young, eligible siblings. Thus, the programme focuses more on 3–6 year-olds than on the more vulnerable 0–3 year-olds, and so attention to growth and health in the first three years of life has been inadequate. Growth monitoring is used by the AWW primarily to determine which children are severely malnourished and thereby entitled to the larger ration of food. It has therefore had little effect on the health knowledge or practices of mothers, or in preventing malnourishment among the children of these impoverished communities.

In the initial stages of ICDS, community preparation and participation were important in establishing *anganwadis*. Villagers were asked to provide the accommodation and participate in the maintenance of the centre, to help with the feeding activity and ensure that all children participated. However, during the programme's rapid expansion, community preparation come to be ignored. Local facilities were first rented, and only later were communities asked to contribute towards rent or provide alternative, free accommodation. The programme calls for *Anganwadi* Workers to be recruited from the communities they serve. But once again, the rush to select workers led to inappropriate choices. Often, preference was given to those with higher educational qualifications or 'contacts', rather than to those who resided in their own villages and had rapport with their communities. Workers who live in other villages or nearby towns find it difficult to be present every day in the village they are allocated, and thus deliver a poorer quality service compared with resident workers.

Strengthening ICDS for All

Recent surveys suggest that children in ICDS areas have similar nutritional status to those in non-ICDS areas despite the purposive selection of more deprived populations for the programme.[4] Improvement in nutritional status seems to accompany participation in ICDS, the actual contribution of food supplements, growth monitoring, nutrition education or other programme components being unmeasured. In general, success in ICDS can be seen more in terms of process indicators (coverage with immunization or vitamin A) than in terms of impact. It is widely acknowledged that the programme has not borne the results it could or should have, given its excellent concept, the infrastructure established and the considerable resources and effort employed. However, given the political support it enjoys, there is little doubt that it is here to stay. Weaknesses in its implementation need to be corrected in order to enhance its impact, and the yield of a substantial social investment.

Decentralization and Community Management. ICDS has been a centrally-controlled programme, with norms and procedures being laid down by the Central Department of Women and Child Development, and all programme costs except those of the food supplement being met by the Central Government. While programme strategies have been revised from time to time, change has been slow, perhaps because of the complex programme design, large numbers covered, geographical spread, socio-cultural diversity, and multiplicity of organizations involved. As the programme has expanded, the Centre has found it increasingly difficult to manage, and performance across project blocks has become increasingly variable. Although various strategies have been suggested to decentralize the programme, such as turning project blocks over to non-governmental organizations to run, few have been implemented. Thus, a significant challenge facing ICDS today is to decentralize management, giving greater autonomy to the state and district levels, increasing state funding, and involving local institutions more effectively. Ultimately, the programme must aim to be 'owned' by communities and managed by them.

Health Care with a Focus on Under-threes. To improve its impact on child nutrition and health, ICDS must focus on children under three years of age, ensuring immunization, control of diarrhoeal diseases and respiratory infections, vitamin supplementation and deworming regularly, and enabling mothers to provide them timely and adequate feeding. In order to do this, *Anganwadi* Workers in new projects should be initiated to their jobs in a phased manner. They can begin by identifying pregnant women and infants in their village, providing them ante-natal and infant services with the help of the female MPW. As these children enter their second year, the relevant modifications can be made in services for them, with a focus on maintaining growth and health, while the original package is provided to newborns and pregnant women. When the first cohort reaches its fourth year, the AWWs could be trained to provide pre-school education and an associated nutritious meal daily. As the *anganwadi* group encompasses all children under six, cared for since birth, the AWW and MPW can focus their attention on infants and toddlers on a 'one day a week' basis. This approach would give the workers and communities a clear indication that ICDS services are meant to begin during pregnancy. It will show that the programme's focus is on maintaining the health and nutritional status of children from birth through the early years, followed by early childhood education. It will also help to streamline management of the AWW's responsibilities.

Improved Training and Supervision. Training in ICDS has been weak and requires considerable attention. Over 300 non-governmental organizations around the country have been running the three-month training courses for *Anganwadi* Workers and Supervisors. While some innovative, participatory approaches have been attempted, most training has been didactic—'lectures' with little discussion, almost no demonstration or hands-on learning, and no team-training of AWWs and MPWs or Supervisors. The training system has not been able to keep pace with programme expansion—many AWWs are 'employed' for a year or more before they receive any training. They are trained for three months at a stretch, and receive little reinforcement or refresher training thereafter. Training them for shorter periods, e.g. three to four weeks at a time, on at least three occasions several months apart, would be more effective. They could be trained specifically for the tasks entailed in the phased approach to their jobs, described above. AWWs must also receive continuous reinforcement of their skills and problem-solving abilities from their Supervisors. This calls for a more manageable ratio of AWWs to Supervisors, ten to one rather then the current 20:1. The selection of experienced AWWs as Supervisors is a potentially-effective strategy to improve relevance, practicality and staff motivation.

Attention to these important issues prior to further expansion of ICDS will be important to ensure that the promise of this comprehensive primary health care programme, based in the community and aiming its major activities at the well-being of mothers and children, is indeed realized.

FALTERING STEPS

In addition to the UIP and ICDS programmes which got under way in the 1980s, there were other health initiatives which faltered, denying India further progress toward Health for All. Foremost among these was the Community Health Workers' Scheme, India's first significant attempt to devolve responsibility for health care to the village level. Another effort was the involvement of non-governmental health organizations in the national health endeavour, and, more recently, of the wider private health sector. These approaches met with varying degrees of success and have important implications for the future.

The Community Health Workers' Scheme

Following reports of successful experiments in the non-governmental sector with lay community health workers (CHWs), the Indian government introduced a CHW Scheme across the country in 1977.*[5] Within five years, some 400 000 CHWs were trained—one for almost every Indian village, constituting the largest health cadre in the world outside of China. But CHWs in India have encountered a number of difficulties stemming from inadequate support from their communities and the health system alike. These have robbed them of their immense potential to date, but could be rectified to revitalize this important approach to primary health care in the future.

One of the main issues enveloping the CHWs was their 'medicalization'.

---

*The names of the worker and the scheme have changed over time—from Community Health Worker in 1977 to Community Health Volunteer in 1980 and (Village) Health Guide in 1981. The most familiar appellation, Community Health Worker, will be used here.

Trained for three months, they focused on providing curative services, to the neglect of preventive and promotive tasks. This was due in large part to their orientation to curative care during their initial training which was conducted by Primary Health Centre doctors and Health Supervisors, who were themselves not instructed appropriately in how to train basic health workers. The CHWs began to perceive themselves as village medical practitioners, often even demanding further training for this purpose. While village communities concurred because their perceived need was for curative services, they usually viewed the CHWs as 'third class doctors', and bypassed their services whenever possible. At the same time, India's powerful medical lobby, the Indian Medical Association, opposed the scheme on the grounds that these workers would indulge in quackery, inflicting inferior or even dangerous care on underserved and unsuspecting villagers.

Indeed, poor role definition led to other difficulties in the scheme. As primary care workers, the CHWs efforts should have been concentrated on the most common, simply-treatable ailments and on preventive strategies

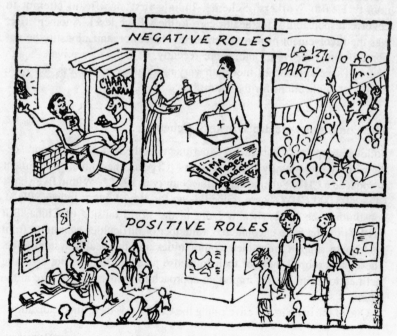

CHWs in India were discredited as 'do-nothings', 'quacks', or political organizers, but they still have enormous potential as basic health workers.

which could be adopted easily by village people. Their work would then have focused on women and children; and given gender relations in Indian society, *women* would have been chosen as village health workers. Instead, CHWs were seen as extensions of the health system, especially to undertake family planning motivation and sanitation tasks. As men were the main targets of the family planning programme in the 1970s and early 1980s, male CHWs were selected. Subsequent realization of the importance and neglect of domiciliary maternal and child health services, and fresh attention to women as the main targets of family planning, led to a change in policy. After 1986 the programme attempted to phase out male workers and recruit females in their place. But the organized male CHWs brought political pressure and legal injunctions against their removal, paralysing the scheme in most states.

The CHW Scheme has been India's most important attempt to 'democratize' health care, to 'place people's health in people's hands'. However, the CHWs' relationship to their communities has been problematic. While the government made it clear at the outset that the CHWs were volunteers, accountable to the communities they came from and served, communities viewed them as government employees because they were subservient to the formal health system which 'paid' them a small monthly stipend (initially Rs 50 or about US $5). The health system personnel also perceived the CHWs as government employees, assigning them additional tasks. This led in turn to CHWs demanding higher remuneration. Although they were willing to come forward for training because it carried a monthly stipend which was five times greater, few CHWs were willing to serve thereafter with any degree of reliability for the small honorarium. On the other hand, providing this stipend for each member of this large corps was a sizeable recurring expense to the government. As a result, in 1981, the Central Government decided to reduce its contribution from 100 to 50 per cent of the costs of the scheme and asked the State Governments to meet the remainder. This led to several States backing out of the programme, demonstrating their lack of commitment to basic health work. Most recently, following the conviction that women should be employed as CHWs, the Central government decided to fund the scheme fully once again—ironically but not surprisingly, from the budget of the family planning programme!

In essence, despite India's early start, the community health worker strategy was not given a fair chance because of administrative and technical confusions. Although there are about 387 000 CHWs 'on the rolls' (about 20 per cent of whom are women), the majority work erratically and are 'paid' irregularly, mostly at the discretion of district or block health administrators. Thus, a lacuna exists in health care at the village level, particularly where there is no ICDS worker. In the decade ahead, the government must revamp the scheme in order to revitalize it. Greater attention must be paid to the contents of the job, the methods of training, support from and supervision by the health system. The CHWs should function as lay first-aid and preventive health workers, focusing on MCH, health education, basic communicable disease control tasks and sanitation—and on family planning only where this is integrated with MCH. A worker must be provided for every village, no matter how small. While female workers are preferable, males could serve where it is difficult for women to function and where *Anganwadi* Workers are already in place. In larger villages, male and female pairs of CHWs could be considered. Most importantly, appropriate mechanisms must be developed to make CHWs accountable to the communities they serve, such as having them managed by community-level institutions.

Seeking Partners to Provide Health Care

In addition to efforts to increase community participation in 'system-managed' programmes such as UIP and ICDS, and to engage private individuals as community health workers, the government sought to involve non-governmental organizations (NGOs) in various aspects of health care during the 1980s. The chapters by Dyal Chand and Mukhopadhyaya in *Practising Health for All* described a number of innovative and successful non-governmental health efforts which came to public notice in the 1970s.[6,7] These had developed new approaches to meeting the health needs of village communities and had brought birth and death rates down within relatively short periods of time. Often, these results were achieved at low cost. These projects were invariably led by charismatic and dedicated persons who had taken up small areas and provided intensive medical and management inputs to achieve their visions of healthy and productive communities.

In the 1980s attention was turned to what these organizations could contribute to the cause of health nation-wide. It was recognized that they were oases in a vast desert of ill-health and deprivation, and ways were sought to widen their impact by involving them in the public health system. In some instances government health facilities and staff have been turned over to NGOs to be run and managed. NGOs have also been involved widely in training workers for the government health system, ranging from CHWs and *Anganwadi* Workers to doctors and health administrators. Through the years, private organizations from grassroots NGOs to national-level institutes of management have been involved in conducting operations research for and assisting in the development of aspects of the public health sector as diverse as management information systems, village-based treatment of ARI, training traditional birth attendants, or cost recovery.

Unfortunately, much of this attempted cross-fertilization has not been as fruitful as expected. The public system has certainly benefited from the training and research inputs provided by NGOs, but this has met a very small proportion of needs. Although NGO projects have been regarded as 'laboratories of learning', the larger governmental sector has been slow to absorb this experience. During the 1980s, there were virtually no new ideas (such as that of community health workers) transplanted from the private to the public sector. Although it is well-recognized that NGOs have particular strengths, for example, in mobilizing community participation—a major reason for the success of their projects, it has also become obvious that the capacity of the large, relatively-inflexible government system to adopt such approaches is limited. At the same time, few NGOs have been able to expand their projects to a scale that is relevant to managers of the government health system.

The attempts to turn government health facilities over to NGOs to run, for example, in the states of Maharashtra, Gujarat and Tamil Nadu, have been somewhat more successful. While there have been tensions between the opposite approaches of the two systems, in several instances these have been overcome. For example, although NGOs consider 'flexibility' to be among their main strengths, they have had to run the public facilities using government norms and procedures. While NGOs can hire and fire staff freely, in the government system the 'easy way out'—dismissal—is not easily achieved. This has led NGOs to try harder to retrain workers or to deploy them in different ways, proving that this can be done. Where NGO leaders have been able to steer the system, they have been able to bring about considerable improvements in performance and effectiveness. On the whole, however, very few NGOs have come forward to undertake such challenges although several states and health programmes (e.g. ICDS) have actively sought them out.

While public–private cooperation will undoubtedly continue in the decades ahead, NGOs do not hold out much hope for the majority of India's people. The entire private voluntary health sector, which may include as many as 5000 organizations, reaches less than five per cent of the country's villages and poor urban communities. An alternative approach mooted, which would also achieve 'community management' of CHWs, is to involve local self-government institutions more widely in health care.

Turning Health over to Local Self-Government

At various times since India's Independence, and particularly at the inception of the Community Health Workers' Scheme, the country has talked of turning the management of health and other social services over to local self-government bodies, known as *panchayati raj* institutions. Indeed, the concept of village autonomy and self-reliance was central to Mahatma Gandhi's vision of Indian self-rule and development; and it has been a recurring, if somewhat tentative, theme in several Health for All documents. While the first few years of the 1980s were silent on this subject, it has been in vogue again since about 1987.

However, India has gained only limited experience of health care managed by village-level government, which has revealed some inherent difficulties. It is widely acknowledged that *panchayati raj* institutions are not representative, being controlled by the dominant socio-economic elites of an area. The poor, socially-backward and women continue to be under-represented—perhaps less so *de jure* because there are quotas for their members on committees than *de facto*. While these vulnerable groups should be the focus of health (and other development) programmes, they lack the power to bring about the reorientation of the system and the redistribution of resources that are required. It is unlikely that the oligarchies that dominate *panchayats* would redress current imbalances unless they can be made to perceive that such decisions are in their own self-interest. Thus, for the goals of Health for All, the process of democratic decentralization would have to be accompanied by efforts to get traditional elites to view 'social goods' such as primary health care, drinking water and education as 'common goods'.

Decentralization would also face some problems which are a legacy of the 'top-down' approach to health planning that India has practised to date. Priorities for spending have been those of the urban-oriented elites. Thus, secondary and tertiary hospital facilities have been established while primary health care services have lagged behind. These priorities are etched deep in the social psyche and are unlikely to be reversed easily by democratic decentralization. The 'mystification' of health care and its control by a medical technocracy have allowed little questioning of these priorities— lay people feel unable to make informed choices and, even more serious, have been misled into believing that 'high technology' medicine will serve them better.

In the Eighth Five-Year Plan (1992–97), village *panchayats* and district-level committees are once again being envisaged as the instruments of social transformation through local area planning. Promises have been made that the necessary development staff and financial resources will be placed under their jurisdiction. The *panchayats* are to have the flexibility to decide how best to use these resources for local development. This is intended to release programmes from standard, centrally-formulated approaches, as well as to reduce the waste and duplication inherent in current fragmented, 'scheme-wise' approaches. To meet these excellent intentions which could generate popular pressure for improvements in health and other social services, local bodies which are currently absent in most parts of the country must first be restored through democratic elections. Through these steps, India could gain some ground that has been lost in the 1980s.

ADJUSTMENTS IN THE 1990s

Focus on the Private Health Sector

There is a large, profit-oriented private health sector in India. This ranges from super-speciality 'corporate' medical centres and sophisticated hospitals to individual private practitioners who are found almost everywhere. There is a wide spectrum of practitioners from modern 'allopaths' (qualified and licensed practitioners of Western medicine), who are largely concentrated in towns, to those who practise one of the several indigenous systems of medicine, primarily in rural areas. About 80 per cent of India's allopathic doctors work in the private sector, along with almost 100 per cent of indigenous doctors. Each of these groups of doctors numbers about half a million, which can be compared with the million or so health workers (including AWWs and CHWs) in the public health system. Because most private doctors run small, out-patient consulting rooms only, despite their large numbers, only about 10 to 15 per cent of urban hospitals and about one-third of hospital beds are in the private sector. The private health sector is largely curative-oriented, preventive health care or promotive services being almost exclusively carried out by government.

In India's mixed economy, consumers can and do exercise eclecticism in their choice of health care provider, turning to whichever system they deem suitable at a given time. A principal consequence of the declining quality of the public health system during the 1980s and of concurrent increases in population was the boom in the use of private health practitioners in both rural and urban areas. The private sector accounts for about 80 per cent of health expenditure in the country. About 75 per cent of all consultations are with private practitioners, only 25 per cent go to the government health sector. In rural areas perhaps one out of four consultations is with an allopathic practitioner, and the balance with traditional practitioners, who may, however, practise a 'mixed' form of medicine.

While the better-off patronize private services almost exclusively, even the poorest 20 per cent choose private practitioners in about 70 per cent of illness episodes. Choices are related to the direct as well as opportunity costs of services and to the perceived quality of care. The reasons given most frequently by respondents in household-level health surveys for not utilizing free government services are the time and cost of travelling to a Primary Health Centre or a district hospital, the long waiting hours at public health facilities, that government workers treat them rudely, or that 'government medicines are no good'.

Ironically, while national health policy holds that the private sector should contribute to governmental health efforts, the reverse actually occurs in numerous ways. For example, the government supports the growth of the private sector through its almost complete subsidy of education for doctors, nurses and paramedics. Despite years of discussion, medical graduates who enter the private sector do not repay the government's investment in their education through any period of public service or even a meaningful public internship. Private practitioners and institutions are subsidized also by tax exemptions, low-interest loans, import concessions and the like. Many institutions also receive grants from the government under a variety of different schemes. Despite this assistance, private sector services remain limited in critical areas such as immunization, MCH services including safe abortion and contraception, low-cost diagnostics and pathology.

Significantly, the 1982 Health Policy Statement was formulated before 'privatization' in the health sector was being discussed with any seriousness in India. It did not pay much heed to the variety that exists in the private sector, nor did it prepare for the sector's phenomenal growth in size and visibility during the 1980s. Indeed, the importance given to the private sector in health planning discussions in India today is an excellent example of how forces other than health policy—notably, the economic trends that have dominated the past decade—are shaping health care in the country. Policy in general, and the roles of the private and public health systems in particular, have been influenced by the new value systems emerging in Indian society. There is generally a gap between public and private goals— but this must be aligned with the needs of society if Health for All is to be achieved through the combined efforts of the public and private sectors.

In the 1990s the health of India's people is likely to be left increasingly to market forces, in contrast with the earlier philosophy that the State

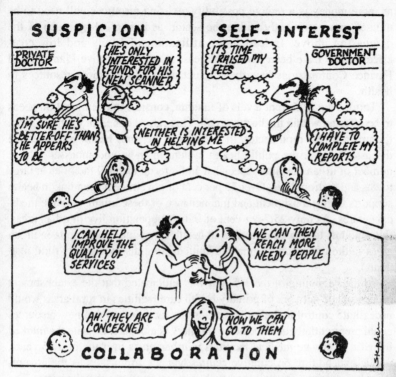

The public and private sectors must overcome self-interest and suspicion of each other to collaborate in a joint quest for Health for All.

should provide health for all. Indeed, as structural adjustment proceeds, the role of the government in health care provision may shrink even further in spite of talk of the government actually increasing spending in the social sectors (health, nutrition, education and family planning) to provide a 'safety net' for the poor.

Reallocation of Public Health Resources

To achieve Health for All even within the next *two* decades will require several simultaneous modifications in public resource allocations to health. First, the size of the annual health budget in the public sector (currently some US $4–5 per capita per year from all government sources) would need to be increased at least four-fold almost immediately. Second, particularly as more money is a remote possibility, existing resources will need to be utilized more efficiently within the sector, as is implied by much of the discussion above. Indeed, poor utilization of funds and low cost-effectiveness have been among the reasons why successive Planning and Finance Commissions have been reluctant to allocate more resources to health.

Third, even at current levels of funding, considerable reallocation needs to be effected within the health sector. This can be done, for example, from the urban to the rural sector. In addition to the rural health infrastructure discussed above, the public health system in India encompasses a large number of urban hospitals, specialist and referral medical facilities in large towns and metropolises. Over 75 per cent of government spending in health supports the establishment and maintenance of these urban, curative medical centres. As only 25.7 per cent of India's population live in urban areas, this amounts to a huge distortion in health expenditure per capita in urban areas (although urban hospitals, admittedly, are also visited by rural residents).

At the beginning of the 1980s it was anticipated that the establishment of a complete network of primary health care facilities in rural areas would necessitate control in the growth of tertiary facilities, so that new resources could preferentially be allocated to primary health care. Despite the marked increase in private medical facilities in urban areas over the past 15 years, public expenditure on curative centres has not diminished as the government has continued to build rather than divest itself of urban hospitals. The number of urban hospitals in the public sector continued to increase during the decade, albeit at a slower pace than they did earlier. By 1987 the urban areas of all major states in the country had exceeded the norms suggested for urban hospitals and beds by the Health for All report,[1] and the national average was 15 times the recommended norm!

The National Health Policy[2] also envisaged that growth in the private sector would take care of demand from the better-off sections of society, enabling the government to reorient its expenditures to care for the poor. But proposals to provide care to the poor in place of 'paying patients' have not been implemented decisively. For example, an experiment in Maharashtra to levy fees at public hospitals on the basis of means' tests was hastily discontinued under political pressure. In general, no reallocation of government spending has occurred from urban to rural, or tertiary to primary facilities, or from the better-off to the poor.

The existing imbalances underscore the need for India to proceed more clearly in accordance with the objectives of national health policy, giving priority to rural primary health care in the 1990s. As the norms for urban health facilities have already been exceeded, less costly functional improvements can be brought about in urban public hospitals to enhance their effectiveness. A system of outreach care to deal with the primary health needs of urban people and a referral system for rural people would help to reduce the burden on tertiary facilities and to increase equity.

Bringing about Synergism for Health

In *Practising Health for All*, John Ratcliffe pointed out that by the 1970s India's southern-most state of Kerala had achieved significantly lower mortality and fertility rates than surrounding populations in other areas with higher economic levels.[8] Despite its poverty, Kerala had surpassed other Indian states in many aspects of social development such as literacy. The link between higher social development and lower birth and death rates gave rise to the 'social justice theory of demographic transition', which held that demographic trends and levels reflect the degree to which political and economic institutions promote social equity. The prevailing theory unifying the experience of Kerala and a few other nations, such as Sri Lanka, Costa Rica and Cuba, led to the belief that smaller and healthier families were possible even in the absence of growth in domestic product, industrial bases, and high per capita incomes.* An important aspect of the Kerala example was that it was a state of a larger political and economic entity and not an 'island' nation. During the 1980s, therefore, considerable attention was focused on Kerala's demographic transition as academics and policy-makers strove to identify influential factors which might be repeated elsewhere in India. Given the country's economic underdevelopment, it became particularly important to examine whether Kerala's achievements provided hope of an alternative route to health in other poverty-ridden areas of the country.

Most analysts have concluded that education—particularly female education—was the basis for Kerala's demographic success. The State had long had education policies which favoured the poor majority instead of the privileged few. After Independence, while other states in India spent 3 to 6 per cent of their budgets on education, Kerala apportioned 15 per cent, allocating it preferentially to primary and secondary schools in contrast with other parts of the country which spent more on higher education.

*See Chapter 17 on Costa Rica by Mohs.

These policies resulted in universal primary education and mass literacy by the 1970s. By 1991, Kerala was 100 per cent literate.

Education increased political consciousness, leading people to demand their rights, including services from the government such as health care. Successive state governments responded and a well-distributed and functioning public health system was built in the state. Consequently, access to and utilization of health services was high. Both were also the cause and consequence of high levels of knowledge about health. Better road communications in Kerala also favour the use of health services. The state has the most extensive medical infrastructure in the country—about four times as many hospitals and nearly twice the number of hospital beds per 100 000 people as the Indian average. Nearly half of these are private. Most significantly, in contrast with the rest of India where public health care caters to the 'few', Kerala's health system responds to a broader and less privileged constituency. Thus, although the level of expenditure per capita in the

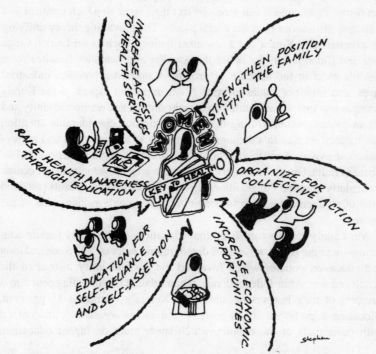

Providing women access to education and health services and economic opportunities is the key to improving health.

health sector is lower in Kerala than in many other Indian states, resources are, once again, more equitably distributed. Ultimately, education and health care work synergistically to influence Kerala's demography.

The more favourable situation with regard to social services in Kerala is also reinforced by the higher status of women. Kerala is the only state in India with more women than men (i.e. a 'female-favourable' sex ratio, which is found in most parts of the world). Women's education has been associated with a higher age at marriage—the average among females in Kerala being 23 years, compared with 17 years nationally. A high proportion of women, particularly those from poor households, are in the work force, which in turn enhances household income. Both female labour force participation and higher income are associated with reduced fertility. Family planning has been successful in Kerala without the compulsion applied in other parts of India. Thus, women are at the centre of the complex web of factors which bring about better health.

Over the past decade, Kerala's demographic evolution has been sustained. By 1991 its life expectancy was 70 years, comparable with 75 years in the US. Its infant mortality rate was 21, significantly lower than the Indian average of 86 and the average of all low income countries, 106. During the 1981–91 decade, Kerala's annual population growth rate was 1.31 per cent, well below the national rate of 2.11 per cent. However, Kerala's economic backwardness and inattention to economic growth has perpetuated low incomes, marked seasonality of employment and inadequate food production, which together have maintained low nutrition levels in the state. The combination of high literacy and low employment in the state led large numbers to migrate to other parts of India and the oil-rich countries in search of work in the 1970s and 1980s. While this helped to raise economic levels, resulting in a decline of about 25 per cent between 1970–71 and 1987–88 in the proportion of Kerala households living 'below the poverty line', the percentage of poor in Kerala still remains above the Indian average.

The paradox of 'social development despite economic backwardness' in Kerala is thus paralleled by a paradox in health: while mortality and fertility are low, malnutrition and morbidity are unacceptably high among large segments of its population. During the 1980s Kerala improved its public food distribution system in order to reduce some of the maldistribution and seasonal fluctuations in food available to households. But in 1989, almost 60 per cent of Kerala households were short of the recommended number of calories. On average, Kerala's households do not meet their daily caloric requirements, although 'mean consumption' improved slightly in the late

1970s and 1980s. The key to better child survival in the state seems to be better intra-household distribution of nutrients despite low overall availability. This is also reflected in lower levels of severe malnourishment in children.

In the 1980s Kerala's high population density and continuous urban-like sprawl showed signs of stressing the environment. Water supplies were increasingly polluted, and agricultural land was relinquished for dwelling and commerce. The combination of inadequate nutrition and declining environmental conditions does not augur well for Kerala's health. Nor do some other effects of its artificially-bolstered economy. A taste for expensive health care has been nurtured by the emigrees' exposure to 'oil-money hospitals' in Gulf countries. Kindled by the influx of large amounts of ready cash, the private health sector in Kerala has grown—perhaps even more rapidly and to more sophisticated levels than in most other parts of India. The cash has fueled inflation in several quarters, including in the prices of food and health care. The situation on the whole calls for urgent attention to employment generation in the state, food production and distribution, water supply and sanitation, and preventive health services. It remains to be seen how Kerala will extricate itself from this declining spiral in the 1990s and improve the quality of life of its people.

Health for Too Many

During the 1980s, developments in other parts of India confirmed what has long been suspected about Kerala: that its achievement is unique—the result of a fortunate confluence of several social, political and infrastructural advancements. These occurred over two centuries as a result of exceptionally progressive policies adopted by a succession of princely rulers and governments. The only recent experience approaching Kerala's has been in Tamil Nadu where, despite persistent poverty, literacy levels have improved and infant mortality and fertility have both declined significantly. In 1990, adult female literacy was 65 per cent, the infant mortality rate was 67 and the crude birth rate was 28. As in Kerala, these improvements can be ascribed to the relatively higher status of women in Tamil Nadu (compared with other parts of India) and to government policies which have promoted 'education for all' and provided nutritional support to the needy. In the states of Karnataka and Maharashtra there are also signs of analogous improvements.

The decade saw a dramatic demographic transition in another tiny state, Goa. But here, in addition to education and higher women's status, rapid industrialization contributed to the decline in mortality and fertility in a population of just over a million! In India's north-east, the death and birth rates of a few similarly small states benefited from the high levels of awareness and more equitable distribution of resources among their distinct tribal populations. On the other hand, mortality and fertility in Punjab, India's most economically-advanced state, did not decline as much as the state's economic development and literacy levels might have predicted. An explanation for this dilemma may lie in the lower status of women in Punjab as demonstrated by a markedly skewed sex ratio (888 females per 1000 males in 1991).

In other parts of India, notably the four large northern states of Bihar, Madhya Pradesh, Rajasthan and Uttar Pradesh, where almost 40 per cent of India's population lives, birth and death rates persisted at unacceptably high levels (e.g. infant mortality over 90 per 1000 live births; crude mortality over 10 and the crude birth rate over 33 per 1000 population). Continued inequalities in the distribution of resources and societal organization perpe-

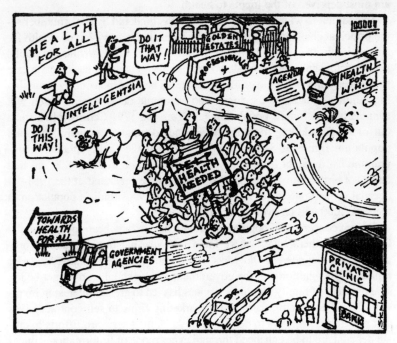

All those working towards Health for All must converge their interests, focusing on the most needy.

tuate poverty and social underdevelopment in these regions. Less than half the population over 7 years of age in these states are literate; less than 30 per cent of their females. Public policies have failed to improve resource or income distribution, or access to health or education services significantly. Feudal politics and the handicaps faced by the bureaucracies in these states exacerbate the difficulty of bringing about change.

In the ultimate analysis, despite Kerala's contrary experience, poverty remains a major reason why health has not improved adequately in these states and many other parts of India. The 1990s have begun and will most probably continue to be characterized by a preoccupation with these large, politically-important states. In fact, the large sizes and backwardness of the four northern states weigh India's development indices down heavily. In 1987–88 about 43 per cent of India's people lived 'below the poverty line', without adequate access to minimum basic needs, including food, clothing, shelter, education and health care. During the decade ahead all those concerned with Health for All in India must focus on the mass of people who are most deprived of the inputs to health.

In addition to widespread poverty, India is hindered by sheer numbers—the principal challenge that the country faces in the provision of Health for All is simply that it must provide health for too many. While the public health sector should concentrate on providing good quality basic health care to the needy, the larger government apparatus bears responsibility for assisting families to achieve the social and economic development which will eventually help India's population stabilize. The 1991 Census jolted India out of its decade-long complacency about population growth. The total population figure of 844 million proved that the family planning programme had brought little relief to the fertility rate in the 1980s and that claims of birth control acceptance were grossly exaggerated. If the 1981–91 decadal growth rate is not reduced during the 1990s, India's population in the year 2000 will be over 1040 million.

Recent concern with population growth has, in fact, been focused on the four large northern states where India's 40-year-old family planning programme has floundered. Old ways of promoting family planning are to be replaced. Recognition that the government can, or should, no longer be the sole provider of family planning services has led to greater interest in involving the private sector, particularly marketing firms to sell contraceptives and private practitioners to deliver family planning services. Efforts to create demand are to be enhanced through every mode of 'information, education and communications', but an increase in the supply of contraceptives and services and greater programme visibility through political support are thought to be the best way of rekindling demand. There is hope that the family planning programme will be less 'vertical' in the future and that measures 'beyond family planning' will be implemented with the utmost seriousness. Else, several of the lessons of the 1980s, and particularly those from Kerala, will go to waste.

India's Experiments with Truth

In India the 1990s have unfolded amid as much political and economic uncertainty as did the 1980s. The Congress Party remained in power through much of the earlier decade, led by Indira Gandhi until her assassination in 1984 and then by her son Rajiv Gandhi. The latter's unpopular policies led to a Congress defeat at the polls in 1989, with a landslide victory for a National Front of parties whose policies were not unlike those of the Janata Government of 1977–80. With this coalition came renewed hope for 'people's government' which had been marginalized over the 1980s. The National Front, however, could not sustain its partnership, with the result that there have been three successive governments between 1989 and 1992. Though all have followed more or less the same health policies, the pace of political change has been too rapid for any significant achievements in health.

At the beginning of this decade the economic scene in India is also troubled. Under pressure from major foreign creditors, the Indian government has initiated structural adjustments. It is feared that worker retrenchment will add to India's already severe unemployment problems, exacerbating the situation of women in particular. The liberalization of an earlier highly-regulated economy has increased inflation, with rising food prices already affecting the poor and middle classes. By the turn of the century the percentage of India's population below the poverty line may reach an all-time high, encompassing a majority of both rural and urban dwellers.

Liberalization is expected to bring in its wake a larger than ever private health sector, including fee-for-service private practitioners and institutions, and a greatly expanded drug and medical technology industry. However, despite this increase in supply, the prices of health goods and services have been rising markedly and are expected to continue to do so. This will mean that the poor will have increasingly little recourse except to the public health sector. Will the social safety nets to be put in place guarantee the poor at least a minimum level of health care?

A spirit of self-rule and self-reliance characterized India's health policy

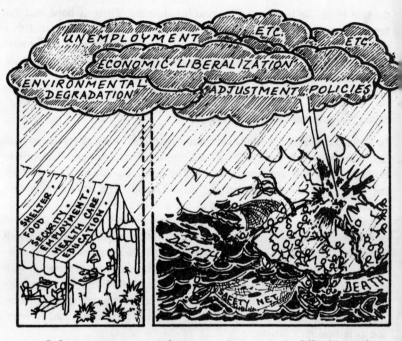

Safety nets must protect the poor against economic difficulties rather than being tardy rescue measures.

at the time of Independence. In the 1950s and 1960s India was a pioneer among developing nations in establishing a rural health care infrastructure which was a model at Alma Ata three decades later, and the first national family planning programme in the world. At the beginning of the 1980s, the country framed a vision of a healthy 'self' which was sorely put to the test during the decade. While India adopted the Alma Ata Declaration with conviction, the decade proved how hard it is to operationalize. Most of the paths that India attempted towards Health for All were littered with obstacles as the country has had to face economic, demographic and political realities.

The dilemma of realizing inner convictions in the face of external difficulties is reminiscent of Mahatma Gandhi's 'experiments with truth'. One can say that India has attempted similar experiments in the health sector, with beliefs such as 'people's health in people's hands', 'health for those most in need', and 'health for all'. But while India pledged to universalize health, she flinched in the face of 'too many', and provided health only for a few; and she failed to allocate adequate resources to health, giving in to competing demands. While she vowed to decentralize health care, the pressures of centralized schemes such as UIP and ICDS took over and efforts to involve communities floundered. A focus on the health of needy people was subverted by concerns with 'hardware', high technology and numerical targets. Unhappily, many other experiments to develop the basic principles of Health for All were also thwarted. Thus, unlike Gandhiji's efforts which harmonized his inward and outward life and led to the development of a strong and purposeful self, most of India's attempts in the sphere of health succumbed to immediate compulsions. On present reckoning, Health for All in India is a dream which will take decades to realize.

References

1. Indian Council of Social Science Research and Indian Council of Medical Research. (1981). *Health for All: An Alternative Strategy*. Institute of Education, Pune.
2. Government of India. (1982). Statement of National Health Policy, Ministry of Health and Family Welfare, New Delhi.
3. Government of India. (1946). *Report of the Health Survey and Development Committee*, Manager of Publications, Delhi.
4. National Institute of Public Cooperation and Child Development. (1992). *National Review of ICDS*, NIPCCD, New Delhi.
5. Bose, Ashish. (1983). The Community Health Worker Scheme: an Indian Experiment. In: *Practising Health for All*, (eds. D. Morley, J. Rohde and G. Williams), Oxford University Press, Oxford, pp. 38–48.
6. Dyal Chand, A. and Ibrahim Soni, M. (1983). Evaluation in Primary Health Care: a Case Study from India. In: *Practising Health for All*, (eds. D. Morley, J. Rohde and G. Williams), Oxford University Press, Oxford, pp. 87–100.
7. Mukhopadhyay, M. (1983). Human Development through Primary Health Care: Case Studies from India. In: *Practising Health for All*, (eds. D. Morley, J. Rohde and G. Williams), Oxford University Press, Oxford, pp. 113–44.
8. Ratcliffe, J. (1983). Social Justice and the Demographic Transition: Lessons from India's Kerala State. In: *Practising Health for All*, (eds. D. Morley, J. Rohde and G. Williams), Oxford University Press, Oxford, pp. 64–82.

CHAPTER 17

Changing Health Paradigms in Costa Rica

EDGAR MOHS

*The author explains how attitudes shaped the Costa Rican health care system and enabled rapid acceleration towards Health for All even in times of fiscal austerity.**

Edgar V. Mohs, *M.D., was Vice Minister of Health in Costa Rica during 1970–71 and Minister during 1986–90. He has been Professor of Paediatrics at the National Children's Hospital, University of Costa Rica, and has held numerous consultancies to WHO and UNICEF.*

INTRODUCTION

Costa Rica has achieved remarkable success in its quest for Health for All. During the twentieth century, infant mortality has fallen more than 90 per cent, from levels of about 200 to 13.9 per 1000 live births in 1989. To understand the process of Costa Rica's present state of good health, I have identified three critical stages through which the country's health pro-gramme has passed during the second half of this century. I have called these phases 'paradigms' because they meet the conditions discussed in Thomas Kuhn's definition.[1] It is these paradigmatic changes in the health system and social structure which have facilitated Costa Rica's quest for Health for All.[2]

ANTECEDENTS

During the first 10 000 years of the history of medicine, the predominant thinking connected illness to magic, attributing it to supernatural origins, thereby generating a totally non-scientific concept of the health–disease

---

*An earlier version of this article appeared in the *Pediatric Infectious Disease Journal*, Vol. 10, No. 6, June 1991.

relationship. In the thousand years that followed, this concept was substituted by an elaborate theory known as the miasma theory, which was a serious effort to find causal mechanisms for disease. Although many creative ideas were conceived by great scientists like Farr, Virchow and Villerme, these very men passionately defended the miasma theory, placing excessive importance on physical elements such as cold and heat, dampness and dryness.

Over the course of centuries, mankind suffered repeated epidemics of plague, typhus, cholera, dysentery and other diseases which often claimed 10–25 per cent of entire populations. Plague wreaked such havoc during the Middle Ages—the time of the Black Death in Europe—that the disease was represented as the first of the Four Horsemen of the Apocalypse. Thus emerged a new character in the realm of public health, an important precursor to the modern epidemiologist, a kind of health inspector who traversed the streets and alleys of villages and cities, seeking out foci of infection and sounding the alarm each time the number of cases of a given disease began to increase in the areas he covered. Unfortunately, this generally resulted only in the flight of population.

The miasma theory ended in the middle of the nineteenth century when Pasteur discovered that each infectious disease is produced by a specific microorganism. This fabulous scientific discovery caused a revolution in health sciences and their application. With the definition of aetiological agents of disease, medicine advanced rapidly and public health was born again based on the Germ Theory, even though some countries had already made significant advances in epidemic prevention and control through empirical measures. With the arrival of the twentieth century, three consecutive paradigms appeared. These we describe as the paradigms of deficiency diseases, infectious diseases and chronic diseases. These three paradigms, the resulting analysis and the strategies evolved for their control describe the process of improved health in Costa Rica over the past fifty years.

COSTA RICA

Costa Rica is a 100-year-old republican democracy with over 92 per cent literacy and without an army since 1948. The three million inhabitants are distributed within 50 000 square kilometres and two ecosystems—mountain and tropical forests. The country's traditional agro-export economy has undergone a process of industrialization and tourism development recently. These activities generated an average gross national product of around US $1700 per capita in 1989, from $500 in 1970.

During the colonial period and the first decades after Independence—from the sixteenth through the nineteenth century—the nation was extremely poor. A large number of infectious diseases affected the quality of life of its inhabitants resulting in a low life expectancy.

Problems in the health sector began to be recorded in the eighteenth century. All records show that in addition to the extreme poverty in which a majority of the people lived, malnutrition, worsened by severe and recurring infections, was the principal cause of death. The high mortality rate among children represented the deplorable health situation of the whole population. A large number of children died during their first year (around 400 per 1000 live births) and life expectancy was very short, at around 30 years.

In the first decades of the twentieth century, it became evident that the fundamental health problems suffered by the population came from the high prevalence of many infectious diseases including malaria, tuberculosis, respiratory infections, diarrhoea, parasitosis, and other diseases preventable by vaccination. As a consequence, it could be deduced that the principal cause of death lay in the lack of control of infectious diseases. However, in the 1940s and 1950s, the widespread diffusion of the discovery of the aetiology of such scourges as beriberi, pellagra and scurvy popularized the belief that nutritional deficiencies were the most important causes of disease and death in the population, particularly among infants. Study and interest turned from infectious diseases to the field of nutrition. This spread to all sectors of the health organization and found root in the designs for understanding, describing and solving problems in public health.

THE PARADIGM OF DEFICIENCY DISEASES

Between 1940 and 1969, deficiency diseases or malnutrition were believed to be the primary determinant of ill-health in Costa Rica. The population's health problems were attributed to poverty, ignorance, exploitation and a lack of food. In addition to malnutrition, infectious diseases and other morbidity were high, resulting in frequent hospitalization. This placed pressures on the few existing hospitals and the limited supply of health services. Among the strategies which developed under this concept was diet improvement through public food distribution, a massive and costly affair. In addition, a large nutrition department was created in the Ministry of Health. The number of hospital beds, doctors and nurses grew extensively. Medicine became highly politicized, with medical schools becoming arenas for discussing national social problems rather than the science and technology of health. The predominant thinking suggested that university classrooms might provide solutions for development, for it was considered that economic growth was the fundamental pillar of improved health. Furthermore, it was held that development could be achieved by nationalizing health services, as well as the nationalization of all means of production. There was a great tendency in universities to evoke, on the one hand, the grandeur achieved in the distant past and, on the other, naively, to expect some miracle in the future. The possibility of doing something tangible immediately and with 'our own hands' was largely discarded.

The philosophical basis for these viewpoints stemmed, in the first place, from the belief that economic growth and industrialization are absolute prerequisites for improved health. A second tenet states that socialization of

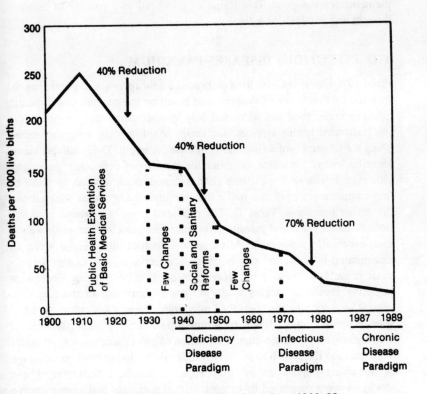

Fig. 1. *Landmarks in infant mortality, Costa Rica 1900–89.*

medicine is a necessary step towards establishing a socialist state and a viable alternative to solving health problems directly. Finally, preventive medicine, the subject of much talk and rhetoric, received few resources and less attention in the system which was still based on curative medicine. The deficiency paradigm was based on a psychological attitude that presumed we were unable to solve our own problems. There was a glorification of the past and a fatalistic attitude towards present and future. In spite of a considerable fall in infant mortality associated with social and sanitary reforms following the end of World War II, the IMR remained largely unchanged at about 80–70 through the two decades preceding 1970 (Fig. 1, p. 381). Most people felt that health problems could only be solved through socio-economic development, that 90 per cent of ill-health was beyond the influence of doctors, nurses, nutritionists and other workers. The other 10 per cent required curative or rehabilitative care, or called for medicines or food supplements for the poor. This frame of mind led to a paucity of creative thought and paralysis of action.

THE INFECTIOUS DISEASES PARADIGM

From 1970 onwards Costa Rica embraced a new approach to public health. Inspired by the theory of systems, and based on the concept that ill-health could be understood and addressed only by a structural reorganization and integration of health services, the entire health system was reorganized along the principles of an infectious disease paradigm. The health problems identified were the same as under the nutritional deficiency paradigm. However, health strategies were now designed to address the proximal or immediate causes of illness rather than the underlying causes which drove the earlier paradigm (Table 1). The problems remained extensive: infectious diseases, intestinal parasites, unwanted pregnancies, low birth-weight and, especially amongst children, severe malnutrition. These were all exacerbated by a limited supply of medical services, which were largely curative and based in hospitals. Having recognized these causes, Costa Rica began to develop strategies totally different from those of the past. The critical strategy was the control of infectious diseases and intestinal parasites. A second emphasis was on promotion of family planning and exclusive breast-feeding as the sound foundation of good nutrition. A third major principle was the switch to primary health care with emphasis on coverage of the entire population using appropriate health technologies. These strategies were supported by extensive legal measures and administrative

Table 1. The contrasting paradigms

Problems	Causes	Strategies	Philosophy	Psychology
The Malnutrition Paradigm				
Malnutrition	Food shortage	Food distribution	Economic growth is prerequisite	Inability to solve own problems
Parasitosis	Poverty	Large nutrition Department in MOH	Socialism is required	Blame on forces outside our control
Infectious diseases	Ignorance	Hospital based curative services	Atomistic approach to problems	Cynicism regarding future change
High mortality	Exploitation	More doctors and specialists	Emphasis on curative medicines	Glorification of the past
High rates of hospitalization		Politicization of medicine	Preventive medicine largely rhetoric	Paralysis and inaction
Low coverage of health services				Dependency
The Infectious Diseases Paradigm				
Malnutrition	Low birth weight	Control infectious diseases and parasitosis	Healthy families contribute most to socio-economic development	Self confidence and belief in progress
High mortality	Artificial feeding	Family planning	Less politicization, more scientific approach to medicine and health	Self reliance and pride
High morbidity	Infectious diseases	Promote breast feeding	Health by everyone	Pro-active approach to problems
High hospitalization rates	Unclean home environment	Universal primary health care	True emphasis on preventive medicine	Urgency to improve
Low coverage health services	Limited supply of health services	Close hospital beds		Future oriented with optimism
	Over-emphasis on hospital care	Appropriate health technologies		
		Legal and administrative reforms		

reforms in the health sector, making Costa Rica's public health system a truly preventive, promotive, and universal self-help programme.

This reorientation did not come about accidentally or arbitrarily. On the contrary, it was founded on a solid philosophical basis that turned the existing paradigm on its head. Rather than maintaining that social and economic development were essential prerequisites for solving health problems, the country embraced the philosophy that healthier families will contribute more to the country's economic and social development. Health interventions took first priority for national resources, substantially impacting the way health care services were organized and offered.

At the same time, efforts were made to reduce the politicization of medicine, emphasizing a more scientific approach to medicine and health. Instead of postulating a socialist revolution as the only solution to health problems, scientific analysis was used to propose a more objective understanding of underlying factors. Simultaneously, a democratic revolution in health was declared in the form of more equitable distribution through an enlarged primary health care system. This new orientation demanded that scientific health care should be available to the entire population. Thus, a commitment to Health for All was articulated in Costa Rica years before the World Health Organization promoted the concept of Health for All by the Year 2000. A final and most fundamental component of this paradigm was the psychological thinking which radically changed the passive and fatalistic thinking of the previous decades, clearly stating that 'In Costa Rica, we can solve our own problems'.

Critical Achievements

The Ministry of Health was reorganized to reflect these principles. A programme for rural health was created to extend coverage of primary health care programmes to the entire population. The interrelationships of various sections of the Ministry were reflected in comprehensive health care in the periphery. A new general health law was enacted which modified the old sanitary code of 1950. The previously disconnected array of institutes, authorities, and various government schemes were brought together in a coordinated National Health System. The Costa Rican social security system, which had previously served citizens mainly in the organized sector, took over the management of all hospitals in the country. The number of admissions to the University of Costa Rica Medical School was doubled and the curriculum reduced from seven to six years. The School of Nursing was transferred to the Faculty of Health Sciences at the same university, and

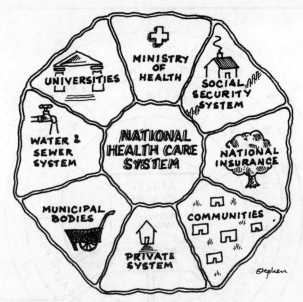

*Previously autonomous and unrelated, all elements of health care
were integrated into an interlinked system by the Ministry of Health
in the 1970s.*

also doubled its number of students. Nursing curriculum was divided into
two tracks: one of two years duration for professional nurses, the other, a
three-year programme providing a bachelor's degree. Courses for training
of nurses' aides tripled their enrolment.

A nationwide safety net of social services to the poor was strengthened
in 1971 with the creation of the Joint Institute of Social Aid with the help
of private funds, and in 1975, with the creation of the Programme of Social
Development and Family Assistance a special fund from payroll taxes.
These interventions, combined with sustained economic growth and a political climate of peace and democratic stability, enabled these previously-
independent and disarticulated institutions to become a truly coordinated
National Health Care system. Interestingly, out of the centralization and
concentration of power at the national headquarters, soon followed an automatic decentralization which placed greater emphasis on local health care
systems. Importance was given to the solution of problems identified by the
people within their own communities. To facilitate this transition, the
country was subdivided into five regions with 81 cantons, each having a

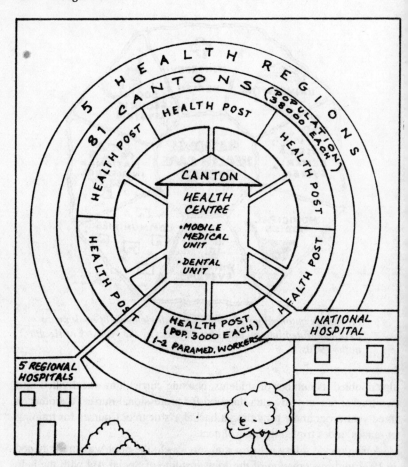

*The health system comprised a uniform pattern of facilities leading
from village health centres to regional and national hospitals.*

population of about 38 000. A health post, staffed by one or two paramedical workers was located within each community of 3000 people. The paramedics were technically supervised and guided by medical professionals at
the canton or municipal health centre. The centre provided mobile medical
and dental services, curative care, and a complete range of preventive and
promotive health activities designed to improve sanitation, public hygiene,
access to family planning, ante-natal care, immunization, and promotive
health education. Efficient referral mechanisms connected each local health
system to regional and national hospitals.

Previously, health programmes had been designed to address specific problems independently. This linear or vertical approach, which had resulted in disarticulated and ineffective programmes, was abandoned for a holistic approach to health and nutrition. With the adoption of more holistic thinking patterns relating to the causes and interrelationships underlying ill-health, far greater attention was given to the synergism that can either make health problems more difficult to solve or, alternatively, can lead to definitive solutions. The interrelationship of infectious disease and malnutrition became more widely recognized along with an understanding that these were related to hygienic health practices, fertility patterns and child-rearing behaviours.

The country began to see health not as a balance of forces but rather as a balance of flows or dynamic behaviours, more like the interrelationships within a living cell. Those of us working in the Ministry of Health found that previously we had identified and isolated problems and designed individual solutions largely in isolation of other programmes. We found that just as there is synergism between problems, so too do solutions which are juxtaposed through interconnected programmes result in greater impact. This concept is best illustrated by the effects on human growth and development of controlling infection, malnutrition and fertility. Growth and development, their monitoring, measurement and promotion, became a central theme of the overall health paradigm.

From the new synergistic perspective, we could no longer separate the health problems of our people. Rather, they were seen as a continuum. While the majority of the population was healthy most of the time, their exposure to unhealthy environments or conditions was recognized to lead to illness, which usually required treatment by a medical worker, less frequently by a doctor, and only rarely required hospitalization. The entire population was seen to be spread across this spectrum—from healthy living to the use of the maximum medical technology available. Each component of health care received the necessary resources in the effort to move the entire population towards the healthy end of the spectrum.

At the same time the nation began to change its interpretation of the relationship between politics, science, technology and development. In less-developed countries, there is a strong tendency for political, bureaucratic, research, service and 'public consumption' activities to be unconnected. Our National Health System enabled a dialogue between political authorities, university and private research centres, health providers and the public at large, bringing greater responsiveness in the application of science and technology to the needs of the people. This improved the efficiency and

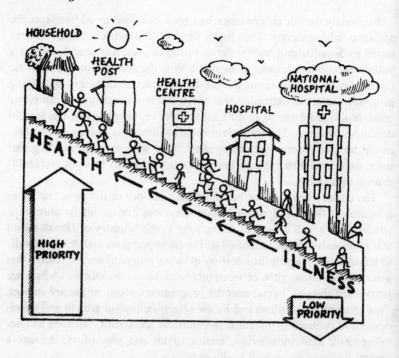

relevance of the two most important institutions in the National Health Care System, the Ministry of Health and the Social Security System. The Ministry has the responsibility of tending to and organizing communities for health promotion activities, disease prevention, and eliminating epidemic foci. Healthy life-styles are promoted along with responsible control of fertility, a healthy environment, and access to the knowledge and practices essential to healthy life. The Costa Rican Social Security System has the task of attending to the population's medical care, starting with simple self-care at home, through dispensaries and clinics, to the highly specialized national hospitals.

Some Results

As a consequence of the development and application of this paradigm, the infant mortality rate in Costa Rica dropped dramatically—by 70 per cent within a decade—from one of the highest rates in the Americas to one of the lowest (Fig. 2a).

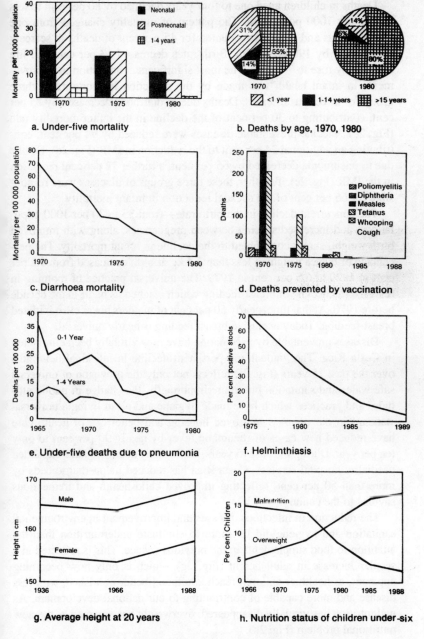

a. Under-five mortality

b. Deaths by age, 1970, 1980

c. Diarrhoea mortality

d. Deaths prevented by vaccination

e. Under-five deaths due to pneumonia

f. Helminthiasis

g. Average height at 20 years

h. Nutrition status of children under-six

Fig. 2. Changes in health, nutrition and disease parameters.

Deaths in children aged one to four years declined by 80 per cent to less than 1 per 1000 population. The pattern of mortality changed from one where infants and children accounted for 45 per cent of deaths to scarcely 20 per cent by 1980 (Fig. 2b). Birth rates decreased 13 per cent and life expectancy rose to 74 years. The most significant contribution to improvements in infant health was made by the reduction in mortality in three groups of infectious diseases. Deaths due to diarrhoea decreased by 85 per cent, contributing to 30 per cent of the decline in the infant mortality rate (Fig. 2c). Vaccine-preventable diseases were reduced by 94 per cent, contributing an additional 24 per cent to the reduction in IMR (Fig. 2d). Deaths due to pneumonia decreased by 65 per cent, a further 12 per cent reduction in the IMR (Fig. 2e). Together, these three groups of illnesses were responsible for 66 per cent of the decadal reduction in infant mortality.

The concurrent decline in the birth rate—from 33 to 20 per 1000 population—and increased spacing between pregnancies, along with improved birth weight, surely contributed to the decline in infant mortality. The percentage of babies weighing less than 2.5 kg at birth decreased from 9.2 per cent in 1970 to 6.5 per cent in 1979. The universal practice of rooming-in reversed the decline of breast-feeding which reached its nadir in the decade before 1970. At that time, nearly 50 per cent of mothers never even initiated breast-feeding. Today exclusive breast feeding is nearly universal.

Diseases preventable by vaccination have now virtually been eliminated in Costa Rica. The gradual and persistent decline in intestinal helminths over the past 15 years (Fig. 2f) reflects not only the provision of universal safe water and sanitation but, more importantly, the change in public attitudes and practices which have made hygiene and clean living a universal standard in our country. Improved housing and better use of health care have reduced new cases of rheumatic fever by nearly 90 per cent to only ten per year. During the past 15 years, while many countries have expanded paediatric hospital services, Costa Rica has reduced its paediatric beds by more than 50 per cent, reflecting improved child health and tremendous savings to the country.

The reduction in infectious diseases and improvement in environmental sanitation and hygiene did far more to eliminate undernutrition than the attention to food supplements in the previous decade. This is reflected in a secular increase in adult height (Fig. 2g), which is only now becoming apparent, as healthier children reach adulthood better nourished, with less disease and more capable of contributing to our national development. As malnutrition has virtually disappeared, overweight has emerged as the new nutritional problem (Fig. 2h).

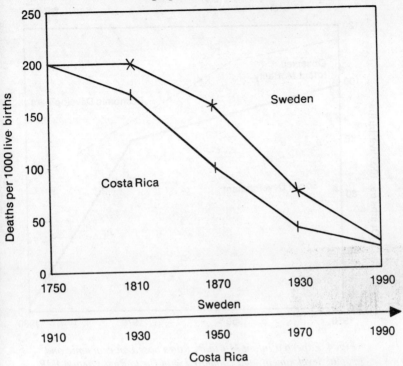

Fig. 3. A comparison of infant mortality in Costa Rica and Sweden.

Today, with a per capita GNP of $1648 (1989) and an IMR of 14, Costa Rica spends $130 per capita on health care. The United States, with a GDP in excess of $15 000 per capita and IMR of 11, spent $2379 per capita for health in 1989. Clearly, Costa Rica has achieved 'good health at low cost'. The health transition of Costa Rica is compared to that of Sweden in Fig. 3. While the trend in infant mortality is identical in the two countries, the transition took nearly two-and-a-half centuries in Sweden but occurred in one-third of that time in Costa Rica.

In an effort to tease out the contribution made by economic, social and health factors, Mauldin and Berelson created a model based on extensive data from transnational studies.[3]

Figure 4 shows the infant mortality expected in Costa Rica on the basis of this model. Were infant mortality to be predicted on the basis of Costa Rica's economic indicators alone, the trend would have followed the upper line. Social indicators, better developed than economic ones in Costa Rica,

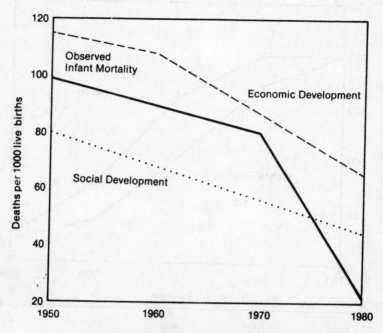

Fig. 4. Expected Infant Mortality Rates based on economic and social development, and compared with Costa Rica's actual IMR.

would predict infant mortality according to the lower (dashed) line. However, the observed infant mortality (solid line) was between these two until 1970 when we adopted the radical, new approach to health described above.

The dramatic impact of the public health policies implemented in the 1970s is shown by the sudden change in the slope of the infant mortality trend-line. The decline in IMR exceeded that predicted by economic or social indicators. From the model, one can hypothesize that about two-thirds of the reduction in infant mortality during the 1970s was attributable to qualitative changes in the health sector, while social and economic development over the same period contributed roughly one-fourth to the decline.[4]

THE CHRONIC DISEASE PARADIGM

Over the past decade, the rapid eradication of malnutrition, control of infections and parasites, and improved environment have brought about a new situation in which chronic ailments predominate. For example, in the field of infant care, perinatal disorders, congenital birth defects, child abuse accidents and poisoning are growing in importance. Our public health services could soon prove unable to deal with this new array of conditions. Thus today a new paradigm with a focus on chronic diseases is emerging. The philosophical basis of this new paradigm and the approach to these diseases must be different from that embraced by the richer countries. We will engender a greater sense of individual responsibility as a majority of these emerging problems are closely related to individual behaviour and are amenable to prevention or early detection and treatment. A growing dependence on science and technology has appeared largely because the prevention, treatment and rehabilitation of the chronic diseases are more complex than those for diseases which characterized the deficiency and infectious disease paradigms. As we have few technological resources and even fewer finances, we must rely on education and behavioural change as our major response to this new paradigm. We need to indigenize science and technology, adapting the most efficient and egalitarian approaches to reducing risk.

We recognize that it is our responsibility to solve our own problems. We have changed so much over the past few years that we now accept change as a part of our lives, and we look to forging a better future with confidence. Although our standard of living is now superior to that at any time in the past, we still have very limited resources. However, we are convinced that with greater effort and efficiency we will find our own way to Health for All in Costa Rica.

RELEVANCE TO OTHER COUNTRIES

Although this experience took place in Costa Rica, it is reasonable to think that it applies to other less-developed countries that are functioning under the first paradigm—deficiency diseases. The malnutrition paradigm condemns a country to a fatalistic approach to poor health even in the face of continued poverty. It is passive and denies the most important scientific and technical advances of our age. But we do not have to follow the example of industrialized countries, who in the course of one or two centuries moved slowly along a path of improved health together with improved economy.[5]

A major difference is that today there is a wide range of appropriate technology at our disposal. Unknown in previous decades, wide-scale affordable interventions can enhance the effectiveness and efficiency of health systems even in the poorest of countries.[6]

The second paradigm of infectious diseases takes a holistic and pragmatic approach to what is possible. It recognizes the importance of education to indicate good personal habits, and fosters the widespread application of affordable technologies through primary health care. A genuine effort to make decentralized, community-responsive primary health care available to all takes pressure off overburdened hospitals and gives full opportunity for the most cost-effective interventions to have maximal impact. This approach empowers people as it enables them to recognize that the major determinants of their own health and that of their family and community are in their own hands.

Our approach must be different from that of developed countries who enriched themselves economically at the time they were overcoming the deficiency and infectious diseases. When they were faced with chronic diseases they had more resources, and hence developed costly approaches. Costa Rica and other less-developed countries which have reached or will soon reach the chronic illness stage lack the riches necessary to meet the high cost of those strategies to avoid or repair the damage caused by the chronic ailments. This disadvantage forces us to base our actions on educating people, on health promotion, and on the development of greater individual responsibility. We must engage in a rigorous selection of priorities and a constant search for efficiency.

Our ability to improve the quality of life and health of people in the less-developed world depends on our ability to correctly interpret the realities which surround us, and to choose and implement adequate health interventions. The history of industrialized nations will not be repeated, and the accumulation of riches will take even longer to occur. As we approach the end of the twentieth century, it would appear that the appropriate decision for the less-developed countries is to abandon the sterile paradigm of the deficiency diseases, whose linear and atomistic approach to individual problems has had inadequate impact and to begin implementing the proactive elements of the paradigms of infectious and chronic diseases vigorously and without any loss of time. In all humility we should avoid rigid or dogmatic prescriptions and admit here that what is proposed in general terms must be enhanced with the unique understanding of each community and with new observations which will continue to add wisdom and relevance in the future, until one day when this paradigm, too, will be abandoned, replaced by the reality of Health for All.

References

1. Kuhn, T. (1970). *The Structure of Scientific Revolutions.* The University of Chicago Press, Chicago, (second edition).
2. Beralanffy, L. Von. (1972). *General Systems Theory.* George Brazillier, New York.
3. Mauldin, W. P. and Berelson, B. (1978). Condition of fertility decline in developing countries, 1965–1975. *Studies in Family Planning.* Vol. 9, pp. 89–148
4. Rosers-Bixby, L. (1986). Infant mortality in Costa Rica: explaining the recent decline. *Studies in Family Planning.* Vol. 17, pp. 57–65.
5. McKeown, T. (1976). *The Role of Medicine: Dream, Mirage or Nemesis?* Nuffield Provincial Hospital Trust, London.
6. Halstead, S. B., Walsh, J. A. and Warren, K. S. (eds). (1985). *Good Health at Low Cost.* Proceedings of a Conference held at Bellagio Conference Center, 29 April–3 May 1985, Rockefeller Foundation, New York, pp. 248.

I V

Interventions on a Global Scale

COMMON GOALS AND APPROACHES

During the 1980s a major development that accelerated progress towards 'Health for All' was the launching of international efforts to combat some important health problems that afflict populations across the globe. The successful eradication of smallpox in the 1970s led to the recognition that other diseases could be controlled by world-wide efforts. The less-developed countries were aided by developed countries which controlled substantial financial and technological resources. Immunization had already proved itself as a technology, and could be applied to several serious diseases—diphtheria, pertussis, tetanus, polio and measles—which were taking their toll of child lives throughout the developing world. Other technologies and treatments began to emerge as candidates for global application—oral rehydration therapy to reduce mortality due to dehydration caused by diarrhoeas, and vitamin A to reduce morbidity and mortality caused by its defi- ciency. Countries also joined together to face yet another universal problem that has been closely related to ill-health and under-development—high fertility. While the prophets of doom continued to predict the dire consequences of population growth on the global environment, scientific developments increased the range of available contraceptive technologies. People throughout the world began to believe in 'social and economic progress through smaller families' and sought contraception of their choice. Epidemiological analysis showed that the spacing of births increased child survival so that those families who believed that they needed to have many children to ensure the survival of a few could be assisted through family planning and other simple technologies to reduce child mortality and thereafter their fertility. This section focuses on four major global efforts which have led to more health for many, and which promise to make still greater contributions to 'Health for All' in the decade ahead.

The Expanded Programme of Immunization (EPI) was the most technocentric top-down public health approach of the 1980s. Built upon the lessons of the smallpox eradication effort, it attempted to provide the benefits of immunization, a highly effective, reliable and modern technology to even larger numbers. As Terrel Hill, Robert Kim-Farley and Jon Rohde discuss, while the EPI effort succeeded in reaching its goal of 80 per cent coverage of infants by the end of 1990, success was due only in part to the centrally-designed top-down approach which had used standardized methods in the choice of vaccines, vaccination schedules, training, supervision, evaluation and so on. Success in reaching the goals of EPI was also due in large measure to the social mobilization which occurred on an unprecedented scale. This mobilization utilized and demonstrated the effectiveness of communication strategies as well as that of people outside the health sector. It also showed the critical role that political forces can play in reaching public health goals. This experience establishes that with careful planning and extensive mobilization some basic health services can indeed be delivered universally.

The chronicle of oral rehydration therapy (ORT), the 'twin engine' with immunization of primary health care technologies, demonstrates the complexity of applying an 'appropriate' health technology in the varied circumstances of many different developing countries. Robert Northrup describes in detail how ORT has become an integral part of every health system. Decision-makers and managers have been faced with difficult choices when wishing to ensure that this life-saving technique is available widely. The involvement of mothers and appropriate training of workers have been central to the effort to provide ORT in homes and health centres alike. While the intricacy of this effort illustrates the wide range of approaches used to operationalize a simple health technology, the overall experience shows, perhaps better than any other, why it is difficult to implement 'everything at once' in primary health care.

TECHNOLOGICAL DEVELOPMENTS AND DIFFUSION

The story of the discovery of the mortality-reducing effect of vitamin A illustrates the difficulties inherent in moving a scientific finding into the realm of an applied technology. When scientists encounter a new and exciting finding they must yet question what weight of evidence is required for its application in the field. Alfred Sommer describes how a well-designed field study led to the unexpected observation that vitamin A supplementation reduced child mortality. He points out the difficulties of obtaining action by programme implementors on the basis of new scientific evidence. The mortality-reducing effects of vitamin A supplements were found to be dramatic—almost 'too good to believe', which occasioned calls for further field trials. But what are the ethics of withholding benefits while further evidence is sought? Is a controlled trial ethical when an intervention is shown to save lives? How does one decide that a new technique should be used? How do we decide to make new investments in public health activities at all?

The issues raised in this chapter have great relevance to future technological developments such as those of new vaccines, some of which are available (such as Hepatitis B vaccine) and others which will come on stream during the decade ahead. At what point should these be included in immunization programmes? What proof should be required of their efficacy, safety and impact? Early results with the Edmundson–Zagreb measles vaccine, which promised protection at a younger age, were obfuscated by further studies which showed a possible detrimental effect leading to increased mortality. When is the evidence enough to go to scale? This difficult question must be faced as scientific advances occur rapidly in areas of new technologies with potential for massive application.

The development of contraceptive technologies has occurred amid many similar concerns. Nevertheless, a wide range of methods is available today. John Rowley and Halfdan Mahler discuss the importance of providing birth spacing as an integral part of health care for the well-being of mothers, children and society at large. Their plea is all the more poignant in the context of the Goals for the 1990s of the World Summit for Children. Each goal would be advanced by effective fertility control, and most of the goals cannot be accomplished unless substantial declines are realized in the rate of population growth. Concerns well beyond the health sector are also dependent upon effective fertility reduction. The strains on the environment, predominantly from pollution and high-consumption Western societies, are being exacerbated at a local level throughout the developing world and threaten to destroy the very ecology that sustains life. Recognition of this evolving disaster has led as notable a public health figure as Maurice King to propose the unthinkable strategy of allowing children to die to offset burgeoning populations.

But family planning services offer a far more effective and humane approach as Haryono Suyono, Lukas Hendrata and Jon Rohde describe in the chapter on the family planning movement in Indonesia. While this experience is that of a single large nation, it has important lessons for global efforts at population control. Based on a communication strategy and a new societal concept—a desire for a small, happy, prosperous family—rather than on a service and technology approach, this family planning programme has mobilized communities at the lowest level. A wide variety of approaches has been used to facilitate the participation of entire communities in the national family planning effort and to encourage widespread adoption of modern methods of contraception. Combined with excellent and reliable service delivery, the 'demand approach' evolved to make Indonesia's family planning programme one of the most effective in the world. The halving of the total fertility rate in only two decades is dramatic. It promises to ensure that Indonesia will continue to progress in other sectors—health and economic—as a result of this effective, community-based nation-wide approach to family planning. Similar success could be achieved if nations across the globe were to join hands in promoting humane approaches to family planning within a context of shared responsibility for our 'one world'.

SOME GLOBAL CONCERNS

These several experiences raise different sets of issues and questions. The achievement of universal immunization occurred in a context of technological diffusion, expert management of health systems, mobilization of many different sections of societies and political will. One might ask:

— What are the conditions that enable the diffusion of technology? How are health systems prepared to receive and disseminate technologies? How much popular support and political will is really required?
— What are the gains and losses to individual countries when they are pressured by international agencies to participate in such global ventures? What are the bases of national independence, dependence and inter-dependence?
— Are there conflicts between considerations of 'scale', 'quality' and 'efficiency' within and across countries?
— How can the experience of a single health intervention be built upon in order to progress towards comprehensive 'Health for All'? What compromises, if any, need to be made? Issues of cost and efficiency need to be considered.

The situation with ORT has been somewhat different. Policy-makers and implementors have been faced with more choices. The involvement of household members is almost a *sine qua non* of the technology. Thus, some key questions are:

— What is the correct mix between fostering people's health education and understanding of health care and 'packaged solutions' which can be delivered by health workers?
— What are the relative roles of the health system and other 'systems' (e.g. education, markets) in spreading 'home-based' technologies? What are the inherent trade-offs of different approaches *or* how can they be made complementary?

Poised for a similar global initiative, vitamin A is still enmeshed in questions regarding the interaction of science, policy and ethics:

— What criteria should be used when deciding whether a technological advance should be made available to people? Who should decide?
— How can health systems implement quick-result, often costlier, solutions efficiently without compromising longer-term, perhaps surer, approaches to a problem?

Finally, about family planning:

— What are the ethics of promoting family planning for global goals given the vast socio-economic differences between countries and between families within countries? Indeed, are smaller families even *possible* without substantially greater equity among families, communities and nations?
— What are the alternatives to an effective family planning effort? Can countries wait for the 'natural' decline in fertility accompanying development? How is this best accelerated?

CHAPTER 18

Expanded Programme on Immunization: A Goal Achieved Towards Health for All

TERREL HILL, ROBERT KIM-FARLEY AND JON ROHDE

The authors describe the global effort during the 1980s that led to the achievement of 80 per cent universal immunization by 1990. They describe the ingredients of this success and draw out the lessons learned from the experiences of many countries that are relevant to the goal of universal primary health care.

Terrel Hill, Ph.D., directed the UNICEF effort in the Expanded Programme on Immunization (EPI) and is now the head of UNICEF health programmes in New York.

Robert Kim-Farley, M.D., was EPI Adviser epidemiologist to the WHO South East Asia Region through much of the 1980s, before moving to Geneva as Global Chief of EPI for WHO.

Jon Rohde, M.D., has worked as Special Adviser in health to UNICEF programmes throughout the world, especially in South Asia.

THE BEGINNINGS OF EPI

Immunization has been practised for the past 200 years but, until the past few decades, had only a marginal effect on the protection of populations against infectious disease. A major breakthrough occurred during the 1960s and early 1970s as the great killer, smallpox, was eliminated by a massive global immunization campaign. The success of this effort was due in part to advances in technology which enabled the vaccine to be freeze-dried and transported without refrigeration, and to be administered simply by the prick of a specially-designed double-pointed needle. It was also due to the important understanding that smallpox could be controlled by rapid and careful identification of new cases, and immunization of those living in the immediate vicinity of any new smallpox case. Thus, in contrast to efforts to immunize entire populations, the eradication of smallpox was accomplished through surveillance and case containment, with vaccination of contacts only.

In 1974, following this success, the World Health Organization established the Expanded Programme on Immunization (EPI) to protect children against tuberculosis, measles, diphtheria, whooping cough (pertussis), tetanus and polio. This programme was led and managed for over a decade by Dr Rafe Henderson whose energy played a major role in its success. It was estimated that approximately five million children died each year during the late 1970s from these six diseases. These deaths, which could be prevented in a safe and cost-effective manner through immunization programmes (Table 1), represented as much as one-third of all deaths occurring among children under the age of five in the world each year.

Table 1. Estimated number of child deaths from EPI diseases, 1980

Disease	Deaths (in '000)
Measles	2700
Pertussis	1200
Neonatal tetanus	1200
Diphtheria	100
Polio	40
Tuberculosis	30
Total	5270

Source: WHO EPI Division, Geneva

It was recognized that successful immunization programmes would require strengthening of primary health care facilities and improvements in the training of health workers. Health services would increasingly need to reach into all communities of the developing world to deliver timely immunization to children and mothers. As vaccines were not heat-stable, an unbroken chain of refrigeration was required to extend from the manufacturer of the vaccine to the clinic or vaccination point. This 'cold chain' includes cold-rooms, freezers, refrigerators, cold-boxes, vaccine-carriers, ice-producers, and an effective management and maintenance system to ensure their continued proper functioning. Safe immunization would require syringes and needles in unprecedented quantities, with greater attention to sterility and safety than previously. Along with an adequate supply of vaccination services, widespread public information was needed to ensure that parents would make appropriate use of immunization services in the first year of a child's life. Thus, a new level of health education and mobilization of communication resources beyond anything previously seen in the health sector was required.

TOWARDS UNIVERSAL CHILDHOOD IMMUNIZATION

Following the establishment of EPI, immunization programmes were initiated in many developing countries in the late 1970s. However, by 1980, global coverage levels of infants and young children were no greater than 20 per cent. In 1977 the World Health Assembly had challenged the countries of the world to provide immunization services for all children, or Universal Childhood Immunization (UCI) by the year 1990.* Many considered this goal unrealistic, virtually unattainable. However, during the following decade, a great international movement was created, giving an entirely new meaning to social mobilization.

In 1982 UNICEF launched the Child Survival and Development Revolution, which included immunization along with other cost-effective, high-impact interventions in its 'GOBI–FFF package'.** Collaboration between international supporting agencies intensified in 1984 with the building of an international coalition called the 'Task Force for Child Survival', which included UNICEF, WHO, UNDP, the World Bank, and the Rockefeller Foundation. In 1985 the United Nations General Assembly affirmed full support for the goal of UCI 1990, and 74 governments, along with more than 400 voluntary agencies, pledged to achieve that goal in commemoration of the fortieth anniversary of the United Nations. International funding was significantly increased, with pledges of more than $100 million each by Rotary International and the Government of Italy. Highly publicized national vaccination days in Colombia and Turkey enhanced the conviction of many other countries that substantial progress could be achieved through major efforts at national social mobilization.

Nearly all countries had established accelerated immunization pro-

---

*The 1990 target towards 'Universal Childhood Immunization' was later operationally defined as 80 per cent coverage of children by their first birthday with the following: one dose of BCG, 3 doses of DPT, 3 doses of polio, and one dose of measles vaccine. The African Ministers of Health set a regional target of 75 per cent, while China selected 85 per cent as its target at national, provincial and county levels.

**GOBI–FFF includes Growth Monitoring, Oral Rehydration, Breastfeeding, Immunization, Family Spacing, Female Education and Food Supplements.

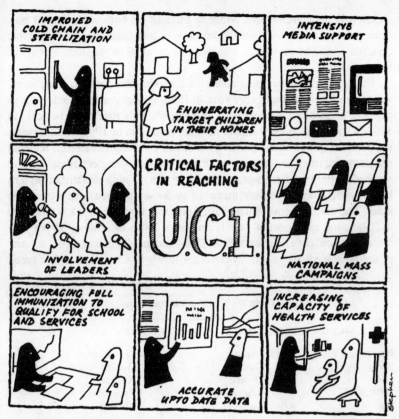

grammes by 1987, utilizing a variety of strategies to improve immunization coverage and strengthen their health care delivery systems and outreach. Strategies were as diverse as: national vaccination days; the involvement of religious leaders, teachers, or politicians; intensive media support; increasing the capacity of health services to give immunization to children at every contact with the health system; identifying and registering eligible children and women in their homes, and careful tracking of each child to ensure completion of the immunization schedule by the first birthday; mandating or encouraging full immunization to qualify for school or other government services, or even before performing religious rites. Immunization was carried out in public by heads of state in Colombia, Turkey, Indonesia and Syria, and by doctors, health workers and volunteers from all levels of society. National days of tranquillity were set aside amidst tumultuous civil conflicts in El Salvador and Lebanon to allow people to protect the lives of children in all communities. Warring factions on both sides ceased hostilities, not just once but annually on three or four occasions, to ensure that children would be protected, whatever the political or religious identity of their parents.

The number of developing countries achieving the immunization coverage targets has increased every year. In 1986, sixteen countries achieved 80 per cent or greater coverage with all antigens. This rose to 34 per cent in 1988, 43 per cent in 1989 and 64 per cent at the end of 1990. With increasing public attention to the global goal, countries strengthened their national programmes, often exceeding even their own highest expectations. Having reached 85 per cent coverage nationally by 1985, China established an ambitious programme to ensure that even under-served areas came up to the mark. The national government called on each province to reach this level by 1988, and each county (numbering over 3000) to achieve 85 per cent immunization coverage by 1990. This immense task has been accomplished—indeed, surpassed, as coverage levels in China currently exceed

Table 2. UCI 1990 achievements

---

64 COUNTRIES REACHED UCI FOR ALL ANTIGENS

Bhutan	Jordan	Saint Vincent
Brunei	Kuwait	Turks & Caicos
China	Oman	Uruguay
D.P.R. Korea	Saudi Arabia	Botswana
Fiji	Syria	Burundi
Hong Kong	Tunisia	Cape Verde
India	Anguilla	C. African Rep.
Indonesia	Antigua	Comoros
Malaysia	Argentina	Congo
Maldives	Barbados	Equat. Guinea
Philippines	Belize	Gabon
Republic of Korea	Brit. Virgin Is.	Gambia
Singapore	Chile	Lesotho
Sri Lanka	Colombia	Malawi
Thailand	Costa Rica	Mauritius
Vietnam	Cuba	Mozambique*
Algeria	Dominica	Seychelles
Bahrain	Monserrat	Sierra Leone
Djibouti	Panama	Swaziland
Egypt	Saint Kitts	Tanzania
Iran	Saint Lucia	Zambia

---

*Achieved in areas under Government control

95 per cent. Tanzania and Botswana achieved high levels of coverage through routine services and have been successful in maintaining these levels for more than two years. Oman, with a well-managed programme which follows all new-borns and catches drop-outs, has maintained greater than 80 per cent coverage since 1987.

By the end of 1990 the global target of 80 per cent was reached for all antigens. The success of this effort served to reduce mortality from EPI diseases by three million deaths and reduce paralytic polio by over 400 000 cases in 1990 alone. An estimated 15 million deaths have been prevented during the decade. Reports from many countries document significant measured reductions in polio cases and pertussis-, tetanus-, and measles-related deaths. Illness and mortality from related diseases such as malnutrition, diarrhoea and pneumonia have reduced as well. A report from Bangladesh documented a 40 per cent decrease in child deaths from diarrhoea and pneumonia following measles vaccine alone.[1] In addition, immunization programmes have substantially strengthened the capacity of primary health care services in numerous developing countries to reach out, in an unprecedented way to under-served populations, providing other essential services on a reliable and regular basis. Health ministries did not achieve this goal alone—whole societies were mobilized. High-level political support and multi-sectoral cooperation helped to marshall the required resources of manpower, money and materials, and more importantly to foster a broad

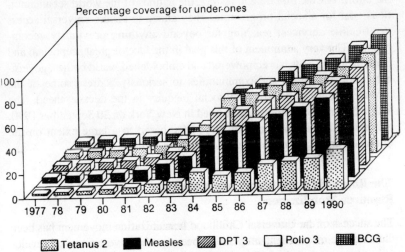

Fig. 1. Immunization coverage 1977–90. Global data from EPI
Information System, August 1991. (Data before 1984 are estimated.)

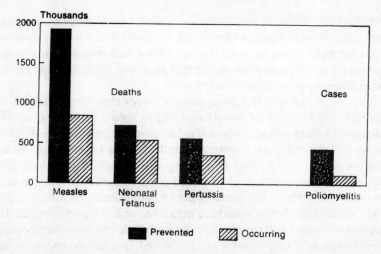

Fig. 2. Cases of and deaths from EPI diseases prevented in 1990 in developing countries. EPI Information System, August 1991.

social understanding and public motivation to ensure full immunization for every child by the age of one year.

The impact of immunization programmes on child deaths and disability alone would justify the effort made, but far more has been accomplished in the effort. For the first time in history, the nations of the world set an ambitious goal for a social programme. They aimed to ensure universal access to effective services, reaching far beyond anything previously accomplished. The very attainment of this goal in the face of great scepticism and overwhelming odds has empowered and emboldened world bodies, governments, organizations and communities to seriously address some of the worst elements of poverty and social inequity in the decade ahead. The World Summit for Children, convened in New York on 30 September 1990, announced ambitious goals for the 1990s, based to a large extent on the optimism arising from the success of EPI.

The Role of International Cooperation and Resource Mobilization

The success of the Universal Childhood Immunization movement has been the outcome of excellent cooperation between the governments of developing countries and the international donor community. During the 1980s, nearly US $500 million were contributed to immunization programmes through UNICEF alone. During this same period, approximately $47 million was contributed by a broad coalition of donors through WHO, in addition to another $56 million provided through the regular WHO budget.

In addition to the UN agencies, major donors for the global immunization programme have been the governments of Canada, Italy, Norway, Sweden, the United Kingdom, the United States, Australia, Denmark, Netherlands, Finland and Japan, and the non-governmental organization Rotary International. The Government of Italy provided more than $150 million between 1986 and 1990, lending major support to 27 African countries and several in Central America and Asia. Sweden has been a significant contributor to countries such as India, Bangladesh, Sri Lanka and Angola both through UNICEF and WHO, and bilaterally. The United States Agency for International Development contributed over $300 million to the global effort. The governments of Sweden, Canada and the United States have been primary donors to India's Universal Immunization Programme. Denmark has contributed significantly to the Kenyan and Tanzanian programmes.

In 1985 Canada launched its special International Immunization Programme managed by the Canadian Public Health Association in cooperation with a wide range of voluntary organizations. This programme, called 'A Miracle in the Making', supported 95 projects in 44 countries with over $40 million. Rotarians world-wide launched their well-known 'Polio Plus' initiative in 1986, with a target to raise $120 million by the year 2005. Over $220 million had been raised by 1990, and donations continue to come in. Perhaps of greater importance, hundreds of thousands of Rotarians have been involved in community mobilization activities in communities throughout the world in support of immunization. In the Americas interagency coordinating committees involving PAHO, UNICEF, USAID, Canada and Rotary, were established by host governments, ensuring a remarkable degree of programme coordination in each country. It has been estimated that a total of $112 million were contributed by external agencies towards the EPI in the Americas in the period 1987–91, of which $34 million were provided through PAHO from regular budget and grant funds.

UNICEF and WHO have worked together to ensure the availability of reliable, safe, low-cost vaccines through international procurement. Through UNICEF alone, a total of over 4.4 billion doses have been procured since 1982 at a cost of nearly US $200 million. Under the new Children's Vaccine Initiative, countries may soon be able to introduce new and improved vaccines developed by the most modern techniques of molecular engineering and purchased at the lowest prices through international tender.

Table 3. Calendar of key mobilization events

1974	EPI established
1977	Last case of smallpox
1977	World Health Assembly set UCI 1990 Goal
1978	Health for All Conference at Alma Ata, USSR
1982	Child Survival and Development Revolution launched
1984	Task Force for Child Survival established at Bellagio
1984	Operation Commando in Burkina Faso
1984	National Vaccination Crusade in Colombia
1985	UNICEF Executive Board and United Nations General Assembly affirm support for UCI 1990 with 'We The People' Declaration
1985	Second Child Survival Task Force meeting at Cartagena, Colombia
1985	Canada launches an international programme for support of immunization
1985	National Immunization Campaign in Turkey
1985	Government of Italy pledges support for immunization
1986	Rotary International 'Polio Plus' programme launched
1986	African Immunization Year
1988	Third Child Survival Task Force meeting at Talloires, France
1990	Fourth Child Survival Task Force meeting at Bangkok, Thailand
1990	World Summit for Children

WHO has provided technical and biological standards for vaccines, and assisted vaccine manufacturers to meet these standards and shipping requirements. In addition, the World Bank and Rotary International have assisted China in domestic production of vaccines, ensuring long-term self-reliant and sustainable programmes. India already produces all vaccines required for its EPI, except for bulk oral polio vaccine for which a national manufacturing capacity is presently being built. Other large countries are increasingly developing their own capacity and independence in vaccine manufacture. It will be necessary to help them enforce good manufacturing practices and to ensure vaccine quality through competent national authorities.

The cost of immunizing a child can be calculated by many methods and has been found to vary greatly from country to country. The lowest estimates measure only the incremental costs of vaccines, transport and supplies, while higher estimates account for the entire range of salaries, vehicles, buildings, sterilizers and the like. An average of $13 per child is generally accepted as a global approximation of the cost of full immunization. This implies that some US $1 billion are required per year to maintain current levels of coverage, about two-thirds of which is borne by the developing countries themselves. The remaining $300 to $400 million will need to be contributed by external sources each year throughout the decade ahead.

In addition to the resources to maintain current EPI operations, additional resources will be required for the activities planned for polio eradication, neonatal tetanus elimination and measles reduction in the 1990s. Furthermore, new vaccines against hepatitis, haemophilus influenza, pneumococcus and perhaps against diarrhoea will require considerably more resources. Funds are needed for their development and procurement, for retraining workers and for the capital and maintenance costs of equipment required to administer them.

THE LESSONS LEARNED

Immunization is now the most widely available health service throughout the developing world. The lessons learned are many, some specific to immunization, many others relevant to achieving high coverage with all primary health services. Starting with the universal objective and clear strategies, the EPI experience demonstrates the crucial roles of political will, social mobilization, innovative use of mass media, and simple, reliable management information systems.

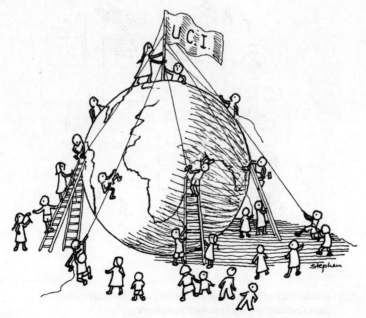

Policies, Goals and Objectives

Clarity in programme objectives and the operational strategy were major factors which facilitated the expansion of this programme in a few years. Unlike malnutrition, diarrhoeal diseases and other illnesses, the immunizable diseases can be prevented by discreet action at specified times. Immunization schedules can be standardized, made precise and uniform everywhere. As preventive action, immunization services can be organized to ensure maximal efficiency, in contrast with curative treatment services which must be ready and waiting to respond to illness whenever it occurs. The technical areas of immunization were developed and refined under the leadership of the WHO Expanded Programme on Immunization Global Advisory Group, so that aspects such as vaccines, immunization schedules and contra-indications became almost universally accepted by the medical profession, programme managers and families throughout the world. The im-

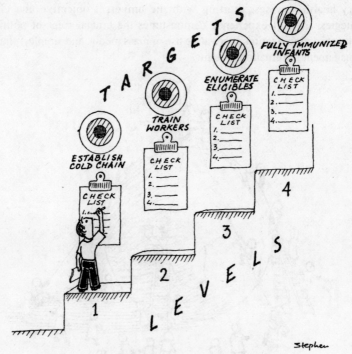

Immunization comprised a concise set of activities enabling standardized work plans and monitoring.

munization process is easily understood by lay persons; and in many societies injections are viewed as 'sophisticated medicine', and are widely popular. The goals of universal coverage were readily understood by political leaders and communities at large and could be translated into local statistics. Accountability for service provision could be demanded at each level. Overall, the clarity and standardization of this programme and its potential for accountability made it an ideal intervention as a first step towards Universal Primary Health Care.

Political Will and Social Mobilization

The drive for Universal Childhood Immunization during the 1980s was unprecedented in that a health programme became a social programme, crossing sectors and levels of society. Beginning with President Betancourt of Colombia in 1984, more than 30 heads of state lent their personal prestige and political support to immunization activities. Their roles varied from publicly launching campaigns and appearing on television or on posters to personally organizing and regularly overseeing the national immunization system to monitor progress. Even in countries where leadership changed midstream, political support transcended personalities and parties as immunization goals were adopted by the new leaders. The high level of central support ensured that political priority for immunization was maintained at provincial, district and community levels. Support has been sustained largely because of the attractiveness and clarity of the message that all children can be protected through an easily-understandable and affordable intervention, its administration can be monitored on a regular basis and workers can be held accountable.

The large-scale national immunization days of the mid-1980s relied upon hundreds of temporary immunization points and thousands of non-health workers to assist in delivery of immunization services. These were useful to initiate the acceleration phase, although many countries which used these strategies eventually had difficulties maintaining high levels of coverage through a routine delivery system. Turkey and Syria utilized temporary immunization sites in mosques or schools during their national campaigns, but later were unable to maintain the level of coverage reached during the campaign year. Continued mobilization was required to reach and sustain high coverage. In contrast, Tunisia, which has a complete health infrastructure, was able to push coverage up quickly with accelerated activities in a single year and maintained nearly 90 per cent coverage during subsequent years. The Philippines, Indonesia and Bangladesh opted to move more gradually, expanding routine access to services, increasing staff training, and extending outreach to each village community. India phased activities over a period of five years, covering groups of districts each year, reaching universal access only in 1990. Late in that year, intensive nation-wide campaigns were launched to augment the regular, reliable, monthly provision of immunization services in each of the country's 600 000 vil-lages. The guarantee of a monthly service in each community enabled India to achieve its goal of 80 per cent coverage by the end of the year.

Very few countries would have been able to reach and maintain 80 per cent or greater coverage without broad promotional efforts. Those few ex-ceptions, such as Sri Lanka, Gambia and Costa Rica, had excellent health care systems which already had the capacity to reach into communities and follow up immunization defaulters. Stories of remarkable effort and inno-vation characterize the EPI in most countries.

Sierra Leone used the period from 1986 through 1990 to completely build a health delivery system in much of the country. Prior to that time the population had almost no access to services, especially immunization. By the end of 1990 more than 80 per cent of infants received the third dose of DPT and polio. Seventy-five per cent received measles immunization.

The Philippines reached more than 80 per cent coverage for all antigens in 1989 and maintained this level in 1990. The programme has expanded to provide universal access as a fully-integrated element of a national PHC programme without using a campaign approach. National success was en-sured through special efforts in lower performing provinces and urban areas.

Indonesia reached the 80 per cent target in November 1990. The infra-structure and capacity to deliver immunization at the village level was care-fully developed during the 1980s. In 1985, the national nutrition and family planning weighing posts were integrated with the EPI programme to form an integrated service point at the hamlet level.* The Government gave high priority to expanding this network to all villages in the country and concur-rently established near-universal access to monthly or bimonthly immuni-zation services. President Suharto gave personal support to the programme and extensive social mobilization has been achieved at all levels.

Bangladesh has made phenomenal progress since 1985 when coverage was less than 10 per cent. UCI was adopted as a high priority by the Gov-ernment and strongly supported by the donor community. The EPI infra-structure was expanded from eight *upazilas* (sub-districts) in 1986 to all 460

*See the chapter on Indonesia's *Posyandus* by Jon Rohde in this book.

by the end of 1989. Extensive social mobilization was the focus of the last year's activities, which emphasized reducing drop-out rates and completing the full series before the first birthday. Many non-governmental organizations (NGOs), in addition to the family planning network, provided extensive support. By 1990 entire areas of the country exceeded global goals and overall coverage exceeded 60 per cent.

In Vietnam a special ceremony was held to celebrate the achievement of 80 per cent coverage on the one-hundredth birthday of the late President Ho Chi Minh. Immense political will resulted in a high priority for immunization at all levels, although a government health infrastructure has not been developed uniformly throughout the country. Remote and mountainous areas still require a campaign approach to reach high levels of performance. Drop-out rates have been significantly reduced through the successful enumeration of children at the community level.

Nigeria implemented a phased expansion of the programme to reach all 400 areas by 1989. Immunization days were first held nationally and then at state and local government levels during 1989 and 1990. Additional initiatives to expand coverage and reduce drop-out rates included house-to-house immunization, enumeration of babies by NGOs and community health workers, and mobilization through primary school teachers and pupils. The costs of cold-chain and social mobilization activities were borne by local governments. The Federal Government has continued to finance most of the EPI vaccines.

Ethiopia, Mozambique and the Sudan were able to achieve high levels of coverage in regions under government control by concentrating on those areas with routine PHC systems. In fact a recent survey in 26 cities of Mozambique found coverage over 80 per cent for all antigens; a remarkable 72 per cent of pregnant women had received tetanus toxoid. The northern regions of Sudan have also achieved 80 per cent coverage for all antigens except measles. Children in the southern areas of Sudan have also been immunized with the assistance of NGOs working in collaboration with UNICEF and with the concurrence of both the Government and the insurgents.

The quest for UCI forced the health systems in many countries to initiate extensive collaboration outside the health sector, often for the first time. Wide and innovative use was made of the influence and goodwill of religious leaders to promote immunization. From Moslem leaders in the Middle East and Asia to Christian priests in South America and Buddhist monks in Asia, religious leaders have played a key role in convincing parents of their responsibility to immunize children. Promotional materials

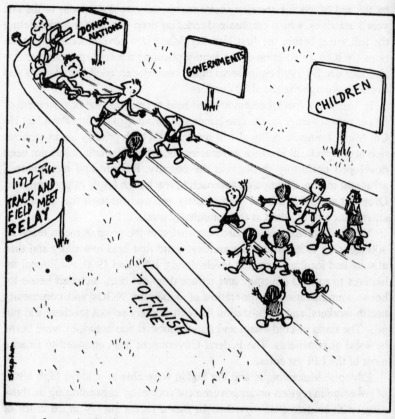

Immunization brought a new degree of donor, government and popular collaboration to accomplish a global goal.

have been developed on the basis of religious texts and teachings. These can now be used to promote other health interventions as well.

Mass media, television, radio, printed materials, puppets and traditional forms of entertainment were used to educate and encourage communities to protect children through immunization. Political commitment to UCI resulted in the allotment of free air-time on television and radio. Widely-known media personalities such as the actress Audrey Hepburn and the cricketer Imran Khan appeared in support of UCI. In many countries immunization messages were aired at prime-time. Innovation has been extensive. Immunization logos, mottos and messages have been printed upon items as ubiquitous as match-boxes, flour bags, cement bags, postage stamps, city buses and food containers.

Worker Outreach and Accountability

The clarity of immunization objectives and the ability to translate national targets into local goals allowed catchment areas to be defined in which health workers had a clear idea of who they were to immunize. This also created important opportunities for community and local government leaders to supervise and coordinate the mobilization of resources which enabled them to provide important support to the usually under-paid health worker. The 80 per cent target also called for a more complete development of outreach systems into communities. The popularity of immunization and the links forged between health workers and communities served to raise the profile and status of health workers.

Information Systems for Management

In 1980 most developing countries did not have adequately-functioning health reporting systems, and consequently could not assess programme performance. The EPI supported the development of national management information systems to record, collect and forward coverage data to higher levels. Computer programmes were written to facilitate this process and were implemented in many countries. The 30-cluster immunization coverage survey technique was developed as a relatively inexpensive method to accurately assess coverage in a defined population and to monitor the validity of routine reporting of immunization. Data collected in a single day under the guidance of one or two experienced field directors was used as a flexible field monitoring tool. In most countries the cost was only a few hundred dollars per survey. In some countries such as India, these surveys have become a routine part of an annual self-evaluation exercise in over 400 districts.

The cluster survey has also been a central tool for more comprehensive programme evaluations carried out periodically with teams from government and donor agencies which support the programme. Following a globally standardized format, these expert teams assisted country managers to identify problem areas in programme operations and regions of the country which were performing less well than desired. They also provided opportunities for donors to witness first-hand the achievements and constraints of the programme, and ways in which they could best provide further support.

The surveys have led frequently to effective micro-planning and problem-solving exercises at district and lower levels of the health system. Decentralized management has been able to identify and solve problems and work towards well-defined goals following established guidelines. The ability to track progress towards clear objective goals and targets for each level of the system fostered a high degree of accountability among workers and their collaborating partners, which contributed to the accomplishment of the 1990 target.

Improved Technology

One of the major challenges to the global immunization programme has been to protect vaccines from heat during the long journey from manufacturer to remote immunization points in each developing country. Vaccines must be kept within a specified range of cold temperatures at all times. The EPI logistics unit at WHO provided specifications for cold chain, sterilization and injection equipment, and assisted a number of countries in the indigenous production of refrigeration equipment reaching international standards and prices. Cold boxes to store and transport vaccines maintaining low temperatures for two to three days were a key factor, especially in the most remote areas. Local production to international standards made them both cheap and available. The EPI and UNICEF have seen exceptional collaboration between governments and the private sector in the development of improved equipment to store and transport vaccines, as well as to provide safe injections.

A number of technological developments have also occurred. Solar-powered refrigerators, though still expensive, have proved their worth in many remote areas of Africa and Asia. Kerosene refrigerators have been improved to function on the lower quality of fuel available in most countries. Special temperature indicators have been extensively used to monitor the status of the cold chain at all levels. Steam sterilization with small portable autoclaves have been promoted along with the use of affordable, reusable plastic and glass sterilizable syringes. Technical support from international organizations to local industries has enabled increasing indigenization of other equipment as well, an important prerequisite for long-term sustainability. Many of these technical innovations in support of immunization have been of relevance and importance to the broader range of health activities conducted at primary health facilities throughout the developing world.

TOWARDS PRIMARY HEALTH CARE

The immunization effort has strengthened other areas of primary health care in many ways. Extensive attention to sterilization of injection equipment has extended to a range of other health centre equipment to protect against the spread of AIDS and hepatitis. Concern over the improper handling and repeated use of disposable syringes led to the development of a single-use disposable syringe which will become commercially available during 1992. These 'autodestruct' syringes will be supplied in a box which doubles as an incinerator, complete with a fuel stick. Acceleration of immunization, pursued over the 1990s, should help to achieve the goals of 90 per cent immunization coverage with all vaccines—eradication of polio, elimination of tetanus, and dramatic reduction of measles cases and deaths. It can also incorporate other vaccines—those already available for use in special populations: yellow fever, meningitis, Japanese B encephalitis, hepatitis B, pneumococcus, influenza; those already under testing: viral pneumonia, rotavirus, dengue; and those being developed against malaria, dysentery, tuberculosis, AIDS and other diseases.

Over the past five years, more than 500 000 health workers have been formally trained in standardized courses for peripheral workers, supervisors, medical officers and programme managers. The approach to training by objectives and establishing competency is relevant to training for many other health interventions to be conducted over the next ten years. The supervision of immunization activities has been increasingly performed by objective checklist assessment. This has led not only to improved accountability but, more importantly, to a supportive relationship between worker and supervisor. This has enabled achievement of specific goals of quality, standardization and coverage. Management by objectives is being practised today throughout primary health care systems in many developing countries.

The outreach developed for immunization can easily be used to deliver other health care. In the best-developed systems, house-to-house enumeration and enlisting of eligible mothers and their children on registers have established a system to identify, trace and follow-up every child born in the community. This basic principle of public health—enumeration of the target population—lays the groundwork for immunization and other preventive services, and for improved monitoring of vital events. It also provides a means to ensure the accountability of health workers to the populations they are serving.

In country after country the status of primary health care workers has improved as a result of their immunization activities. In some places these workers previously had focused major attention on a single disease or programme such as tuberculosis, malaria or family planning. With the provision of reliable immunization they are now seen as having more comprehensive skills, medical credibility and interest in community well-being.

In many countries immunization services are provided on a daily basis at 'fixed' health facilities as well as through outreach efforts to each village or community on at least one fixed day every month. The establishment of a reliable and regular service, conveniently located in the community, provides an opportunity for a full array of primary health care activities. By the end of 1990 approximately 80 per cent of the world's infants had at least five contacts with the health care system, totalling approximately 500 million contacts. While such contacts provided an excellent opportunity for health workers to offer additional services, both preventive and curative, the nature of the services has varied widely. Some outreach systems delivered vitamin A and other nutritional supplements on a periodic basis. They taught family members about diarrhoea and distributed oral rehydra-

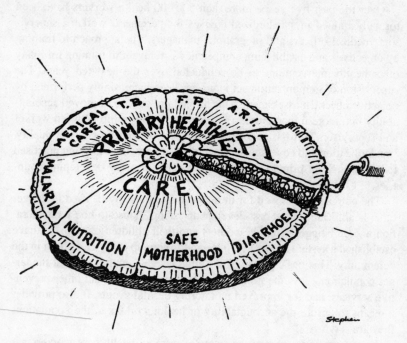

EPI—an important portion of the Primary Health Care pie.

tion packets for home use. Interacting with village midwives or volunteer community health workers, pregnant women were screened for ante-natal risk factors and were provided with tetanus toxoid immunization and also iron-folic acid tablets to overcome anaemia. They received information and guidance on nutrition, and referral for obstetric care during delivery.

During the past seven or eight years extensive debate has occurred over the issue of 'comprehensive' versus 'selective' primary health care. Some argue for a broad set of activities encompassing the entire array of health programmes and moving to scale only gradually as worker capacity, logistics, community demand and funding grow over the years. Others favour rapidly accelerating highly cost-effective interventions such as immunization programmes to serve as a 'cutting' or 'leading edge'. In fact the ultimate vision of both approaches is the same—a comprehensive health system. It is really only the timing that is at issue. Given that resources are finite, social justice and equity demand that all people should have access to at least the selective services that can provide significant reductions in suffering, disability and death. Immunization programmes have provided experience of simplicity, generating a critical mass of political will, achieving wide coverage with a preventive service, reaching the previously unreached, setting up management information and logistics systems, and developing an overall system which can progressively support a wider range of goals and services.

Following their positive experience with immunization promotion, several countries have initiated intensive social mobilization activities for diarrhoeal disease control and other health interventions. The wide use of modern mass media has lead to a greater appreciation of its potential for social marketing. The range of marketing activities, including research into knowledge and behaviour patterns made this a comprehensive marketing endeavour. The research provided deeper understanding of the population and enabled carefully-adjusted communication strategies, linked to regular feedback and redesign of messages. The result has been the creation of wide-scale behavioural change. The potential for applying this experience to a broad range of socially-desirable behaviours, even beyond health, is now obvious in many countries.

The World Summit for Children, in which over 150 countries participated, called for a wide array of new goals for the 1990s: reduction of infant and child mortality by one-third; reduction of maternal mortality by one-half, and halving of malnutrition rates, in addition to goals in the fields of education, water and sanitation. The experience of immunization in the 1980s has not only established a precedent for the enunciation of such ambitious goals but has also emboldened the leaders of the world, participating agencies, NGOs and communities to attempt to accomplish the impossible. The achievement of 80 per cent immunization coverage has convinced many that these goals, far broader in scope and ambition, can and must be reached. Their broad range will require an even greater level of dedication, higher degree of community involvement and even stronger political will. The success of UCI is the promise that even these ambitious and worthwhile goals can be accomplished before the world enters the next millennium.

Reference

1. Koenig, M. A., Khan, M. A., Wojtyniak, B. *et al.* (1990). Impact of measles vaccination on childhood mortality in rural Bangladesh. *Bulletin of World Health Organization*, Vol. 68, pp. 441–7.

CHAPTER 19

Oral Rehydration Therapy: From Principle to Practice

ROBERT NORTHRUP

The author describes the numerous strategies and steps involved in expanding access to and the use of oral rehydration therapy for diarrhoea. ORT has been used world-wide with considerable success and its story reveals the numerous challenges inherent in providing primary health care to all.

Robert Northrup, M.D., was involved in initial laboratory and clinical studies which led to the development of oral rehydration therapy in 1968. He was Technical Director of the USAID-sponsored PRITECH project to encourage ORT, and is presently Professor of Community Medicine at Brown University, Providence, Rhode Island, USA.

INTRODUCTION

Oral rehydration therapy for diarrhoea (ORT), the miracle discovery of the 1960s, is perhaps the single technology which best embodies the principles of primary health care. ORT is both a curative and preventive intervention. It involves both the health care system and the community. It is both an action that a health worker takes for a patient and an action which a child patient's mother can perform. ORT can be carried out with packets of Oral Rehydration Salts (ORS) from the commercial market or with ingredients found in the home. Thus it can be an important tool in implementing the principles of comprehensive Primary Health Care which stress empowering individuals and families to manage their own health problems.

ORT is a new technology. In its present form it was discovered less than 25 years ago.[1] In this short period it has made the transition from the laboratory to national programmes and widespread use by mothers and health workers in the developing world. This chapter reviews the steps of that transition and consequent achievements. It identifies tasks yet incomplete or not done and seeks lessons in this experience which are applicable to

Table 1. Steps to take ORT to scale

---

1. Laboratory animal and *in vitro* studies: elucidate principles of ORT.[2]
2. Clinical studies: demonstrate that ORT principle works in humans.[3]
3. Initial field studies: show that it can be applied in field situations.[4]
4. Clinical studies of home ingredient-based ORT.[5]
5. Pilot studies in communities.[6]
6. Formation of WHO Control of Diarrhoeal Diseases Programme.
7. Formation of national CDD programmes.
8. Spread of ORT to mothers and practitioners.

---

other health technologies and so potentially useful in solving large-scale public health problems.

A list of the steps involved in taking ORT from a laboratory finding to a massive public programme is given in Table 1. Each of these is itself the summary of a detailed process.

TAKING ORT TO SCALE

Initial laboratory research studies documented the basic principle of ORT, that intestinal sodium and water absorption is enhanced by glucose. By 1968 the correct proportions of these ingredients had been empirically devised and ORT was shown to be effective in cholera. Application of ORT in field hospitals and refugee camps demonstrated the life-saving effectiveness of ORT in the simplest clinical circumstances. Subsequent studies used solutions made from home ingredients (sugar and salt) in place of the complete formula. ORT was shown to be effective in replacing fluid and electrolyte losses in diarrhoea from all aetiologies in all age groups. The wide applicability of this robust technology led to the formation in 1979 of a special division within WHO, the Control of Diarrhoeal Diseases Programme. Over the past decade, as national CDD programmes have been established in 100 developing countries, people's access to ORS packets and to practitioners trained in ORT has gone from near zero to 58 per cent. In some countries and regions it is over 70 per cent. ORT is now estimated to be used in 32 per cent of diarrhoea episodes world-wide.[7] Evaluations in Egypt suggested that ORT was responsible for a 36 per cent reduction in infant mortality and a 43 per cent reduction in child mortality.[8]

In this brief period, ORT has truly 'gone to scale', reaching a level of acceptance and effective use able to produce an impact on entire countries. This wide application of scientific principles to a pressing public health problem is a modern demonstration of 'taking science where the diarrhoea is'.[9] The issues in this expansion have been technical, sociological and political, involving scientists, bureaucrats, trainers, health workers, communicators, community leaders and mothers everywhere. From international meetings to village gatherings, from government bureaucracies to private commercial enterprises, the story of taking ORT to scale touches all elements of the development process itself.

Defining the Technology

A critical initial step in making it available to all was to define it clearly. What was ORT? What exactly was to be promoted?

ORT was defined differently by different groups and the definition kept changing. There were many who saw ORT as a *product*, a packet of oral rehydration salts (ORS). For these persons the challenge of ORT programmes was primarily that of production and distribution. In contrast others saw ORT as a set of *behaviours*, ideally involving commonly-available home ingredients. They believed that the challenge was primarily one of public education and behavioural change. A third group—among them many medical workers—saw ORT as *a medical procedure* to be performed by well-trained doctors or nurses. However, others viewed ORT as a prime example of technology which could be de-medicalized, performed by mothers, thereby facilitating people's independence from medical and commercial systems.

Initially ORT meant fluid therapy for rehydration only. However, as understanding of effective diarrhoea treatment grew, the phrase 'oral rehydration therapy' was extended by some to include other elements of good clinical case management of diarrhoea, particularly feeding. Thus, it became 'oral therapy' more broadly. Various cereal starches could effectively replace sugar, adding more calories at less osmotic cost to the solution. Continued feeding during diarrhoea not only hastened recovery but was found to reduce the nutritional impact of illness and to lessen the likelihood of an acute diarrhoea episode evolving into the more dangerous persistent diarrhoea.

Packet or Home Solution—Promoting a Product or a Behaviour

The complete ORS formula incorporated into packets was the foundation of many national programmes. Egypt's National Control of Diarrhoeal Diseases Programme (NCDDP) was the most visible one using this approach.

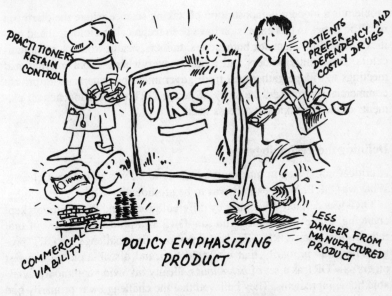

POLICY EMPHASIZING PRODUCT

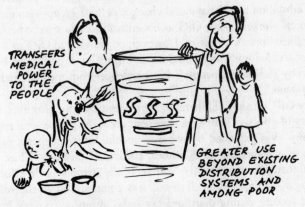

POLICY EMPHASIZING BEHAVIOUR

Top-down and bottom-up policies for ORT.

Packets of *Rehydran* were distributed through official government channels to government health centres and hospitals, and through a parastatal drug company to private pharmacies for sale directly to consumers. Although

some attention was given to home fluids, the programme primarily promoted use of solutions made from these packets. As a result, packet use
skyrocketed, covering as many as 70 per cent of diarrhoea episodes
throughout the country.

Pakistan intensified its national ORT efforts in a similar way. The EPI
Programme's vaccinators placed two packets of ORS in every home and
taught mothers how to mix and use the solution. This approach worked in
those parts of the country where the immunization programme was running
well. Millions of packets were distributed and mothers' use of ORT was
high. However, a year later when the need to resupply mothers arose, the
Ministry of Health realized that the recurrent cost of the large numbers of
ORS packets exceeded their budget. Foreseeing reductions in donor subsidies for ORS packets, the Ministry announced a new policy: that fluids
made from home ingredients, not packets, should be used by mothers at
home.

The approach emphasizing home-made ORT emerged from research
which showed that a solution made from household sugar and salt, if prepared accurately, was nearly as effective in preventing or treating dehydration from diarrhoea as the official ORS solution.[5] Indeed, much of the
enthusiasm for ORT of community-oriented PHC experts such as David
Werner in Mexico and David Sanders in Zimbabwe was based on the potential to empower families and communities to control diarrhoeal disease
themselves by just this mechanism: preparation of fluids from simple materials available in almost every home.[10,11] In Nigeria, O. Ransome Kuti had
observed that the availability of ORS packets in the early 1970s led mothers
to stop using the sugar–salt solution (SSS) which they had previously been
taught to make. SSS had lost its perceived value. This led to a policy decision in Nigeria to forbid the distribution of ORS packets from government
health facilities. All patients were to be encouraged to use SSS prepared
from home materials. The more complete ORS solution prepared from packets would be administered only *at* health facilities to those children who
had not responded to the simpler SSS given at home. The educational emphasis was to be on instructing mothers how to prepare and give SSS at
home.

The Bangladesh Rural Advancement Committee (BRAC), a non-governmental development agency, realized that it would be logistically very
difficult and prohibitively expensive to provide packets throughout the
country. Accordingly they launched a programme based on SSS which
reached all 13 million homes in the country within a decade (see the chapter
by Lovell and Abed in this book). Field-workers hired by BRAC visited

each household and taught seven critical points about diarrhoea, including the preparation of 'lobon-gur'.[12]*

The BRAC programme was particularly unique because it utilized a house-to-house teaching approach, but was able to cover the entire population of Bangladesh in ten years. Mothers were taught to mix ORT in their own homes by workers using a set lesson which was repeated until the main points were readily recalled. More than a thousand field-workers taught mothers to demonstrate their competence in the mixing and use of SSS. Workers were paid on the basis of the results of a follow-up 'test' of a 5 per cent sample of mothers who were asked to recall the seven messages and demonstrate correct preparation of the solution. Follow-up of households as long as four years after training showed a high degree of knowledge retention and ability to mix SSS.

A number of countries in Africa, such as those in the Sahel, Ruwanda and others, adopted the home-use of sugar–salt solution as their primary approach. Given that most of these countries are rural and that their people have limited access to shops or health facilities, this orientation towards behavioural change and the use of home-made solutions rather than towards promoting the use of a product is appropriate, even necessary.

However, most countries have adopted a 'mixed approach', promoting both packets and behaviour modifications/home solutions. Indonesia supported the use of home fluids as the first step for a mother to take when her baby begins to have diarrhoea, reserving ORS packets for children presenting at health centres with dehydration. While this substantially reduced the demand on packets, mothers seeking treatment early in the course of illness were frequently offered inappropriate drugs as ORS was saved for dehydration cases only. Recently the government has recommended ORS packets to be given to any mother seeking care for a child with diarrhoea, whether dehydrated or not. Inappropriate drug use is now falling.

What is the desirable balance between home solutions and ORS packets in national CDD programmes? Emphasis on the ORS packet may be most suitable for countries such as Egypt where family incomes are comparatively high, where most of the population is urban or suburban with easy access to both health facilities and commercial pharmacies, and where purchasing a commercial product is a standard response to illness. However, the product approach can run into problems, as it did in Pakistan where the government could not sustain the free provision of packets to the entire population on its own budget and also was reluctant to depend on private

*The Bengali names for crude salt and sugar.

pharmaceutical manufacturers and shops to provide packets. In any case the rural character of Pakistan would make access to such sources of ORS packets difficult for most of the population.

The approach promoting the home sugar–salt solution led to a different kind of problem, related to the ineffectiveness of much of public health education. While literate health workers may more easily remember the appropriate measures of salt and sugar and can identify a one litre or 200 millilitre container, many rural, often illiterate, families cannot. BRAC's home educational programme overcame this difficulty with extremely intensive teaching and demonstration techniques, but most other programmes have been less effective. Often, home prepared solutions have too much salt or sugar or too little water. Such hypertonic (overly concentrated) solutions are potentially dangerous to the child with diarrhoea. A study in Ruwanda found more than 75 per cent of mothers preparing potentially dangerous solutions;[13] and in India it was one-third or more.[14] Such experience led WHO to propose that solutions requiring recipes and measurement for preparation should be avoided.

The choice between promoting the ORS packet or the home solution is both a technical and philosophical one. The appropriateness of the choice made will strongly influence the ability of a national programme to take ORT to scale in an effective and sustainable fashion. A policy which emphasizes the ORS packet—a product—takes advantage of the commercial nature of health care even in developing countries, the desire of practitioners to retain control of technologies, the tendency of many patients to dependency and preference for purchased remedies, and the potential for greater efficacy and reduced danger from manufactured products. A policy emphasizing the home-made sugar–salt solution—behavioural change—transfers medical power to the people and thus makes the technology useful beyond the reach of existing distribution systems (governmental) and among the poor, also reducing pressures on government budgets.

PROMOTING ORT: FROM PILOT TO PROGRAMME

The process by which ORT has spread from research centres and pilot projects to government and non-government programmes is an excellent example of the methods of promotion needed to disseminate any new medical technology, particularly one not inherently attractive commercially. The early stages of this process benefited from some man-made as well as natural disasters, specifically the Bangladesh Liberation War in 1971 which led to massive refugee movement across the country's borders, and the Ethiopian famine which took place at approximately the same time. Faced with an immense diarrhoea problem, medical workers had almost no choice but to use the new method in whatever form they could manage.[15] The results were dramatic and convincing. Clearly this was a technology which could save thousands of lives in these critical circumstances.

This bolstered the confidence of those involved, who then began to spread the idea to more routine circumstances. Ransome Kuti and David Morley began to use sugar–salt solution in managing diarrhoea in their paediatric clinics in Nigeria. Interest in Indonesia was stimulated further by Jon Rohde who had used ORT in the Calcutta refugee camps and had seen case fatality lower than in hospitals using intravenous solutions. Leading paediatricians formed the Indonesian Coordinating Board for Paediatric Gastroenterology in 1974 which focused on diarrhoea as its major concern and began to work with the government to spread the ORT concept.

The WHO CDD Programme

Meanwhile the WHO Cholera Control Programme began to include ORT in its cholera and diarrhoea courses at training centres in the Philippines, Egypt and elsewhere. The Cholera Control section at WHO headquarters was reorganized in 1979 to become the Control of Diarrhoeal Diseases (CDD) Programme, with its own advisory council and biennial budget. Diarrhoea case management by health workers and mothers, focusing on ORT, was accorded top priority. Under the directorship of Michael Merson, CDD set as its first critical target the establishment of national CDD programmes—structured working units in ministries of health with one or more persons responsible only for diarrhoea—in every developing country. CDD reviewed policies related to every aspect of diarrhoea case management, training, communications and ORS production, and formulated standardized and succinct guidelines, manuals and training modules. These standards and materials provided the basis for action by the newly-organized national CDD units. Technical consultants from the WHO CDD Programme became familiar callers in every country, running courses in case management, programme management and supervision, based on the policies and manuals of the programme, and providing advice on every aspect of CDD. They supported national CDD programme assessments and field surveys every three or four years, which identified and solved problems. At WHO headquarters in Geneva the CDD Programme monitored progress and supported practical CDD research through its scientific working groups. In this fashion the CDD Programme had a remarkable stimulating as well as unifying impact on the spread of ORT and correct management of diarrhoea cases.

Primary Health Care

In 1978 national and international interests in affordable community-based health efforts culminated in the Alma Ata Declaration which codified the fundamental principles of comprehensive primary health care (PHC), including ORT. However, even with broad interest, it was evident that the health impact of PHC would not be quick to appear. Some observers felt that the PHC approach was too broad, and was not likely to have a measurable short-term impact on health status. What was needed was to focus efforts both on technologies that worked and on diseases that were major causes of mortality. This concept was the basis for selective primary health care and of the UNICEF Child Survival and Development Revolution.[16] Concentrating on four technologies UNICEF promoted 'GOBI' (Growth monitoring, ORT, Breast-feeding, Immunization), thus making universal ORT a goal of UNICEF in every developing country.

The United States Agency for International Development (USAID) chose an even shorter list of priority interventions: the 'Twin Engines of Health Development'—ORT and immunization. USAID began to pay for the training, communications and management activities of host country health ministries which would spread ORT and CDD. A project focused on diarrhoea, PRITECH, was established in Washington to support these USAID activities overseas. Its role was to provide technical experts in ORT and CDD who, along with WHO consultants, could help countries plan their programmes and make the policy and operational decisions needed to implement the many different types of activities required.

International Conferences on ORT

In the early 1980s ORT was still more the darling of developed country scientists and international assistance agencies than the child of developing country health ministries. The first International Conference on ORT (ICORT-I), held in Washington D.C. in 1983, may well have been instrumental in convincing developing country officials that ORT was worthwhile, something they should want to do.[17] At ICORT-I developed country clinical investigators described the merits of ORT to their developing country counterparts, specifically pointing out its effectiveness in individual patients with diarrhoea. Many of the officials returned home with a personal commitment to take definitive action in CDD/ORT.

By 1985 many national CDD programmes had been initiated but leaders were wondering what activities should be emphasized and what operational approaches would make them successful. ICORT-II responded by featuring programme implementors and specialists in training, communications, ORS manufacture and distribution, and other CDD programme components, who shared detailed experiences with national CDD programme representatives.[18]

By 1988 the tables had turned. ICORT-III featured developing country managers who shared with each other and their donor agency supporters the

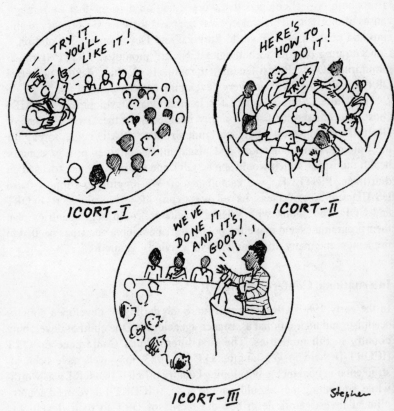

International ORT conferences reflected the evolving transfer of this technology to developing countries.

approaches that had been useful in overcoming problems and the successes they had achieved.[19]

Though expensive and time-consuming, these ORT conferences played a major role in stimulating action and fostering persistent commitment to CDD/ORT by host governments. The presentation exemplified the evolving relationships between international donors and experts and counterpart national CDD programme managers and policy-makers. ICORT-I said: 'Try it, you'll like it!' ICORT-II said: 'Here's how to do it.' ICORT-III said: 'We've done it and it's good!'

The Role of PVOs

Parallel to the progress of ORT at government level was the rapid spread of ORT among private voluntary organizations (PVOs), both national and international. Yayasan Indonesia Sejahtera, a local private development agency in Central Java, was already teaching community health workers how to prepare sugar–salt solution in 1974. They even popularized a double-ended plastic spoon with which to measure the correct amount of salt and sugar for a glassful of ORT, a measuring device eventually circulated to many other countries by David Morley. Similar groups in other countries recognized the power over disease which this remarkable technology could give to ordinary people and adopted it as a central component of their health programmes, almost always emphasizing home-made sugar–salt solution. The most prominent example of this was the BRAC programme but they were joined by international agencies such as CARE, CRS and Save the Children Fund as well as a host of national NGOs. While this grass-roots spread of the ORT idea led to a confusing multiplicity of recipes and instructions for use, it played an important role in making ORT available to health workers and communities not reached by government programmes.

National Research and Evaluation

National research has also played an important role in the spread of ORT. In the early stages of the ORT effort it was not uncommon to hear the comment: 'Well, ORT may work in country X but the situation is different here.' Research carried out by local paediatricians on topics such as ORT effectiveness in diarrhoea of different aetiologies and on the lack of effectiveness of antibiotics in most diarrhoeas helped to counter this argument. When key paediatricians or decision-makers had seen ORT's effectiveness for themselves, with data collected under their own control, they became promoters. Because of this, WHO, USAID and other donor agencies supported many small local research projects which confirmed findings from elsewhere. This emphasis on locally-relevant applied research was a forerunner of the 'essential national health research' now recommended as an integral part of all developing country health systems.[20]

National programmes were evaluated by field surveys of ORT usage in households and health facilities, especially carried out to assess whether previously set targets had been met. These became important motivators of managers and ministries to change operational approaches and policies or to provide additional resources. Initially those responsible for implementation often felt that there was neither time nor manpower available for field monitoring or evaluation. As a result field problems were not being detected, much less dealt with, and it was not possible to say whether progress was taking place or not. Thus, making funds available for monitoring and evaluation became a critical promotional approach adopted by multilateral agencies. This mechanism has served to improve the quality and effectiveness of CDD programmes.

CHANGING PRACTITIONERS' BEHAVIOUR

The WHO CDD Programme began to train doctors at health facilities, reasoning that they would in turn spread the message to their staff and patients. Paramedics, drug stores and other providers were to be taught only after all health facilities in the country had high use rates and effective case management and only then would home therapy be actively promoted. However, while this sequential approach seemed both logical and manageable it was followed strictly by only a few countries, if any. In most, efforts to train practitioners and to communicate directly with parents proceeded simultaneously. While this combined approach may be more difficult to manage, it is believed to be more appropriate because it aims at empowering people as well as medical practitioners. Through demand for ORT an informed public has proved to be a major determinant of medical practice.

In some countries such as the Sahelian nations of Mali and Niger, leading paediatricians did not promote ORT, continuing to use intravenous infusions for dehydrated children and Ganidan, a sulfa antibiotic, and activated charcoal for ambulatory diarrhoea cases. Because of this resistance, diarrhoea programmes in those countries chose to emphasize public communication as their first major effort. They undertook mass campaigns to promote the use of sugar–salt solution in the home rather than training doctors in hospital diarrhoea wards. These communication efforts used both mass media and person-to-person approaches. By working through the public health system, with its emphasis on public education, these communication efforts also reached health practitioners working in peripheal areas. Many were encouraged to use ORS packets, even though they still prescribed Ganidan and charbon as well.

To convert a practitioner to using ORT regularly and effectively was found to be much more difficult than expected. One enthusiastic educator in Pakistan, who had trained scores of physicians with a dynamic lecturing technique, found that almost none of them were actually using ORT regularly in their practices when he surveyed them some time later.

However, many physicians responded after a 'conversion experience'. Personally rehydrating a lethargic child with decreased skin turgor, seeing that child come to life and begin to play and eat after being given ORT, had a dramatic effect on these physicians, an effect which lectures were unable to produce. In the manner of enthusiastic religious converts, these physicians became 'apostles' of ORT, promoting it among their colleagues as well as giving it to their own patients.

Such experiences led to the principle of 'hands-on' training which was eventually recognized as fundamental for effective training in diarrhoea treatment. It led further to the development of Diarrhoea Training Units (DTU) in teaching hospitals where correct diarrhoea case management emphasizing ORT is being practised. DTUs and training supported by WHO in a few key places, (e.g. ICDDR,B in Dhaka, Lahore, Jakarta, Manila, Cairo) 'converted' leading paediatricians and CDD programme managers from other countries. Some returned home to establish their own DTUs. For example, teams consisting of a paediatrician and a nurse from eight Indonesian medical schools returned home after intensive training at ICDDR,B with missionary zeal. In collaboration with the national CDD programme and PRITECH/USAID, they established DTUs and revised the curriculum for training medical students and paediatricians from the 16 other medical schools in the country. A similar sequence of events has occurred in Pakistan, Egypt and the Philippines. The Zaire DTU has provided excellent experience for French-speaking African physicians.

The strategy of establishing DTUs has been more effective in standardizing good case management training than previous efforts which only provided training direction and materials. It has led to the clarification of standards at diarrhoea treatment facilities for patient screening, equipment and supplies, and the use of space. Wall-charts and forms to be used in evaluating diarrhoea patients have helped to standardize and broaden the information to be collected. Supervisory check-lists have clarified standards for clinical methods and provided means to measure them. With these standards in hand, national CDD programmes can distinguish good training and good diarrhoea treatment. While most training efforts so far have concentrated on doctors already in service, WHO has recently released a book with text and exercises for medical students which will play the same role in medical schools as earlier manuals and with practitioners.

Even a 'conversion experience' may not result in the desired changes in diarrhoea treatment once a trainee returns home. A range of problems there must be overcome. Mothers often expect prescription drugs. Physical arrangements in the places where diarrhoea patients are seen often make it difficult to educate mothers. In addition to managing dehydrated children with ORT, trainees must convince and teach parents and other health staff, establish ORT corners in their facilities, and deal with local supervisors. As these actions often fail to occur, additional steps have been developed to enhance the effectiveness of training in changing treatment practices. These include the following.

Table 2. ORT-related publications: Evidence for the range of issues to be addressed in scaling up a major public health effort

Title/Authors	Source of publication	Description
CDD Programme Management: A Training Course	CDD/WHO	Training course for programme managers of national CDD programmes.
Supervisory Skills (CDD): A Training Course	CDD/WHO	Training programme for middle level supervisors in national diarrhoeal disease control programmes.
Diarrhoea Training Unit, Directors' Guide and Teaching Materials	CDD/WHO	Detailed lecture notes and teacher's guide for a training unit to teach clinical management of diarrhoea in a large hospital training centre.
Diarrhoea Management Training Course: Guidelines for Conducting Clinical Training Courses at Health Centres	CDD/WHO	Adaptation of clinical training in diarrhoea case management to the needs of small facilities and small hospitals.
Readings on Diarrhoea: Student Manual	CDD/WHO	The first portion of a set of materials for faculty members teaching medical students about diarrhoea.

Title/Authors	Source of publication	Description
Training for the Control of Diarrhoeal Disease Intermediate Level	PRITECH	Modules to train middle-level workers such as nurses in CDD.
Field Implementation Aids	PRITECH	Practical guidelines for programme managers to address each of the necessary components of a national CDD programme.
Improved Nutritional Therapy of Diarrhoea: A Guide for Programme Planners, Brown & Bentley	PRITECH	Guidelines for programme managers specifically in the nutritional management of diarrhoea.
Improving Young Child Feeding During Diarrhoea: A Guide for Investigators and Programme Managers, Griffiths, Piwoz *et al.*	PRITECH	Protocol and instructions regarding field investigations leading to improved recommendations for child feeding during diarrhoea.
Communication for Child Survival, Rasmussen *et al.*	Healthcom	Manual for developing communications in ORT and other child survival projects.
Communication: A guide for Disease Control Programmes Planning Management and Appraisal of Communication Activities	CDD/WHO	Guidelines for programme managers in communications regarding diarrhoea, particularly mass media.
Talking with Mothers about Diarrhoea: a Workshop for Physicians, Smith *et al.*	PRITECH	Module to teach physicians and other health workers about communication techniques in diarrhoea case management.
Oral Rehydration Salts: Planning, Establishment, and Operation of Production Facilities	CDD/WHO	Manual for local producers of oral rehydration salt packets.
Rational Use of Drugs in the Management of Acute Diarrhoea in Children	CDD/WHO	Case management policy regarding drugs in the treatment of patients with diarrhoea.
Manual for Assessment and Planning of National ORT Programmes, Lesar *et al.*	PRITECH	Manual for comprehensive assessment and planning of programmes, for use by consultants and national programme managers.
Health Facility Survey Manual: Diarrhoea Case Management	CDD/WHO	Guidelines and survey forms for assessing the competence of health facilities in providing diarrhoea care.

Providing special instruction in needed additional skills. For example, the training materials for medical students provide practice in convincing mothers that anti-diarrhoeals or antibiotics are not needed. The West Java ORT programme used the same interactive teaching methods to train health centre doctors as they wanted the doctors to use in training VHWs at home.

Including planning in the training course. Pakistan, Indonesia and the Philippines included time in the training for trainees to make detailed plans. Trainees together identified the problems and persons they would need to deal with, then planned the steps needed for each. In Pakistan the trainees' supervisors were invited to participate in the final session where each trainee presented his plan so that any issues could be resolved on the spot. This approach is formalized in the WHO/CDD DTU Director's Guide.

Providing follow-up and support after the course. In Pakistan a physician from the DTU visited each trainee in his home institution at least once to help the latter train other personnel at his own base, facilitate needed action from the trainee's supervisor, help set up the ORT corner, or solve any other problems, as well as to monitor the treatment which the trainee was providing.

Regathering trainees to report progress. In West Java, Indonesia, VHW trainees knew that a month after their day-long training they would report together on their community promotion activities. Nearly all carried out their assignments. In addition to motivating the trainees, the second training day helped to clarify methods and solve problems through a sharing of experiences. Such split courses—two days of teaching with a month of practice in between—influence behaviour more strongly than the usual one-session strategy.

Changing the environment in which the trainee works. Easy availability of anti-diarrhoeals makes their use much more likely but making them unavailable to the practitioner increases the prospects that ORT will be used. Some programmes in the Sahel were successful in having 'Ganidan et Charbon' removed from the list of drugs which could be ordered by physicians working in the government health facilities. This led to a substantial increase in ORS use. In Pakistan combinations of antibiotics and anti-diarrhoeals were de-registered and withdrawn from the market. In Bangladesh the government removed all anti-diarrhoeals from the approved list of essential drugs for their national formulary. These actions make other treatments less available and also give a strong message to physicians about the appropriate treatment.

Monitoring what happens after the course. Problems are uncovered through field visits, including discussions with health workers and community people, and formal surveys carried out at regular intervals. An 'epidemic' of hypernatraemia seemed to be occurring in Egypt. The first indication that a problem existed came from anecdotal reports from hospital physicians. An objective study of the serum sodium values of children admitted to hospital confirmed that hypernatraemia was occurring. These and other studies suggested that incorrect mixing of ORS was probably responsible. By increasing the emphasis on mixing techniques in the television campaigns, the incidence of hypernatraemia was reduced.

The WHO/CDD Programme estimates that 17 per cent of all government health workers have been trained in the past 12 years and that usage rates of ORT by practitioners now exceed 50 per cent and in some places have reached 80 per cent of diarrhoeal cases.

CHANGING PARENTS' BEHAVIOUR

To reach parents with a new technology, the most effective channels of communication must be chosen.

Educating when Sick: The ORT Corner

Parents are best educated when they bring their sick children to a health facility for treatment. This is a time when they are both interested and attentive to advice, although they may be distracted by the sick child and unable to remember. Establishing 'ORT corners' for diarrhoea has helped to make such encounters more effective by allowing parents to rehydrate their child themselves as they wait in the clinic. An ORT corner is a space in any health facility—a corner of the waiting room or a separate area— where the equipment and supplies for teaching and actually giving ORT are ready for use. There may be samples of local containers to demonstrate how much fluid is to be used, mixing spoons to demonstrate the correct quantity of sugar and salt (in places where SSS is recommended), clean water, posters and take-home pamphlets. When the ORT corner is established in an out-patient waiting area, parents can hydrate their child while waiting for medical consultation. If the practitioner determines that further hydration is needed, the child and parent are sent back to the ORT corner. There a health worker demonstrates how to prepare the ORT solution and the mother actually rehydrates her child herself. This allows health workers to see immediately if the mother is having any problems, and to correct any misinformation or faulty behaviour. Health workers can also instruct mothers about breast-feeding and other feeding during and after diarrhoea.

Health workers, especially doctors, may not be skilful in teaching. A special training module has been developed to teach health workers how to talk more effectively with mothers about diarrhoea. The module emphasizes the use of checking questions, demonstrating rather than just talking, praising the mother when she has done something correctly, and obtaining the mother's agreement that she will give ORT and feeding. It was used enthusiastically in Pakistan. To help further, 25 small multi-coloured instruction sheets have been packaged in every box of 50 ORS packets by the manufacturer. This makes them automatically available at the health facility along with ORS, and every mother can be given one as a reminder. It avoids the problem found in many countries of educational materials being unavailable with ORS packets because they are distributed through other

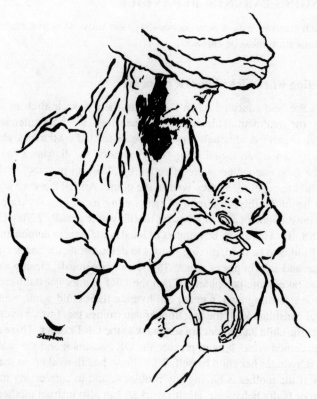

When a father learns to rehydrate his sick child, the lesson can have long lasting impact.

channels. In Nigeria a catchy ORT song has been extremely effective in teaching mothers how to mix sugar–salt solution. It is quite impressive to visit a clinic and find that every mother in the waiting room can sing the song and perform the mixing and feeding motions which accompany the words!

Educating when Well: Mass Media Communication

Mass media channels aimed directly at families have the potential to reach a much larger proportion of the population and messages can be carefully controlled. By using radio or TV, ORT programmes can leap-frog over the many practitioners who are either not fully converted or not yet trained. For these reasons most national CDD programmes initiated ORT communications through these channels, beginning with 'social marketing' of ORT. In the early years of ORT promotion when WHO encouraged the establishment of national CDD programmes, communications messages were designed around conference tables in capitals, or even in other countries. They were often inconsistent with the words mothers used for diarrhoea and with prevailing practices and beliefs. As a result, they were often not effective. The single most important activity related to the eventual success of communication programmes has been the field anthropological and ethnographic studies done to identify existing beliefs and practices related to diarrhoea and to test alternative messages with mothers.

The utilization of market research techniques in the communications effort has strengthened the credibility of messages given by health workers and made rehydration a household word and procedure in many societies. Marketing people have also brought their concern for monitoring behaviour into the programme. Companies promoting commercial products constantly monitor sales and change their advertising strategy if it is not working. Similarly, promotional campaigns for ORT are monitored to enable rapid correction of errors or deficiencies in messages. In the Gambia an intensive promotional campaign for sugar–salt solution led to rapidly-increased use. When active promotion stopped, monitoring showed that use of SSS fell off rapidly. It was concluded that continued promotion was necessary to maintain high ORT use rates and a new promotional campaign was begun.

The Egyptian programme allowed a full flowering of the social marketing approach. With adequate funds for marketing research and the development and broadcasting of brief 'spots', the Egyptian CDD programme emphasized television (available in over 90 per cent of households) to reach nearly the whole population. With mothers demanding ORS from doctors and pharmacists, ORS use rates rose to 70 per cent or more of diarrhoeal episodes.[8] In contrast to the Gambia, the media campaign in Egypt was accompanied by widespread intensive training of health workers which, reinforced by popular demand, succeeded in making ORS the accepted norm for diarrhoea case management among both practitioners and mothers.

A critical question in the design of media campaigns has been whether mothers need to understand what they are doing as opposed to merely following instructions. A prescriptive approach may be fine for usual medical encounters in which the only instructions needed are 'take one three-times a day'. For use of fluid or continued feeding in diarrhoea, however, an educational effort to produce real understanding, to provide a logical basis

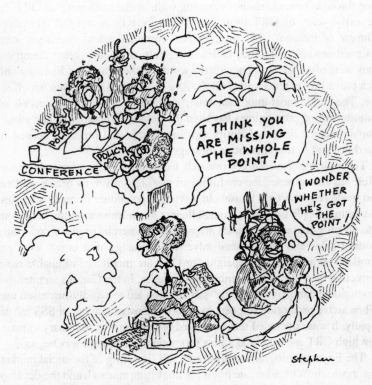

Research with careful attention to cultural concerns is critical to successful design of mass media and even to policy-making.

for the desired behaviour, may be critical to its acceptance. Both the Egyptian and Philippine campaigns began by promoting the concept of a 'new' disease, dehydration, as a frequent or common complication of diarrhoea.[8] By emphasizing that dehydration could kill and yet could be prevented, the Egyptian programme produced a three-fold increase in consultations at health facilities for diarrhoea. Acceptance of the concept of dehydration became so widespread that children who were asked to discuss drought* in a school examination discussed diarrhoea, dehydration and ORT instead of agriculture and hunger!

Doctors have long pursued the ethical principle of *primum nul nocere,* 'above all, do no harm'. Large-scale efforts in ORT communications have taught us that the recommended formulas as well as teaching methods used must be assessed carefully. Good training and good communications can lead to practitioners and patients using ORT effectively. Poor training or poor communications can lead to error and failure. An approach which might be quite effective and safe when administered by health workers directly can become ineffective and potentially dangerous when translated into a media message. Communication, like medicine, has to be used judiciously and correctly.

REACHING THOSE OUTSIDE GOVERNMENT SERVICES

To influence the behaviour of all those who treat diarrhoea, programmes must reach private practitioners as well as those who work for governments. In fact diarrhoea care for most of the world's people is provided outside the government sector. For example, a large rural study in India found that only 7 per cent of those seeking care obtained it from government sources.[14] In Pakistan, the figure was 16 per cent. Yet CDD programmes in most countries have confined their attention largely to the government health system. Important participants beyond the government sector include commercial firms, NGOs and professional organizations of practitioners.

ORS SALES THROUGH THE COMMERCIAL SECTOR

In many countries commercial pharmaceutical manufacturers have been slow to adopt ORS. In part this may be due to the failure of ORT to halt diarrhoea. Patients and practitioners alike seek a 'cure'. It may also have been the result of direct public promotion by governments of ORT and ORS

*The Arabic word for drought—*gaffef*—is the same as that for dehydration.

as an inexpensive home remedy. Manufacturers fear that free distribution by governments will reduce sales of ORS. Often there is price control and low profit margins for the product. Where governments have sought to collaborate with commercial firms, the partnership has often been a reluctant one because commercial firms have feared entanglement with slow bureaucratic decision-making as well as pressure to keep prices and profits low.

Furthermore, pharmaceutical companies primarily utilize an 'ethical' approach in which drugs are promoted only to physicians who will either provide them directly for a fee or prescribe them to be purchased by patients from a pharmacist. Many drug companies do not have a marketing and distribution network aimed directly at consumers and would have to make significant investments to develop these. Manufacturers of popular products such as soap flakes, matches, packaged foods and popular drugs like aspirin who have such activities have not perceived the potential of ORS. Some wish to avoid the liability inherent in a health product while others who sell anti-diarrhoeal preparations (such as Woodward's gripe water or Enterostop) do not wish to impede the success of these 'cash cows' by introducing competitive products.

Numerous strategies have been used to facilitate commercial ORS production and sales within this set of constraints. These have ranged from 'doing nothing' to attempts to eliminate competitive drugs from the market, to working with companies, manufacturers' associations and pharmacists to actively promote ORS.

Doing Nothing

The Fair Deal Corporation (FDC) in India was among the first corporations to make a major effort to sell ORS for profit, beginning in the early 1970s. India may have been a supportive environment for such an effort as the national CDD programme was comparatively inactive through the 1980s and thus restrictive regulations constraining the ORS formula, price, profit margins or allowable promotional techniques were not developed. In this environment, FDC responded to its own perceptions of the market and developed creative ideas regarding sales strategies. The company presently sells 40–50 million packets of ORS annually!

'Do nothing' really means 'Don't erect barriers'.

Setting Treatment Standards, Emphasizing ORT and Non-use of Anti-diarrhoeals and other Drugs

Eliminating Competitive Drugs from the Market by De-registration or an Essential Drugs Programme

These two strategies are additive. The first has been done in nearly every country. It is necessary but not sufficient. By adding the second step the first strategy acquires operational meaning and begins to have effect. As already noted such changes of the environment worked well in Pakistan, the Sahel and Bangladesh.

Strengthening Pharmaceutical Company Capabilities to Produce and Sell ORS

WHO, USAID and others have provided expert engineering and production consultancy to companies to assist in developing or improving facilities for local production of ORS. In Pakistan consultants from the PRITECH project assisted companies which had not previously had substantial experience or skills in promotion, specifically in 'detailing'—the promotion of products to physicians and pharmacists through the use of direct presentations by field representatives. PRITECH provided training for managers in planning promotional campaigns and in training detail men to give convincing presentations.

Allowing Product and Price Variations, Market Segmentation

The Fair Deal Corporation in India began with an ORS with a lower sodium content and more glucose than the standard WHO formula, to which were added calcium and magnesium. These variations were intended to make ORS more attractive to physicians. From this beginning Fair Deal developed a 'health drink' (Beoral) which became popular as an after-sport drink as well as for diarrhoeal hydration. Recently they have marketed a 200 ml packet of standard WHO formula ORS (Poonarjal) directly to consumers. Prices for these products range from the easily-affordable to higher-priced 'ethical' items. Because it has been allowed to present a mix of products and prices aimed at both the 'ethical' market (doctors) and ordinary consumers, FDC has found ORS sufficiently profitable to aggressively promote and expand sales and to take on the economic challenge of developing a consumer-oriented marketing and distribution system.

Funding Market Research and Generic ORS Promotion

The Egyptian CDD Programme discussed above is an excellent example of an extensive market research effort. Rather than using an existing private pharmaceutical corporation, the programme established a parastatal corporation which could take on the task of distributing ORS to private pharmacies. This corporation was supported by an intensive promotional campaign over public television and radio. The impact of this approach on sales was quite dramatic. Despite the free distribution of ORS through government health facilities, 60 per cent of the country's packets were purchased directly from pharmacies.

In Pakistan the government's advertising campaign for its brand of ORS (Nimkol) brought broad public awareness of ORT, enhancing sales of the many other commercial preparations as well. In West Java the combination of advertising by the government through mass media and promotion by an ORS manufacturer in pharmaceutical shops was so successful that the government began to fear it would run out of ORS. It requested the pharmaceutical company to stop its promotional effort!

Contracting to Purchase a Guaranteed Amount of ORS Every Year

This strategy encourages companies by ensuring at least a minimal return on their ORS activities. In Pakistan the government contracts with Wilson, a local pharmaceutical manufacturer, for a large supply of ORS annually. This has encouraged the company to promote ORS actively, with the effect that they sell the most ORS of all manufacturers, over and above their sales to the government.

Subsidizing a Particular ORS Marketing Activity

In Bangladesh USAID has supported a Social Marketing Project which promotes and distributes ORS. In the Philippines the national programme, with USAID support, has been seeking to contract with a local private manufacturer to produce and distribute ORS with an initial large subsidy. This approach has the disadvantage of producing an organization dependent on outside funding subsidies. It may be necessary, however, to initiate commercial interest.

Promoting Participation of Companies and Manufacturers' Associations in National ORT Programmes

Many companies are anxious to be well thought of by the Ministry of Health so that when they need approval for other activities it will be forthcoming. This may be particularly true of multinational pharmaceutical firms which frequently must obtain licenses to import materials and equipment and seek registration of new products. One firm indicated to a consultant that it would be prepared to make minimal profit or even take a small loss on ORS if its efforts to promote ORS would help get the support of the MOH for other activities. Many multinational firms have active public service programmes and budgets.

Supporting Medical Society–Pharmaceutical Firm Collaboration

UNICEF has supported collaboration between the Indian Medical Association (IMA) and the Association of Pharmaceutical Manufacturers in which the IMA has made it clear to the manufacturers that they want the companies to support national treatment policies, to standardize ORS composition to meet WHO recommendations, and to adopt uniform packaging and instructions.

Supporting Efforts to Improve the Efficacy of ORS

Pharmaceutical manufacturers have watched the studies of rice-based and alanine-containing ORS closely as both seem to reduce stool output (i.e. an anti-diarrhoeal effect). Indeed, one company is already marketing a liquid premixed rehydration solution based on rice starch with promotional material which stresses the reduction in stool output which is expected from use of the product (Ricelyte TM, Mead-Johnson). This reduction in stool is, of course, the main concern of the mother.

Working Directly with Pharmacists and Drug Sellers

In most cases interaction with the sellers of ORS is best left to pharmaceutical firms, as dealing with the 'point of sale' is an area in which they excel. In addition to detailing, the firms are masters at adjusting payment terms, securing a visible place on the shelf, providing posters to advertise the product and, above all, at effective distribution—ensuring that the seller does not run out of the product. Those that do not excel are quickly out of business.

However, in some cases CDD programmes or donors have collaborated with national or international pharmacist associations to develop policies or to present updates at annual conferences. The potential for working with schools that train pharmacists is largely untapped.

Unfortunately there are more failures than successes in stimulating commercial firms to produce and promote ORS. For example, while Nigeria has a strong commercial drug sector, national policy restricts ORS to use within health facilities and sends a strong 'hands off'! message to any prospective ORS manufacturer.

There is constant tension between keeping prices low in order to ensure access of the poor to ORS and allowing prices which include profits to

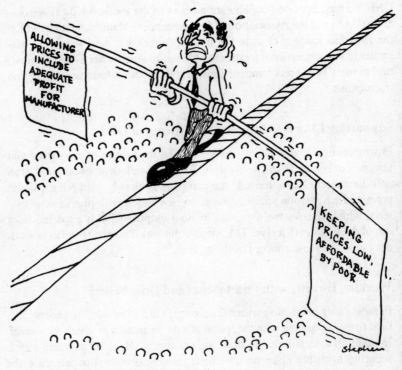

A dilemma faced by ORT and potentially by other primary health technologies.

encourage manufacturers' participation. Dealing with this tension is an important part of the challenge to take ORT to scale in a sustainable fashion. A country-wide study in India in 1988 found that the average rural family spent a comparatively large sum of money on diarrhoea treatment—Rs 27 per episode.[14]* Most governments are unable or unwilling to support the cost of the ORS needed for all diarrhoea cases in their country but they could provide free ORS to families who are unable to pay. If ministries encourage commercial firms to become active promoters of ORS, this will shift the cost of ORS to those users who prefer private or commercial providers, releasing government supplies for the poor.

REACHING NGOs AND INDIVIDUAL PRIVATE PRACTITIONERS

NGOs and individual private practitioners present yet another challenge. The Indian study mentioned above found private practitioners (some certified, others not; some well trained, others without any formal training) provide the vast majority of diarrhoea care for children in rural areas.[14] Treatment of diarrhoea may comprise a quarter or more of the income of practitioners, most of whom charge only for the injections and medicines they dispense. In many African countries NGOs provide significant proportions of all health care. Influencing such practitioners and NGOs to adopt ORT and standardize their ORT techniques and communications messages is critical. Yet the task is difficult because of the large number of individuals and organizations that must be reached.

Two types of approaches have been used with success in addition to supporting commercial promotion of ORS to practitioners by manufacturers. The choice among these depends on whether ORT use has been constrained by a lack of information or by other factors such as convenience, profit or time available.

Direct Training of Practitioners

In 1986 the Indian Medical Association (IMA) undertook an ambitious programme to retrain its 60 000 members in the correct use of ORT. To avoid variations in training content they used video recordings of lectures by well-known Indian paediatricians and a WHO film which dramatically portrayed the recovery of dehydrated children treated with ORT. One hun-

---

*This was equivalent to twice the minimum daily wage, and to US $2 at the time.

dred and thirty-five facilitators were trained in four national DTUs. They were provided with the video cassette and answers to sets of expected questions. In turn, these facilitators conducted more than 1000 two-to-three-hour workshops, training more than 30 000 IMA members. Pre- and post-test evaluation showed a substantial improvement of knowledge; and follow-up after several years showed that more than 80 per cent reported using ORT in practice. While hands-on experience during training would probably enhance ORT adoption, it is almost impossible to provide this for such large numbers. In addition it would be difficult to attract practitioners away from their practices for the three to five days usually required for such hands-on training.

Using a similar approach, the Philippine Paediatric Association (PPA) has conducted one-day training-of-trainer sessions. When these trainers returned home they conducted two-to-three-hour seminars for other PPA members as well as non-paediatric physicians in their communities. They also established ORT corners and began to use a special clinical form for diarrhoea in local hospitals. These innovations influenced the behaviour of those who had attended the seminars as well as those who had not. The PPA has also developed a correspondence course on diarrhoea case management.[21]

Mass Media Communication

Mass media promotion of ORT which is aimed at families also reaches practitioners as they watch or listen to the same programmes. In addition, when a mass media campaign influences mothers to request ORT from their practitioner or to question the appropriateness of drug treatment for diarrhoea, it will have a substantial indirect effect on practitioner behaviour. Some mass media campaigns have already begun to implement this strategy explicitly, using messages like 'The modern doctor treats diarrhoea with ORT', or 'If your doctor gives you a prescription for drugs, ask him if they are really necessary. They can be dangerous to your child.'

Individual ORS Promotion

Using sales representatives to call on individual practitioners in their offices—'detailing'—is the core promotional technique used by most pharmaceutical companies. Strategies by such companies to stimulate ORS sales usually involve ORS detailing. In many countries firms are already detailing ORS, giving free ORS samples, pamphlets, etc. Such promotion to individual practitioners is reinforced by company sponsorship of professional meetings, providing speakers, meals, brief-cases and other items. Detailing is an effective promotional technique, as evidenced by drug firm profits. Since the cost of detailing must be recovered from sales, the price of ORS will include these costs. Thus, restrictions on ORS prices may interfere with companies mounting promotional campaigns.

A similar approach has been used in the U.S. to discourage inappropriate clinical behaviour. Called 'counter-detailing', it has incorporated standard detailing techniques but it markets the idea of *not* doing a particular thing, e.g. not using an expensive antibiotic but a cheaper and equally effective one.[22] This approach is being tried in Indonesia to discourage drug use as well as encourage ORT. It will probably be effective but its cost may be difficult for government CDD or health education programmes to sustain within their scanty budgets.

Pre-service Training

Most of the activities of CDD programmes aimed at practitioners have been directed at those already in practice. Recognizing the long-range need to avoid producing doctors or nurses who do not use ORT, some countries and donor agencies have directed attention to influencing how diarrhoea management is taught to student doctors and nurses. In conjunction with the Association of Philippine Medical Colleges the Philippine Paediatric Association produced a special textbook on diarrhoea stressing ORT. It was distributed widely to medical schools who signed a commitment to teach ORT effectively.[21] A series of workshops was conducted to train faculty members to use teaching modules on diarrhoea prepared by PRI-TECH/USAID and WHO. An evaluation of the first six medical schools participating in this programme showed that all had well-functioning DTUs and were using many of the teaching activities for students and residents. The workshops have now been extended to the remaining medical schools. A similar approach has been successful in Indonesian medical schools. PRI-TECH/USAID consultants have also worked with ten nursing schools in Sahelian countries to develop and implement a special diarrhoea curriculum for French-speaking nurses. It is now also available in English for use elsewhere.

Critical to the effectiveness of these efforts has been the development of DTUs at these schools. The most important parts of these efforts to improve diarrhoea teaching have been, first, to ensure that the facilities and methods for treating diarrhoea are correct and meet DTU standards; and second, to ensure that students get actual hands-on experience in rehydrating patients, seeing 'real doctors'—their professors—doing the same. A major task remaining to take ORT to scale is to develop DTUs and good diarrhoea treatment and teaching in every medical school.

FACING THE CHALLENGES

Perhaps the most important element in the success achieved so far in taking ORT to scale has been the establishment of national diarrhoea programmes which focused on ORT. This has helped to concentrate the funds and attention of governments and donors on diarrhoea and ORT, and has provided a team of workers able to devote their attention to this area.

But now other causes of diarrhoeal mortality such as dysentery and persistent diarrhoea which are not curable with ORT alone are attracting attention and support of national programmes away from ORT, especially in places where ORT has begun to reduce mortality from acute watery diarrhoea. This is facilitated by the improvements in reporting which ORT programmes have brought about. The relative success of ORT and resulting reduction in deaths from acute dehydration must not be allowed to distract programmes from the importance of continuing and strengthening those efforts.

Many stress the fact that ORT is curative and does not prevent diarrhoea. They urge more activity in hygiene education, promotion of exclusive breast-feeding, sanitation and water supply and measles immunization. This translates into demands to displace the television spots on ORT or feeding during diarrhoea with spots about hand-washing or breast-feeding, to take time from training courses for prevention-related activities and to move ORT funding into prevention.

In some countries a philosophical commitment to integrated primary care has begun to interfere with the CDD programme holding courses devoted exclusively to diarrhoea, making supervisory field visits in which only diarrhoea-related activities are reviewed, or planning a focused diarrhoea communications campaign. In heavily-integrated activities ORT/CDD is combined with immunization, acute respiratory infection control, nutrition and breast-feeding, with consequent shrinkage of the diarrhoea content.

The integrationists are joined by the supporters of comprehensive primary care. They argue that most national ORT/CDD programmes are top-down and emphasize medical personnel and use of ORS packets. Thus, the proponents say, they do not adequately empower the community to control its own health care. They want to shift the emphasis and resources away from centralized, governmental, technical CDD programmmes towards grass-roots efforts which would give first priority to community organization.

These diversionary forces are aided by the impending termination of several five-to-ten-year donor projects begun in the early 1980s which supplied funds to start national ORT programmes. As those funds disappear many national governments have not identified indigenous funds to take their place, even though the programmes have not yet achieved their targets.

More broadly, both donors and governments tend to lose interest in any initiative after a few years. Each begins with enthusiasm and hope that a particular strategy will solve the problems created by poverty and ignorance. When, as in all programmes, the strategy encounters difficulties, the decision-makers begin to seek the next potential panacea. When ORT did not immediately eliminate all mortality from diarrhoea, planners and funders began to question whether it was an appropriate continuing investment. The shift in national and international CDD attention away from acute dehydrating diarrhoea and ORT towards dysentery, persistent diarrhoea and diarrhoea preventive efforts, that is, towards problems and interventions which are even more complex, has further worsened government and donor disenchantment. The current new fads in donor funding include alternative modes of financing health care and planning for adequate care of adult medical problems such as cancer and heart disease. The commitment to maximum reduction of mortality, which was the basis for the Child Survival and Development Revolution, appears to be losing strength.

Yet much remains to be done in ORT. Despite its successes in going to scale, there are many practitioners and mothers who still have not adopted ORT as their primary response to diarrhoea, and each new generation adds a cohort of medical workers and mothers who need to be convinced. The basic reasons which attracted the world to ORT remain valid. ORT became part of the Child Survival and Development Revolution because it was an effective and feasible intervention against a major cause of childhood mortality. We have learned that the process of taking ORT to scale has not been as simple as ORT itself, nor as simple as we had hoped. Yet ORT remains simpler, cheaper and more effective than the interventions needed to attack persistent diarrhoea or run an integrated and community-based primary health care programme. The full impact of this life-saving technology will only be felt when it more widely and completely pervades general knowledge and practice in the treatment of all cases of diarrhoea. The lessons learned from taking this technology to scale provide not only important

A RANGE OF REHYDRATION METHODS FOR CHILDREN WITH DIARRHOEA

intravenous solution (I.V.)	factory-prepared oral solution	factory-prepared packets of 'rehydration salts' for mixing in water	bags with salts, prepared at the health centre for mixing in water	homemade drink made with plastic measuring spoons	homemade drink made with spoons found in the home	homemade drink made with homemade spoons	homemade drink with salt & sugar measured with the fingers or by another traditional way
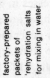	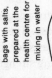	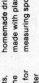		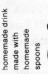			

MORE DEPENDENCY control in the hands of institutions and professionals

MORE SELF-SUFFICIENCY control in the hands of the family

ADVANTAGES AND DISADVANTAGES

Control and responsibility mainly in the hands of professionals, institutions and drug companies

Measurements more precise and 'controlled' (at least in theory)

More magical; acceptance may be quicker but with less understanding

More dependency—on high technology, on outside resources, on centralized services, and on local and international politics

More expensive

Easier to gather data on, and prepare statistics about

Reaches fewer people; supply often uncertain and inadequate

Sometimes causes delay in treatment, because special materials have to be obtained; effect is more curative than preventive

Focus is on materials and supply (so cost goes up each year)

May give better (safer) results for individuals treated in time, but has worse results overall since many children never receive the liquid, or are given it too late

ADVANTAGES AND DISADVANTAGES

Control and responsibility mostly in the hands of the family

Measurements less precise, less 'controlled'

More practical and easier to understand

More self-sufficiency; uses local resources (whatever is available in the home or in stores)

Cheaper

Harder to gather data on, and prepare statistics about

Reaches more people; supply is local and almost always available

Treatment can begin at the first sign of diarrhoea; more preventive than curative

Focus is on people and on education, so the people's capacity for self-care increases over the years (cost goes down)

May be less safe in individual cases due to the possibility of errors in preparing or giving it, but it probably saves many more lives—since it reaches more children more quickly directions for CDD programmes in the years ahead but also give valuable lessons in the process of making appropriate modern health technologies available to all.

References

1. Van Heyningen, W. E. and Seal, J. R. (1983). *Cholera: The American Scientific Experience 1947–1980*. Westview Press, Boulder, Colorado.
2. Love, A. H. G. (1965). *The effect of glucose on cation transport*. Proceedings of the Cholera Research Symposium, Honolulu, January, 1965. Washington D.C., U.S. Government Printing Office, p. 144.
3. Hirschhorn, N., Kinzie, J. L., Sachar, D. B., *et al.* (1968). Decrease in net stool output in cholera during intestinal perfusion with glucose-containing solution. *New England Journal of Medicine*, Vol. 279, p. 176.
4. Cash, R. A., Nalin, D. R., Rochat, R., *et al.* (1970). A clinical trial of oral therapy in a rural cholera-treatment center. *American Journal of Tropical Medicine and Hygiene*, Vol. 19, p. 635.
5. Nalin, D. R. (1975). Sucrose in oral therapy for cholera and related diarrhoeas. *Lancet*, Vol. 1, p. 1400.
6. Rahaman, M. M., *et al.* (1979). Diarrhoea mortality in two Bangladeshi villages with and without community-based oral rehydration therapy. *Lancet*, Vol. 2, pp. 809–12.
7. World Health Organization. *Programme for Control of Diarrhoeal Diseases: Seventh Programme Report 1988–1989*. CSHO/CDD/90.34, World Health Organization, Geneva.
8. El-Rafie, M., Hassouna, W. A., Hirschhorn, N., *et al.* (1990). Effect of diarrhoeal disease control on infant and childhood mortality in Egypt: Report from the National Control of Diarrhoeal Diseases Project. *Lancet*, Vol. 1, pp. 334–8.
9. Rohde, J. E. and Northrup, R. S. (1976). Taking science where the diarrhoea is. *Paediatric Diarrhoea*. In: *Acute Diarrhoea in Childhood*, CIBA Foundation Symposium 42, Elsevier/Excerpta Medica/North Holland, pp. 339–66.
10. Werner, D. (1977). *Where there is no doctor*. Hesperian Foundation.
11. Northrup, R. S., Sanders, D., Taylor, C., Werner, D., *et al.* (1990). Implementing ORT programmes at community and district levels: Reaping the benefits of cereal-based ORT. In: *Cereal-based oral rehydration therapy for diarrhoea*, (ed. Elliot K. Attawell). Report of the International Symposium, Aga Khan Foundation, International Child Health Foundation, Geneva.
12. Chowdury, A. M. R., Vaughan, V. P., Abed, F. H. (1988). Mothers learn to save the lives of their children. *World Health Forum*, Vol. 9, pp. 239–44.
13. Control of Childhood Communicable Disease Project: Unpublished Report.
14. Viswanathan, H. and Rohde, J. E. (1990). *Diarrhoea in rural India—A nationwide study of mothers and practitioners*. Vision Books, Delhi.
15. Mahalanobis, D., Chaudhuri, A. B., Bagchi, N. G., *et al.* (1973). Oral fluid therapy of cholera among Bangladesh refugees. *Johns Hopkins Medical Journal*, Vol. 132, p. 197.
16. Rohde, J. E. (1983). Why the other half dies: The science and politics of child mor

tality in the Third World. The Leonard Parsons Memorial Lecture, Birmingham, U.K. 1982. *Assignment Chila en* 61/62; pp. 35–7.

17. Proceedings of the International Conference on Oral Rehydration Therapy, Agency for International Development, in cooperation with ICDDR,B, UNICEF, and WHO, 7–10 June 1983, Washington, D.C.

18. Proceedings of the International Conference on Oral Rehydration Therapy, Agency for International Development, in cooperation with ICDDR,B, UNICEF, and WHO, 10–13 December 1985.

19. Proceedings of the Third International Conference on Oral Rehydration Therapy, Agency for International Development, Washington D.C., 14–16 December 1988.

20. Commission on Health Research for Development. (1990). *Health research: Essential link to development.* Oxford University Press, New York.

21. Ocampo, P. S. (ed). (1985). Acute diarrhoeas, their management and prevention. The Ministry of Health, The Philippine Paediatric Society and the Kabalikat ng Pamilyang Pilipino Foundation.

22. Aurora, J. and Sourmerai, S. (1983). Improved drug therapeutic decision through educational outreach. A randomized controlled trial of an academically based detailing. *New England Journal of Medecine*, Vol. 308, pp. 1457–63.

CHAPTER 20

Vitamin A for Child Survival: Science and Politics

ALFRED SOMMER

The author records the discovery of the mortality-reducing effects of vitamin A. While scientific difficulties have been surmounted, incorporating the scientific findings into international health policy has been equally challenging and often more frustrating.

Alfred Sommer, M.D., M.P.H. has lived in Bangladesh and Indonesia conducting field epidemiological research on vitamin A deficiency. He is presently Dean of the School of Public Health at Johns Hopkins University, Baltimore, Maryland, U.S.A.

THE BACKGROUND

The relationship between vitamin A deficiency and increased childhood mortality is now widely accepted, and the importance of improving vitamin A status is rapidly gaining a central place in primary health care and child survival strategies. This turning point in the story of vitamin A came during 1990–91 after seven years of intense controversy. The delay had more to do with sociology and politics than with science. The story would possibly have been much longer and less controversial if the original investigators had not taken a pro-active stance based on their perceived need to pursue the policy implications of a discovery which they believed had enormous potential for children's health and survival.

Astonishingly, the benefits of vitamin A were readily anticipated on the basis of animal and clinical data which were 40 to 60 years old. During the first two decades of the present century, vitamin A was identified as an essential element for the normal growth and health of laboratory animals.[1] When made deficient, the animals ceased growing, developed overwhelming sepsis and died prematurely. The ocular signs of vitamin A deficiency (xerophthalmia) were late manifestations in those few animals who could be kept alive. Similar observations were made on deprived European children, where night blindness and Bitot's spots were associated with growth retardation and urinary tract and respiratory infections.[2,3] By the end of World War I, European governments virtually eliminated the problem by ensuring adequate consumption of vitamin A-rich dairy products.

The potential public health significance of vitamin A deficiency in the developing world was poorly appreciated, probably because the disease disappeared from the Western world as a result of government legislation and improved living standards, and because physicians focused on the dramatic ocular manifestations (xerophthalmia) as a cause of blindness. The medical and nutritional problems of the developing world appeared so complex that few scientists or health workers could consider a single nutrient capable of profoundly affecting children's health and well-being.

Interest in preventing nutritional blindness rose in the early 1970s with the recognition that vitamin A deficiency was widespread in the developing world and probably accounted for a significant number of sightless children. Patwardhan in Jordan and Swaminathan among others in India advocated periodic administration of large doses of vitamin A (200 000 to 300 000 IU) every six to twelve months as a means of building liver stores and protecting children against nutritional blindness.[4,5] Indeed, a number of countries such as Bangladesh, India and Indonesia implemented these suggestions to varying degrees, while pursuing alternative strategies for improving vitamin A nutrition.

At the 1972 World Food Conference in Rome, Henry Kissinger pledged that the United States would provide assistance in controlling this blinding disease, and brought new attention to the problem. This provided the stimulus and funds for an International Vitamin A Consultative Group (IVACG), which has served ever since as a forum for periodic exchanges of scientific data, for sensitization of policy-makers, and as a source of authoritative guidelines on specific aspects of the problem.

As countries and voluntary agencies began to mount efforts to improve vitamin A status, largely built around periodic supplementation of young children with large doses of vitamin A, and to treat active eye disease by intramuscular injection of water-miscible vitamin A, it became apparent that too little was known about the epidemiology and causes of vitamin A deficiency, its classification and diagnosis, and its optimal treatment and prevention. Helen Keller International, which was then assisting a number of governments in assessing the severity and magnitude of the problem and in mounting large-dose capsule distribution programmes, provided me with the opportunity to address these issues in a large-scale research project. Given the absence of suitable data upon which to base rational recommendations, I proposed a large and complex series of inter-related studies to answer questions ranging from the epidemiology of vitamin A deficiency through the pathogenesis of xerophthalmia and its clinical manifestations and management. USAID proved willing to fund the research programme, and a capable group of Indonesian colleagues were eager to tackle the problem.

EARLY INDONESIAN STUDIES

There were three basic, inter-related scientific investigations conducted in Indonesia between 1976 and 1979. The first was a hospital-based study of children with clinical xerophthalmia which enabled us to document the various clinical stages of disease, their pathogenesis, optimal treatment and, importantly, to identify various risk factors associated with the development of ocular signs and symptoms through case-control techniques.

An early and practical observation related to treatment. Existing WHO recommendations were based upon limited animal and human studies and not on controlled clinical trials among children with active xerophthalmia. The recommendations called for immediate intramuscular injection with 100 000 IU of water-miscible vitamin A of any child with evidence of xerophthalmia. It was only after arriving in Indonesia and attempting to treat xerophthalmic children that I discovered *water-miscible*, injectable vitamin A was not available anywhere on the world market except perhaps in India. We immediately conducted a controlled clinical trial in which half of the children with xerophthalmia received 200 000 IU of oil-miscible vitamin A orally, and the other half received 100 000 IU of (specially-prepared) water-miscible vitamin A intramuscularly. There was absolutely no difference in the clinical or biochemical response of the two groups of children.[6]

The practical implications of this simple trial were important as intramuscular vitamin A (if available) was more expensive than the oral preparation, and also required needles and syringes for administration. Further, injections delayed treatment and raised the risks of hepatitis and other communicable diseases. Oral dosing was not only cheaper and safer but could be administered by teachers, primary health care workers and others in immediate contact with affected rural children. Given the urgency of treatment, particularly when the cornea was already involved, the health implications were enormous.

Despite the striking clinical and biochemical results of this trial, published in the *Lancet* in 1980, it was four years before IVACG and WHO officially recognized that injectable preparations were unnecessary. It was more than ten years before they were relegated to a footnote in the WHO recommendation schedule. Although it was not the major publicized reason for the delayed response, it was argued that 'physicians like to give injections, and people like to receive them'. This dubious rationale has had the expected negative effects: foreign-aid workers, principally physicians, travelling to vitamin A deficiency areas repeatedly and urgently request injectable vitamin A. As a result, the most widely available and largely useless form, locally manufactured oil-miscible vitamin A, has been difficult to remove from the market.

COMMUNITY-BASED STUDIES

A large community-based study was conducted simultaneously with the hospital-based investigation. Preschool-age children were examined every three months and children with corneal involvement were enrolled for treatment. The community study examined these children on seven occasions, three months apart, providing 18 months of observations during which factors present at the time of each evaluation could be related to past and future events. Methods and results were examined as the study progressed in order to alter techniques where necessary, adopt additional components to answer questions we had not originally conceived, and employ approaches validated in the course of our work.

One such insight was that a mother's verbal history of her child's night blindness (based upon a locally-appropriate and well-recognized term) was as sensitive and specific a test, or more so, than the objective tests we had devised for detecting its presence.[7] During the first round of evaluations we collected clinical data on all children and estimated serum vitamin A levels on those with active xerophthalmia, as well as for neighbourhood controls and a random sub-sample of the entire population. In every instance in which objective tests demonstrated that a child suffered from night blindness, the mother or guardian had provided a positive history. In the few instances of a positive history where our objective clinical tests were negative, the children's serum vitamin A levels were as depressed as those in whom our objective tests were positive. Subsequent studies in Indonesia and elsewhere in Asia and Africa have confirmed the value of a simple history of night blindness in assessing xerophthalmia in the population.

These biochemical data provided our first insight into the community clustering of vitamin A deficiency. Serum vitamin A levels were lowest in children with active xerophthalmia (14 µg/dl); they were highest in children from other communities or elsewhere in the village who were clinically normal (20 µg/dl). Children who appeared to be normal but lived next door to children with xerophthalmia had serum vitamin A levels between these two extremes (17 µg/dl), an observation which has been made also subsequently in a number of other communities. This indicated the need for 'treating' communities or neighbourhoods, not just children with obvious clinical disease.

This community-based study provided the first solid estimates of the incidence, severity and magnitude of vitamin A deficiency and xerophthalmia for Indonesia in particular and, by extrapolation, for the rest of the developing world.[8] These estimates have formed the basis for world-wide calculations made subsequently by the World Health Organization—five to ten million new cases of xerophthalmia and half-a-million going blind annually. They also served as the basis for the 1980 revision of the 'criteria for a public health problem'.[9]

The community-based studies also identified factors that increased the risk of a child developing xerophthalmia (moderate vitamin A deficiency)—poor dietary intake of vitamin A, or frequent diarrhoea and respiratory disease. This longitudinal data provided true incidence rates (the rate of *development* of the disease in relation to a pre-existing risk factor), and confirmed associations that had been made in cross-sectional prevalence surveys. The advantage of the longitudinal studies was that one could tell which was 'the chicken' and which 'the egg'. The presence of xerophthalmia and a recent history of diarrhoea in a prevalence survey did not distinguish whether the diarrhoea led to the vitamin A deficiency, or vitamin A deficiency led to the diarrhoea. This study demonstrated that diarrhoea (and respiratory disease) increased the risk of subsequent xerophthalmia.[10]

It was Pasteur who claimed that 'chance favours the prepared mind'. While analysing the above-mentioned studies to identify risk factors leading to xerophthalmia, it was noted that children with existing xerophthalmia had a higher rate of subsequent mortality and morbidity than those with normal eyes. Not only was pre-existing xerophthalmia associated with a higher risk of subsequent mortality, but the risk of dying increased with the severity of pre-existing xerophthalmia (Fig. 1). This relationship was internally consistent, and led to the conclusion that vitamin A deficiency might play a major role in determining child survival. The same 'dose–response' relationship existed after adjusting for other factors that could affect the outcome, such as age, anthropometric status (protein–energy malnutrition), and even pre-existing infections.[11]

A subsequent paper provided a partial explanation for this phenomenon:

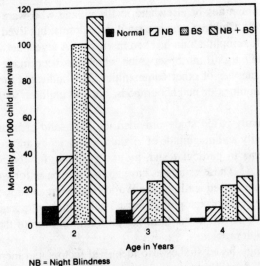

NB = Night Blindness
BS = Bitot's Spots
NB + BS = Night Blidness and Bitot's Spots

Fig. 1. Mortality among children by clinical findings.[11]

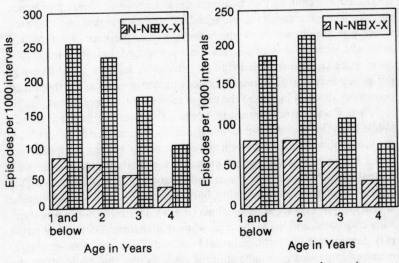

Fig. 2. Incidence of diarrhoea and respiratory disease by age in children with (X-X) and without (N-N) mild xerophthalmia at both start and end of interval.[12]

children with pre-existing xerophthalmia also had an increased risk of developing respiratory disease and diarrhoea subsequently (Fig. 2).[12] Indeed, mild xerophthalmia was a better predictor of illness than was anthropometric status. Both publications elicited little response: a single letter to the editor wondered whether the same results were true if we adjusted for a different anthropometric index. Neither observation led, as far as could be told, to interest on anyone's part nor to follow-up investigations by others. These were to follow much later.

RANDOMIZED TRIAL

We felt these observations warranted further investigation. If vitamin A supplementation could change childhood mortality it would have enormous implications for primary health care and child survival efforts. A large-scale, controlled trial which was then being planned in Northern Sumatra to test the effectiveness of vitamin A supplementation on the incidence of xerophthalmia was broadened to include the impact of vitamin A on mortality. While the Indonesian government was supportive of the project, it did not believe that it was ethical to provide some children with high-dose vitamin A and others with placebos. However, it was in the midst of expanding the xerophthalmia prevention programme through semi-annual distribution of vitamin A. We were able to take advantage of this expansion simply by randomizing the order in which new villages were included in the programme. By the end of the first year of follow-up, the results were striking. Children living in vitamin A-programme villages died at only one-third to one-half the rate of children in the control villages.

These preliminary findings were provided to the United Nations Administrative Coordinating Committee's Subcommittee on Nutrition (ACC/SCN), which concluded that there was sufficient reason to believe that vitamin A distribution in deficient populations would reduce mortality. The results of the original observational study and the randomized community trial formed the basis for a World Health Assembly resolution which requested that the WHO initiate global efforts to control vitamin A deficiency and its attendant blindness and mortality. When the scientific paper was published in the *Lancet* it was accompanied by an editorial entitled 'The Fall and Rise of the Anti-Infective Vitamin'.[13]

THE EFFECTS OF CONTROVERSY

The response of much of the scientific community was disbelief and distrust, despite the earlier animal and human data, the consistency of our various studies, and their biological plausibility. The lack of disinterested neutrality was striking. One investigator announced that he was re-analysing Indian data to 'disprove' the association between xerophthalmia and subsequent risk of infectious disease. The team that actually conducted the analysis ultimately proved the opposite.[14] Indeed, our publications seemed to generate more alarm than enthusiasm.

The controversy reached such proportions that, at the request of USAID, the U.S. National Academy of Science formed a committee to critique our work and provide recommendations for further trials. The results of their deliberations were, at best, disappointing. The senior statistician expressed frustration with the other members' lack of understanding of randomized trials and their focus, instead, on identifying inevitable (but, in his opinion, irrelevant) weaknesses. The Committee took over a year-and-a-half to publish its conclusions recommending further studies, but ethical issues of replicating our work raised so much concern that at least two members of the Committee wrote independent, dissenting reports on the morality and necessity of performing future studies. The main authors focused solely on the intervention trial, ignoring virtually all other available data as well as the problems of carrying out massive investigations under field conditions (the North Sumatran study had involved almost 30 000 children in 450 villages). The NAS panel also made much of the absence of placebos in the Indonesian study, although the basis for such concern was limited. Placebos are useful when attempting to distinguish an outcome related to an active agent (e.g. vitamin A) from a non-specific effect of the consumption of that agent. 'Placebo effects' are frequently encountered with subjective outcomes (e.g. whether the recipient 'feels' better or worse), but placebos are hardly likely to affect an outcome as objective and definitive as a child's death. The pains with which we had detailed all observations were used against the study. Our publication reported every conceivable baseline parameter that might have affected the outcome, with two minor differences between study and control group being pointed out by us and adjusted for in the analysis. The Committee held these to be important confounding variables that placed the conclusions in serious question! A subsequent replicate study in India, published in 1990, confirmed our results and was greeted by many as employing major methodological advances, yet it did not provide the important baseline comparisons.[15]

The negative reactions to the North Sumatran controlled trial seemed to emanate from numerous sources: an unwillingness to break with preconceptions concerning the potential value of a single micronutrient; failure to recognize that no single epidemiological study is ever 'perfect' in all regards and that the strength of available data comes from its consistency with other observations; and strongly held prejudices against scientists promoting the policy implications of their own findings.

THE PHILIPPINES STUDY

The impact of supplementation is likely to vary from one culture to another, depending upon the severity and extent of vitamin A deficiency, the causes of mortality, frequency and severity of infections and the dose of the infectious agent, along with other contributory conditions like general nutritional status and access to and utilization of health services. We therefore planned and initiated a large-scale study in Albay Province in the Philippines, in collaboration with the Ministry of Health and The Nutrition Centre of the Philippines. The ethical dilemma previously raised by members of the NAS Committee was to our minds irrelevant: the Government of the Philippines was not prepared to launch a vitamin A intervention programme on the basis of xerophthalmia alone or of the theoretical impact of vitamin A on mortality without evidence that such an impact would be forthcoming. Their hesitation was not unreasonable: while vitamin A is inexpensive (less than 2 U.S. cents per dose), delivering it to every pre-school child is no easy task and would call for a significant diversion of limited health resources. Determining the actual benefit would provide a rational basis, if any, for initiating a major public health intervention programme.

This second population-wide investigation in pre-school children contained a number of refinements over the original study. The most important were having adjacent data-processing facilities (which allowed more frequent, timely follow-up, with near 'real-time' results) and a placebo control. After two years of preliminary work, field-testing, census and enumeration, and a successful transition to a new government following the overthrow of the Marcos regime, the Philippine trial was destroyed three days before its start, when an irresponsible political activist alleged on the radio that the purpose of the study was to determine whether large-dose vitamin A would kill Filipino children! Paradoxically, the ethical issue was thus turned on its head—it was the intervention, not the placebo, to which he publicly objected. It was not that some children would be denied the potential benefits of vitamin A but rather, he speculated, that some would be killed by its use. This was an extraordinary accusation considering that not a single death has ever been traced to pure vitamin A toxicity even from *far* larger doses.[16] Subsequently the Philippine study was transformed into a multicentric hospital-based trial of the impact of vitamin A on children admitted with moderate to severe measles and respiratory infections in Metro-Manila hospitals. It is still going on. The community study was redesigned and moved to the *terai* region (foothills) of Nepal.

THE TURNING POINT

A turning point in the vitamin A story came at the 1989 IVACG meeting in Nepal where investigators from half-a-dozen countries reported the early findings of their morbidity and mortality studies. Most confirmed our observations, creating a critical mass of data from different settings that could not be ignored. Subsequently published results from the Nepal study demonstrated a dramatic fall in mortality, from 6 months of age through childhood.[17] A fortification trial in West Java by Indonesian scientists yielded almost identical results to those of the Sumatran study.[18] In south India, weekly supplementation of vitamin A showed mortality reduction starting at 6 months of age, just as seen in Nepal.[15] In an entirely independent investigation in the mountainous regions of Nepal, Daulaire and colleagues have further confirmed these results with a study design similar to that used in North Sumatra.[19]

However, one published study from India reported only a 7 per cent reduction, and the most recently reported results of a large trial in North Africa found no beneficial effects.[20,21] Implementation difficulties were experienced by both groups. But inability to demonstrate an effect does not prove the absence of an effect. Furthermore, one expects variation in the size of an effect, depending upon many local factors. Large field investigations will inevitably suffer from methodological shortcomings. As studies are often conducted in primitive and impoverished rural settings with limited budgets, logistic difficulties, and sometimes even in the midst of civil war or famine, it is not surprising to find that some fail to demonstrate a significant impact. While mortality would seem to be an easily measurable end-point, it is, in fact, an extremely difficult parameter to measure, as the absence of children at follow-up may be due to a number of factors: migration, temporary absence or death.

ISSUES AND LESSONS

Ethical Research

The question of ethical behaviour in the conduct of public health research

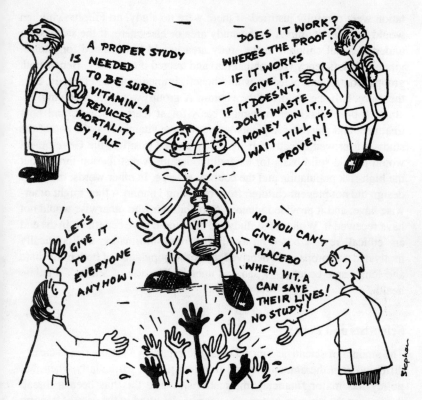

The scientists' quandary: when to study and when to act.

is clearly crucial. We have observed that it operates for and against studies that need to be undertaken. As there is no absolute 'ethics', each group of investigators must address the problem in their unique context. For instance, the original intervention trial in Indonesia could not use a placebo because it was considered 'unethical' as the Ministry of Health was already planning widespread distribution of vitamin A in the area in which the investigation was to be conducted. What made that investigation 'ethical', was that no one was deprived of the vitamin A that they would otherwise have received. Rather, since the Government could not cover all 500 new villages simultaneously, they allowed us to randomize the order in which the villages were included. In contrast, in the Philippines ethical considerations concerning the withholding of vitamin A from half the study population were carefully justified: if there were no study, no Filipino children would receive vitamin A in the study area or elsewhere; if the study were undertaken, all children in the study area would be screened for clinical vitamin A deficiency (xerophthalmia) and treated if necessary. Hence, both groups, control and placebo, would benefit immediately and directly. Furthermore, half the children (the vitamin A group) would be receiving vitamin A prophylaxis on a regular basis for at least one year, and both treatment and placebo recipients would receive vitamin A at the end of the study if it proved effective. If the study proved positive, the Government would have a solid basis for extending vitamin A distribution throughout the high-risk population and the country at large. In other words, the study design did not prevent children from receiving vitamin A they might otherwise have; and it provided vitamin A to children who otherwise would not have received it. Without the study, no one would have benefited. In the end an 'ethical' review based on totally incorrect information and politically motivated and propagated deprived the entire population of both immediate and long range benefits—a sad and unethical misuse of 'ethics' in public health.

Scientists and Policy

The amount of scientific data necessary to establish a simple fact is clearly different from the amount needed to affect policy, particularly when that policy has major financial implications. While this has been a thread throughout the vitamin A story, it is easily identified in the case of treating children with moderate to severe measles with vitamin A. Our first investigation in Tanzania demonstrated that providing large-dose vitamin A on two successive days to measles cases reduced mortality by 50 per cent compared with children who received routine hospital treatment.[22] This too resulted in a *Lancet* editorial and in a joint recommendation from WHO and UNICEF that vitamin A should be a standard part of treatment for all children with measles in countries in which vitamin A deficiency was recognized as a problem, or in which measles case fatality rates exceeded one per cent. However, few if any countries complied with this recommendation. Presumably they felt that a single hospital-based study in Tanzania was inadequate data upon which to adopt sweeping policy changes.

Four years later a similar study from Capetown, South Africa, was submitted for publication. The editors accepted the manuscript on its scientific merits, but had great reservations about publishing it in view of our earlier studies and the resulting joint WHO–UNICEF recommendations. Some felt the South African study should never have been done—the answer was already known. They felt it unethical to include a placebo group amongst whom mortality was once again shown to be double those given vitamin A. Fortunately the editors decided that in the absence of a demonstrable policy impact from the earlier work, *failure* to publish the South African study would itself be unethical, while publication might well lead to the health practice intended.[23] Such seems to have been the effect.

To affect policy decisions, particularly if these require alteration of previously held concepts and practices, requires a good deal more evidence than would ordinarily be necessary simply to establish an esoteric scientific 'fact'. While the weight of evidence from laboratory, clinical trials and controlled community studies has demonstrated the mortality reduction impact of adequate vitamin A in deficient populations, it remains to be seen how many more studies, meetings and workshops, discussions amongst experts, data and evidence will be necessary before consensus emerges and wide-scale action is taken to eliminate unnecessary deaths and illness from vitamin A deficiency.

Between the reports of the North Sumatran study and the subsequent replications, a great deal of time was spent travelling about the world, setting up our own studies, stimulating other researchers to undertake independent efforts and assisting governments interested in mounting intervention programmes on the basis of available data. Very little energy was expended in arguing with detractors. It was considered far more appropriate and productive to expand the research base and disseminate it widely than to engage in polemics. This is not an accustomed role for scientists nor a particularly comfortable one, though perhaps it should be. Those working in molecular genetics do not face the same problems of moral immediacy as those working at the interface of relevant and immediate public health issues. The public health investigator and policy-promoter must be entirely open and objective about the strengths and limitations of their studies, and advance their cause through repeated and improved methodological approaches and disinterested facilitation of other people's work.

An insightful examination of research results will often lead in directions quite different from those anticipated. These new directions may be far more important than those originally posed. Our original work and interest was related to the effect of vitamin A deficiency on the eye and the means to prevent blindness. The impact on susceptibility to infection and mortality, especially in the very young, emerged before us as a result of carefully-designed field investigation methodologies. An investigator must always be open to recognizing results which were never envisioned.

THE FUTURE

At the Global Summit for Children in September 1990 world leaders endorsed the goal to eliminate vitamin A deficiency during the next decade. As a result interest has risen among international agencies, particularly WHO and UNICEF, in taking more immediate and visible action. During 1990–91 the frequency of scientific and policy meetings on child survival increased as further data supported the impact of vitamin A. Yet at the same time, a small number of persistent sceptics, no longer able to deny the impact shown by the well-designed studies, have objected to the large-scale use of vitamin A to reduce child mortality for other reasons. They consider dietary changes more desirable than supplementary dosing, opposing a realistic mixed strategy to deal both with urgent needs as well as long-term sustainability. They decry dependency on multinational pharmaceutical producers of synthetic vitamin A, even when this is far less expensive than local production. They fear the spectre of vertical programmes, even though most methods of improving vitamin A status can be integrated into primary health care. They even object on the grounds that vitamin A may be toxic in some yet-unidentified fashion in infancy. Studies are already under way to address the serious scientific reservations and there appear to be no immediate or long-term side-effects from doses of 50 000 to 100 000 units given to children even in the earliest months of life. Obstacles related to a fear of foreign influence or the effect of vitamin A supplementation on socio-political systems are hard for a scientific worker to understand and deal with. Nevertheless, from a small handful of scientists in the early 1970s, the field is now rich in the creative energies of scores of dedicated investigators and interested policy-makers.

By mid-1992, vitamin A mortality research and programmes had become major, mainline health initiatives. Further studies from South Africa have demonstrated that treatment of measles reduced acute and long-term (six-month) morbidity, and some from Ghana showed that high dose, periodic community-wide supplementation reduced mortality by approximately 20 per cent and the severity of infectious episodes among pre-school children.[24,25] Thus the basis for policy and action seems securely established. All available published data were reviewed by a group of concerned scientists and health policy-makers at the Rockefeller Study Center. After considered discussion they issued the 'Bellagio Brief' which concluded that improving the vitamin A status of deficient children would significantly reduce their mortality and the severity of their infections.[26] At the same time, it raised the important issue of the need for addressing the risk of increased mortality and morbidity in marginally-deficient populations where xerophthalmia is not common.

The political apogee took place in Montreal in October 1991 at a meeting on micronutrient deficiencies hosted jointly by the Director General of WHO and the Executive Director of UNICEF. The 300 health leaders from around the world debated not whether vitamin A programming was important and valuable, but how best to get on with the job of preventing vitamin A deficiency world-wide by the year 2000.

The vitamin A story is not yet fully written. At the level of basic research, we need to understand *how* vitamin A affects growth, haemopoiesis, resistance to infection, and mortality. At the level of programmes, we need to identify successful, culturally-specific approaches to improving vitamin A status, whether through changes in diet or a multiplicity of methods for supplementing natural dietary sources.

Who knows what other scientific facts may hold the prospect of dramatic improvements in child health and survival simply by their wider dissemination, confirmation and application? The quest for 'Health for All by the year 2000' is contingent upon a more rapid adoption and application of proven effective interventions that can be affordably integrated into existing health care systems to improve the lives of common people.

References

1. McCollum, E. V. and Davis, M. (1913). The necessity of certain lipins in the diet during growth. *Journal of Biological Chem*istry, Vol. 15, pp. 167–75.
2. Bloch, C. E. (1921). Clinical investigation of xerophthalmia and dystrophy in infants and young children (Xerophthalmia et dystrophia alipogenetica). *Journal of Hygiene (Cambridge)*, Vol. 19, pp. 283–301.
3. Sommer A. (1982). *Nutritional blindness: Xerophthalmia and keratomalacia.* Oxford University Press, New York.
4. Patwardhan, V. N., Kamel, W. W. and Pharaon, H. (1966). Studies on vitamin A deficiency in infants and young children in Jordan. II. A pilot trial of vitamin A prophylaxis in Jordanian infants. Project Report, World Health Organization, pp. 103–37.
5. Swaminathan, M. C., Susheela, T. P. and Thimmayamma, B. V. S. (1970). Field prophylactic trial with single annual oral massive dose of vitamin A. *American Journal of Clinical Nutrition*, Vol. 23, pp. 119–22.
6. Sommer, A., Muhilal, Tarwotjo, I., *et al.* (1980). Oral versus intramuscular vitamin A in the treatment of xerophthalmia. *Lancet*, Vol. 1, pp. 557–9.
7. Sommer, A., Hussaini, G., Muhilal, *et al.* (1980). History of night blindness: A simple tool for xerophthalmia screening. *American Journal of Clinical Nutrition*, Vol. 33, pp. 887–91.
8. Sommer, A., Tarwotjo, I. and Hussaini, G. (1981). Incidence, prevalence and scale of blinding malnutrition. *Lancet*, Vol. 1, pp. 1407–8.

9. World Health Organization. (1982). *Control of vitamin A deficiency and xerophthalmia.* Technical Report Series, No. 672, World Health Organization, Geneva.

10. Sommer, A., Tarwotjo, I. and Katz, J. (1987). Increased risk of xerophthalmia following diarrhoea and respiratory disease. *American Journal of Clinical Nutrition,* Vol. 45, pp. 977–80.

11. Sommer, A., Tarwotjo, I., Hussaini, G., *et al.* (1983). Increased mortality in children with mild vitamin A deficiency. *Lancet,* Vol. 2, pp. 585–8.

12. Sommer, A., Katz, J. and Tarwotjo, I. (1984). Increased risk of respiratory disease and diarrhoea in children with pre-existing mild vitamin A deficiency. *American Journal of Clinical Nutrition,* Vol. 40, pp. 1090–5.

13. Sommer, A., Tarwotjo, I., Djunaedi, E., *et al.* (1986). Impact of vitamin A supplementation on childhood mortality: A randomized controlled community trial. *Lancet,* Vol. 1, pp. 1169–73.

14. Milton, R. C., Reddy, V. and Naidu, A. N. (1987). Mild vitamin A deficiency and childhood morbidity—An Indian experience. *American Journal of Clinical Nutrition,* Vol. 46, pp. 827–9.

15. Rahmathullah, L., Underwood, B. A., Thulasiraj, R. D., *et al.* (1990). Reduced mortality among children in Southern India receiving a small weekly dose of vitamin A. *New England Journal of Medicine,* Vol. 323, pp. 929–35.

16. Bauernfeind, J. C. (1980). The safe use of vitamin A. A report of the International Vitamin A Consultative Group.

17. West, K. P., Pokhrel, R. P., Katy, J. *et al.* (1991). Efficacy of vitamin A in reducing preschool child mortality in Nepal. *Lancet,* Vol. 338, pp. 67–71.

18. Muhilal, Permeisih, D., Idjradinata, Y. R., *et al.* (1988). Vitamin A-fortified monosodium glutamate and health, growth, and survival of children: A controlled field trial. *American Journal of Clinical Nutrition,* Vol. 48, pp. 1271–6.

19. Daulaire, N. M. P., Starbuck, E. S., Houston, R. M., *et al.* (1992). Childhood mortality after a high dose of vitamin A in a high risk population. *British Mediical Journal,* Vol. 304, pp. 207–10.

20. Vijayaraghavan, K., Radhalah, G., Prakasam, B. S., *et al.* (1990). Effect of massive dose of vitamin A on morbidity and mortality in Indian children. *Lancet,* Vol. 336, pp. 1342–5.

21. Herera, M. G., Nestle, P., El Amin, A., *et al.* (1992). Vitamin A supplementation and child survival. *Lancet,* Vol. 340, pp. 267–71.

22. Barclay, A. J. G., Foster, A. and Sommer, A. (1987). Vitamin A supplementation and mortality related to measles: A randomized clinical trial. *British Medical Journal,* Vol. 294, pp. 294–6.

23. Hussey, G. D. and Klein, M. (1990). A randomized, controlled trial of vitamin A in children with severe measles. *New England Journal of Medicine,* Vol. 323, pp. 160–4.

24. Coustsoudis, A., Broughton, M. and Coovadia, H. M. (1991). Vitamin A supplementation reduces measles morbidity in young African children: A randomized, placebo-controlled, double-blind trial. *American Journal of Clinical Nutrition,* Vol. 54, pp. 890–5.

25. Arthur, P., Kirkwood, B., Ross, D., *et al.* (1992). Impact of vitamin A supplementation on childhood morbidity in northern Ghana. *Lancet,* Vol. 339, pp. 361–2.

26. Sommer, A. (1992). Vitamin A deficiency and childhood mortality. *Lancet,* Vol. 339, p. 864.

CHAPTER 21

Family Planning can Contribute to Health for All

JOHN ROWLEY AND HALFDAN MAHLER

The authors argue that family planning is a neglected practical measure, critical to enhancing the status and health of women as well as the overall well-being of families and communities.

John Rowley is Assistant Director of the International Planned Parenthood Federation heading the Publications and Communications Services.

Halfdan Mahler, M.D., was Director-General of the World Health Organization from 1980 to 1988. He is now the Executive Director of the International Planned Parenthood Federation from where he enthusiastically continues to support comprehensive health care for all.

INTRODUCTION

Forty years ago in November 1952, a group of well-meaning—and as it turns out, far-sighted—social reformers met in Bombay and set up a federation of eight family planning associations. These pioneers of the International Planned Parenthood Federation, as they called it, were internationalists. They spanned the rich world and the poor. Their concern was not only to extend the rights of planned parenthood to all couples, but to help bring about a balance between population and natural resources. In both respects they were ahead of their time.

It was another decade before the United Nations began responding to calls for help with family planning. In the mid-1960s the World Health Organization began to grasp the health implications of unplanned pregnancies. It was not until 1969 that the United Nations Fund for Population Activities (UNFPA) was formed and began helping governments set up national family planning programmes.

We recall this, not only because 1992 was IPPF's fortieth anniversary year but because an historical perspective is helpful in looking forward to the last fateful years of this millennium and into the next century. It is easy to be overcome by the absurdities of a world which wastes resources on a gargantuan scale but fails to invest more than a pittance on the long-term health of human populations, or to safeguard the health of the earth's precious air, soils, forests and water, on which all species depend.

Our pioneers in Bombay made slow progress at first. In the early 1960s fewer than 15 million couples in the developing world outside China were using contraception. Today, some 380 million couples in the developing world are taking charge of their fertility—over half of all couples in the child-bearing years. Over 90 per cent of the world's population lives in countries with positive family planning policies and programmes.

THE DEMOGRAPHIC TRANSITION

There is now no doubt that the world is in transition, social and demographic. We are on the way to creating a world in which mankind's success in reducing death rates is matched by a move towards fewer, healthier, planned births. Such a world will be one in which women everywhere have a right to control their own fertility. It will be one in which reproductive health is a matter of universal care and concern. It will be a world where population growth rates no longer fuel urban and environmental pressures which help perpetuate gross disparities of wealth and poverty and which lead to continuing destruction of the 'spaceship in which we travel'. Hopefully, it will be a world where the commitment to future generations is matched by the concern that all children are wanted children.

But we have yet to reach the fulcrum of the demographic transition when, some time in the early years of the new century, fewer children will be born in a year than in the year before. At that point, the annual population addition, now running at 90 million will begin to slow; and the human race—now totalling 5.3 billion—will be on the way to stabilizing its numbers at somewhere between 11 and 14 billion. This will occur in the second half of the twenty-first century. In the years until that turning point we face our greatest challenge, with the largest generation of young people ever known soon to be in need of information and services to plan healthy sexual and reproductive lives.

THE CHALLENGES

There are 1.7 billion people under the age of 15 in the world today. During this decade, many of them will become sexually active. The 15–25 year

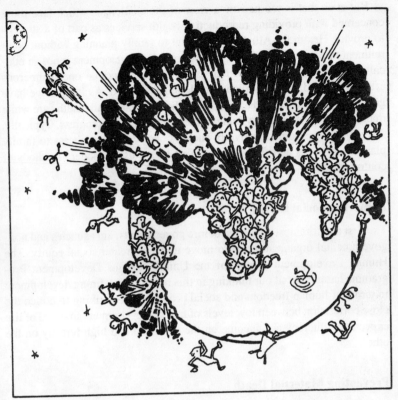

With a world bursting with people can we reach Health for All?

age-group will grow by a quarter in the 1990s and the number of married women in the fertile age-group in the developing world outside China will almost double in the 20 years up to 2010. All this presents a tremendous challenge to those charged with providing reproductive health care, including sex education, contraceptive counselling and services.

In theory, demographic targets set by the United Nations can be met if contraceptive prevalence in the developing world is increased from today's 51 per cent to 59 per cent by the year 2000. This would mean extending services to 567 million couples—an additional 186 million above today. In reality the challenge is even greater since most of those practising contraception in the developing world are not well served with a choice of the most suitable and reliable methods. A quantum leap in the *quality* of services is needed.

But even that is too narrow a view of the challenges which face those concerned with providing reproductive health services as part of a strategy to provide Health for All. A commitment to family planning without commitment to personal health and socio-economic development is not an ethically acceptable proposition. Nor is it really a workable one. Numerous efforts confined to family planning alone have failed. As long as we have governments which spend a mere $1 per head a year on all health care while maintaining a vast military budget, there will be slow progress. Typically, fewer than one woman in five in such a country has any access to family planning services and fewer than one in 14 are using modern methods of contraception.

Achieving Social Equity

The first and foremost challenge before governments, aid agencies and non-governmental organizations is to move towards greater social equity. The Human Development Report of the United Nations Development Programme has advanced our thinking in this respect by defining development in terms of human freedom and social progress. It is striking to notice the close correlation between low levels of human development in terms of life expectancy, literacy and income on the one hand and high fertility on the other.

Preventing Maternal Death

The second challenge relates directly to the healthy survival of families, particularly mothers and children. Thankfully, since the Safe Motherhood Conference in Nairobi in 1987, a great deal of attention has been given to the tragedy of maternal death and morbidity. Pregnancy-related deaths, which kill at least 500 000 women each year, have been neglected because those who suffer them are neglected people. They are people with the least power and influence over how public resources are spent. They are the poor, rural peasants and, above all, women.

Very often the road to maternal death has its beginning deep in a woman's past life. It may be in her own infancy or even before her birth that deficiencies of calcium or vitamin D or iron begin. Continued through childhood and adolescence, they result in contracted pelvis, and eventually in death from obstructed labour; or they can lead to chronic iron-deficiency anaemia and result in death through haemorrhage. The train of negative factors goes on through the stages of a woman's life especially where re-

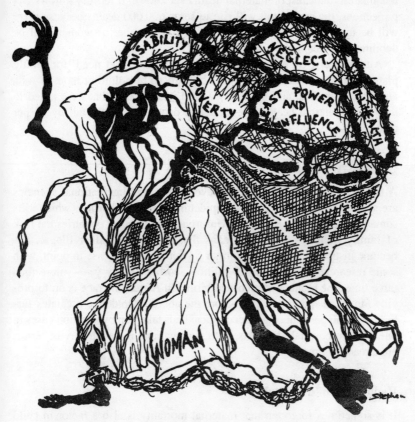

Women carry an undue burden of negative factors which makes their reproductive risks even greater.

productive and family planning services are absent. There are the special risks of adolescent pregnancy, maternal depletion from closely-spaced pregnancies, the burden of heavy physical labour in the reproductive period, the renewed risk of child-bearing after age 35 and worse, after 40, the compounding risks of grand multiparity, and throughout these years, the ghastly dangers of illegal abortion to which women may be driven in sheer desperation. All these are like links in a chain from which only menopause or the grave offer hope of escape—hope that could be realized by family planning.

Sadly, the last decade of this century of technological wizardry may see the greatest holocaust of maternal death ever known. If fertility follows UN projections, the annual toll will rise to some 600 000 deaths because there will be many more births. And 16 times this number of women will be debilitated or maimed, some of them for life.

Alternatively, by meeting even the existing 'unmet need' for family planning, maternal death rates could be reduced by a third or more in Asia and Latin America, and by nearly a fifth in Africa. If this were allied to improved maternal health care, maternal death rates could fall by 50 per cent.

Curbing Abortion

A third challenge which national governments and international agencies are slow to tackle is the growing epidemic of illegal abortion, which kills some 200 000 women each year. Unfortunately, in many countries the lack of family planning services means that abortion, legal or illegal, has become institutionalized. The former Soviet Union is a case in point, with some researchers estimating 20 million abortions every year—more than three times the number of recorded births. In Africa, the race is on to provide family planning services before the abortion epidemic escalates further. With 60 per cent of gynaecological beds taken up by abortion cases in one African hospital, the costs, both personal and in health service terms, are already enormous.

Reducing Child Mortality

It is sometimes forgotten that maternal mortality is also a factor in child mortality. UNICEF's report, *The State of the World's Children 1991*, provides a compelling chapter which analyses the effects on both mother and child health of simultaneous action to bring about fertility decline—improvement in the lives of women, reduction of child deaths, and improved availability of family planning. The report says that all of these interventions make an important contribution to improving the lives of millions of people: 'The fact that they also make a strong synergistic contribution to solving the population problem, and that they can all be accomplished at a relatively modest cost, add up to what should be an irresistible case for simultaneous action on all these fronts in the decade ahead.' UNICEF rightly points out that the potential for reducing child deaths is especially compatible with the need to reduce births. This is because 'three of the most important strategies now available for reducing child deaths—the education of women, the well-informed timing of births, and breast-feeding—also happen to be among the most direct methods of reducing child births'. UNICEF readily acknowledges that 'the well-informed timing and spacing of births is one of the greatest of all opportunities for improving the health and saving the lives of women and children'.

Apart from its benefits to women's health in reducing maternal illness, disability, death and abortions, 'for the children, a responsible planning of family size can mean better levels of health, nutrition, education, and is one of the most powerful means of achieving many of the most basic human development goals adopted for the year 2000'.

Empowering Women

This document is another testament to the consensus that has now been achieved on the goals which those concerned with real human development are promoting. These goals include one which we would stress above all others: the empowerment of women.

Women represent a resource that is both grossly abused and under-appreciated, to the detriment of us all. Within IPPF our aim is both to increase the contribution of women among family planning and health volunteers and staff, and to find ways of empowering young women with the knowledge, skills and opportunities for increased participation in decision-making, to improve their status socially, economically, and in terms of health for themselves and their children.

A BROADER ROLE

This is certainly one of the contributions that the non-governmental sector can make. But there are others. Of prime importance is the lead which NGOs can take in pioneering high-quality family planning. By this we do not mean glossy clinics—but caring services which meet people's needs and give them informed choices. A second priority is community outreach and involvement—the harnessing of 'people power'—using flexible approaches that respond to local needs and opportunities. A third is the involvement of young people. A fourth is reaching out to men, who have been excluded too long from a process which they often misunderstand. Finally, we have to think beyond family planning services to the broader goal of sexual and reproductive health for all, a concept that will embrace the AIDS pandemic but not treat it as an isolated phenomenon.

SUPPORT TO FAMILY PLANNING

This decade began with many hopeful signs of commitment to family planning. Donor governments acknowledged the scale of the need for information and services for the 900 million couples who will be on earth by the year 2000. Meetings of spiritual leaders reinforced the widespread conviction that optimism about the future would add to success in meeting that need. The cost has been estimated at some $9 billion a year by the century's end—perhaps $3 billion of which will come from international donors. This is not a huge sum. A tripling of today's spending will be equivalent only to six-tenths of one per cent of what the world spends on armaments every year—two or three days worth of arms. We need to spend more, too, on reproductive research which today receives $53 million less in real terms than it did in the 1970s.

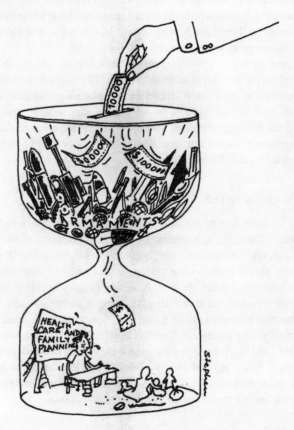

In some countries, consumers will be prepared and able to pay more towards their contraceptive services. In others, governments must take a lead in manufacturing supplies and improving services. But the international community must also help in the crucial period of transition to a better, more stable world.

ETHICS AND HUMAN RIGHTS

There are still some who question the ethics of family planning. But who can question the ethics of promoting the well-being and saving the lives of millions of women and children, and perhaps also saving the environment on the way? What has happened to the ethics of our contemporary world if we are compelled to debate whether or not to leave sick and starving children to their fate? Is human life worth so very little?

And what of human rights? The 1968 International Conference on Human Rights, held in Teheran, endorsed the view that access to family planning information and services is a basic human right, and should be available to couples, to individuals and to the young world-wide. What mockery it makes of human rights if women and children are condemned to death when life-saving family planning is a do-able proposition worldwide!

IPPF and its member associations have never practised so-called 'population control', but through information and education we encourage millions to be responsible parents and to understand the social and economic carrying-capacity of the land their children will inherit.

And so we steer our spaceship earth onward and upward to that distant planet where every child is a wanted child, a child who can be loved, nurtured, and kept alive at any cost. Let us rise to the challenge of which Eddah Gachukia from Kenya spoke at a women's leadership conference in Vienna in January 1991: 'We want to get to the position where a woman jumps for joy when she is pregnant.' On that day, the world will jump for joy with her.

References

1. Draper, W. H. (1990, 1991, 1992). *Human Development Report*. Oxford University Press (for UNDP, New York).
2. Grant, J. P. (1991). *The State of the World's Children 1991*. Oxford University Press (for UNICEF, New York).

CHAPTER 22

The Family Planning Movement in Indonesia

HARYONO SUYONO, LUKAS HENDRATA AND JON ROHDE

The authors describe how Indonesia's family planning programme has evolved to become a national movement focusing on quality of life and planning for a better future among families and communities and at the national level.

Haryono Suyono, Ph.D., is the Director of the National Family Planning Coordinating Board of Indonesia and has been a prime architect of its strategies since its inception 20 years ago.

Lukas Hendrata, M.D., helped formulate the early family planning communication strategies and has continued to work as a consultant to Indonesia's family planning programme as Director of the Prosperous Indonesia Foundation (YIS).

Jon Rohde, M.D., worked in Indonesia for nearly ten years and has returned frequently as a consultant in health, nutrition and family planning.

INTRODUCTION

In the late 1960s demographers projected the population of Indonesia in the year 2000 as 220 to 230 million, a prospect which promised to lay waste economists' plans for national development. With a life expectancy of 54 and an infant mortality rate of 140 or more, the total fertility rate was 5.6 and fewer than 50 000 couples practised family planning. Soekarno's earlier pro-natalist policy was not consistent with the emerging technocracy's plans for economic and social development. In 1970 President Soeharto initiated the National Family Planning Coordinating Board (*BKKBN*). Since then the fertility rate has fallen by over 40 per cent and today more than 18 million couples practise some form of family planning, with 15 to 20 000 new participants inducted every day. The infant mortality rate has dropped to under 60 and life expectancy in Indonesia is now a respectable 63 years. The country's population was 179.3 million in 1991, 5 to 10 million lower than predicted, and the nation expects to achieve its planned growth rate of 1.6 per cent by 1995. The story of this success revolves around the *BKKBN*, but in reality it is the tale of a successful national development effort. Family planning in Indonesia is a dynamic mix of political commitment, inter-sectoral organization and collaboration and modern participatory management. It combines successful information, education and motivational campaigns, innovative training approaches for development, the use of a simplified and streamlined information system for measured accountability, wide availability of contraceptives and relevant health care, and, above all, an entrepreneurial bureaucracy committed to decentralization and innovative approaches to involving the community. Today the Indonesian Family Planning Programme is an integral part of the national development strategy. It continues to evolve as it faces new challenges which are the hallmark of a maturing and developing country.

EARLY CLINICAL SERVICES

Prior to 1970, contraceptive services were provided largely through the private sector, particularly the Indonesian Planned Parenthood Federation, founded in 1957. IPPF provided clinical services and information to individual clients through many urban branches. Following the signing of the World Population Declaration by President Soeharto in 1967, the Ministry of Health began to offer contraceptive pills and IUDs through their fixed clinic services. Initial acceptors were limited largely to the educated elite, who often obtained their information and motivation from personal interactions with the small group of pioneers dedicated to family planning or from abroad.

As improved public health brought crude death rates to less than 15, birth rates hovered above 40 and population growth in the 1960s approached 3 per cent. While vast unsettled spaces remained on the outer islands, the population density on Java and Bali, where two-thirds of Indonesia's people resided, was already amongst the highest on earth (600 per square kilometre). Demographers from research and development institutions both at home and abroad recognized that the rapidly growing population would substantially reduce the benefits of the expanding economy, raise the costs of necessary social programmes, and bring ecological and social disruption in the future. One prominent demographer-economist, Widjojo, became the Chairman of the powerful and prestigious National

Planning Board (*BAPPENAS*), bringing the concern for population to the top of the national development agenda.

NATIONAL FAMILY PLANNING COORDINATING BOARD (*BKKBN*)

In 1970 President Soeharto established the National Family Planning Coordinating Board, *BKKBN*, an agency designed to make family planning more than just a clinical service available through the Health Department. It would endeavour to increase nation-wide acceptance of a smaller family norm for the sake of the health and well-being of the family, the community and the country. From the outset *BKKBN* did not confine itself either to the motivation and recruitment of new acceptors nor to the provision of family planning services. In addition, its Division of Population was concerned about educating the public on the entire range of issues emerging from the growing population. A Research and Development Division was established and adequately funded to take initiatives, not just on a pilot basis but often covering large populations to develop innovative ways of motivating and involving communities. As a coordinating body it was *BKKBN*'s responsibility to be sure that concerns for population and family planning were extended throughout the government system.

As before, the Ministry of Health provided clinical services and dramatically increased the training of doctors and paramedical workers in the use and problems of modern contraceptives. The Ministry of Religious Affairs was consulted at the very beginning to ensure that public approaches were consistent with religious beliefs and enjoyed the active support of religious leaders. Islamic scholars, social organizations and, eventually, individual *imams* (head priests) gave major support and guidance to the programme. Christian and Hindu organizations played an important role in the populations where these religious persuasions prevailed. The Ministry of Information and Broadcasting was an integral partner from the outset, using modern methods of mass communication to make the concept and technical details of family planning common knowledge. Family planning was moved actively out of the realm of private, unspoken behaviour and placed squarely in the public domain, a point of community conversation and concern. The Education Ministry modified curriculum to emphasize the desirability and benefits of small families, starting from primary school. Adult literacy classes also included more explicit information on family planning services. The Ministry of Industries was one of the first to motivate and provide regular services to workers employed in the formal sector, exhorting employers to educate and encourage their staff to avail of modern contraceptive services. The armed forces provided strong motivation and convenient services to all its members. The Home Ministry began to monitor local birth rates and family planning use, asking civil leaders to encourage and support family planning.

In a land where large families were considered desirable and often necessary, the campaign initially proposed limitation of family size to four, then three and eventually, embraced the 'two-child norm'. Important to the acceptance of this concept was the support of the nation's President and, through him, of civil leaders at all levels, including the village *lurah* or headman. During the early years, the programme concentrated its efforts on informing and educating people in the community about the benefits of planning one's own family. This effort was supported by the provision of services in health clinics, particularly in areas with high population densities on the islands of Java and Bali. While these two islands represent a mere seven per cent of the country's total land area, they contained two-thirds of the national population.

OUTREACH WORKERS—*PLKB*

The next phase began in 1972 when *BKKBN* developed a core of family planning field-workers (*PLKB*) whose primary function was to motivate and provide services to eligible couples. Working out of government clinics, the workers tended to reach clients who were already motivated, in touch with the system. In 1974 a critical decision was taken to base the *PLKB* in the villages they served (each covered 3000 to 5000 people). Only their supervisor (group leader) was given a desk and chair at the sub-district office (population 30 000). This seemingly simple decision to deprive a worker of a seat, as it were, in the health centre, placed the *PLKB* squarely in the heart of the community. Family planning users increased rapidly with the introduction of the oral pill, the most popular method. *PLKB*s delivered contraceptives in the privacy of each home, combining personalized information and a convenient service. To cater to the rising numbers of acceptors, outreach medical teams provided consultation, especially to those new acceptors who encountered problems with a method. By the mid-1970s 7000 *PLKB*s were spending an increasingly large part of their time servicing current users, leaving less time to motivate new acceptors. A new approach was necessary.

VILLAGE ACCEPTOR CLUBS—*POS KB*

The Research and Development (R&D) Division had been exploring a number of community-based approaches to both acceptor recruitment and contraceptive resupply. They had found that satisfied acceptors in the community enjoyed gathering as a 'club' to discuss their experience, their commitment and their expectations. For a small stipend, some community members had been willing to distribute the monthly supply of contraceptives to each participating household. This rapidly led to a fully volunteer force throughout Java and Bali. Indigenous community organizations grasped the opportunity to provide a useful, desired community service and established community-based family planning clubs called *kelompok akseptor*—acceptor clubs, or *Pos KB*—FP posts. There was no cost to *BKKBN*. Initially asked only to assist the government in providing resupply services, these community-based women acceptor groups took over the family planning programme and thus started its transformation to the national movement it is today.

Throughout the 1970s community acceptor groups were responsible for recruiting new acceptors and for encouraging the continued participation of

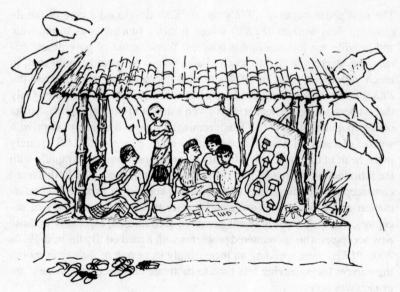

Village clubs are a key to recruiting new acceptors and resupplying current contraceptive users.

their own members. Over half of all new rural acceptors were recruited through village groups and a majority of pill and condom users were supplied through them. Each group maintained records of all couples in their village, acceptor and continuing-user status, accounting for the distribution of contraceptive commodities. This gave each acceptor club a sense of being in charge, of calling on the government workers for services and supplies rather than the reverse. Community ownership led to commitment.

For its part, the government had to provide reliable, regular and free supplies of contraceptives and back-up medical services. The evolution of acceptor groups varied from community to community. Because these groups came from the wide range of the country's socio-cultural and economic groups, they understood people's problems better and were more responsive to the needs of their neighbours. Their involvement and demands brought new perspectives to and opportunities for service delivery improvement which became a major concern of the national programme.

In this time the *BKKBN* had developed a simple postcard-sized information system which recorded the particulars of each new acceptor including age, parity, education and method of choice. Processed within weeks at a central computer unit in Jakarta, feedback was given telegraphically to each province, district and sub-district. Even village heads rapidly became conversant with the jargon of family planning. All knew their number of eligible couples (PUS), current users (CUs), new acceptors in the past year, contraceptive mix and, eventually, even the average parity, age of users and duration of use. Innovative means of motivating entire villages emerged. In Bali at the monthly *banjar* (hamlet) meeting a village map was displayed with the contraceptive choice of each participating household clearly indicated. Village sign-boards showed what proportion of the village population was using contraception and competition ensued between neighbouring villages, sub-districts and even districts in a province. This competition became a major driving force in the programme. Recognition was given by civil leaders to those communities which were participating most fully. At no time were any incentive payments made to induce new acceptors. The only promise was that of a 'Small, Prosperous and Happy Family' to those who became regular programme participants. However, communities did receive special farm credit, hybrid coconut seedlings and other material bonuses for high performance. The Home Ministry incorporated the current user rate among the parameters by which villages were evaluated in the national village classification scheme. By the late 1970s family planning was universalized in Java and Bali, with acceptor rates often exceeding 50 per cent of eligible couples in many districts.

BEYOND FAMILY PLANNING TO CHILD NUTRITION—*KB-GIZI*

Having succeeded in popularizing the small family concept, *BKKBN* was faced with a rising demand for a broader array of welfare services. The slogan 'A Small Happy Prosperous Family' threatened to be an empty one if only contraceptive services were provided. Again, the R&D wing had explored a number of approaches 'beyond family planning' and recognized the potential of village-based child health and nutrition services to sustain the family planning effort. Women Family Welfare Clubs (*PKK*), present in almost every village, not only formed the core of many acceptor clubs but had also begun monthly weighing of children in an effort to improve nutrition and child health. The *BKKBN* recognized that this recurring activity was an opportunity to provide an array of services, as well as to continue motivating mothers to use contraception, focusing on the health of their youngest child. Started in 1979 the family planning–nutrition programme (*KB-Gizi*) initially aimed at family planning acceptors but grew to embrace all families in almost 30 000 villages during Indonesia's Third Five-Year Plan period (1979–84).* The key to this extension was the role of the *PLKB* who were retrained in procedures to assist and encourage mothers' groups to conduct monthly village-based child nutrition activities. Based on the Health Department's Family Nutrition Improvement Activities (*UPGK*), the *KB-Gizi* programme grew faster and larger as it built on the existing network of acceptor clubs, guided by the 7000 field-workers who were well-equipped with weight charts, weighing scales and other materials necessary for the monthly-weighing activity. Contraceptive resupply was a convenient part of the monthly focus on young child nutrition and growth.

During the 1980s the many lessons in community involvement generated by the *PLKB* in Java and Bali were extended to all 27 provinces in the far-flung outer islands of the Indonesian archipelago. Lessons of the previous ten years were put to work in communities far less compact, socially coherent, and often far less educated. Over the decade 20 000 *PLKB* were recruited and trained locally for these culturally-diverse islands. The high fertility rate and low use of health services in these remote areas became a major challenge to the expanding family planning programme.

---

*See the chapter by Jon Rohde and Lucas Hendrata in *Practising Health for All* (D. Morley, J. Rohde and G. Williams, eds.), Oxford University Press, Oxford, 1983, pp. 252–71; and the chapter by Jon Rohde in this volume.

THE INTEGRATED SERVICE POST—*POSYANDU*

In 1984 at the inception of the Fourth Five-Year Plan, the potential for village-based, volunteer-run nutrition and family planning services was well-established. The Health Department, recognizing the tremendous potential for its many outreach programmes, took over responsibility for the village integrated service-delivery post, now renamed *Posyandu*. (This programme is discussed more fully in the chapter by Rohde in this volume.)

The monthly gathering run by village volunteers was now joined by a worker from the nearest health centre who provided, in addition to the baby-weighing, a resupply of contraceptives and essential nutrition commodities, immunization services, ante-natal screening for pregnant women, and a modicum of medical care with a limited number of essential drugs. By the end of the decade there were nearly a quarter million *posyandus* run by volunteers in each of Indonesia's 67 000 villages. During 1990 *posyandus* provided full immunization to more than 80 per cent of the children

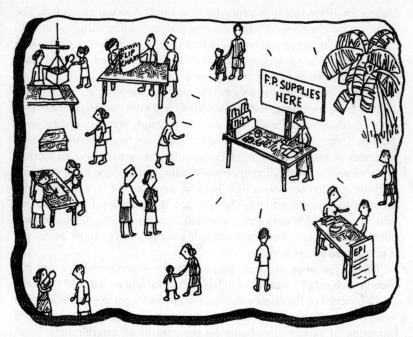

The monthly 'posyandu' in the village provides a convenient opportunity for replenishment of family planning supplies.

born in Indonesia. Some 18 million immunizations were provided, over four million family planning users continued to receive contraceptives at these monthly meetings and 25 to 35 per cent of new acceptors were recruited there.

There was considerable variation in activity from village to village based on local leadership and popular demand. In many the approach became more encompassing, including literacy programmes, income-generating activities, buying and selling cooperatives, and agricultural extension services for small animals and home-gardening. A broad range of government services relevant to young families became part and parcel of acceptor group activities. People recognized that by becoming family planning acceptors they could have access to more tangible benefits that would improve the quality of their lives, their families' welfare, and the development of their community.

A NATIONAL MOVEMENT FOR FAMILY PLANNING

During the 1980s family planning became a truly national movement. The President gave regular and consistent support, providing adequate funds to the family planning programme even during difficult economic times when the budget for other government activities had to be reduced. He often made public statements in support of the programme and constantly cited its positive impact on Indonesian society. He held his ministers accountable for support from their departments. Governors and civil employees were promoted partially on the basis of the success of family planning in their jurisdictions. Every two years the President recognized model family planning acceptors by inviting them to the Presidential Palace to receive his congratulations and an award directly. Family planning has come to be seen as a patriotic activity, not only a right but also a responsibility, a positive contribution to national welfare. The message that planning for the nation's future starts in each and every home, and includes not only family fertility but also availability of education, reliable health services and a decent job is propagated and believed widely.

The performance of the Indonesian family planning programme has been the subject of a number of independent evaluations. The 1987 Indonesia Contraceptive Prevalence Survey found that 94 per cent of Indonesian women knew about modern contraceptive methods and strongly supported limitation of family size. Some 50 per cent of all eligible Indonesian couples were using modern contraceptives to plan their families. On Java and Bali almost 80 per cent of couples are practising family planning currently. Some 18 million current users and 15 to 20 thousand new acceptors every day place considerable demands on clinical services, calling for quality and sustainability. Counselling remains an integral part of the programme. All new acceptors receive a careful medical examination. An increasingly broad range of contraceptives is available free through family planning posts and health centres.

Concern for women's welfare is expanding continuously. One strategy strongly emphasized in the current Plan is 'Safe Motherhood'. Properly-spaced pregnancies are important to overall maternal welfare but, in addition, peri-natal care is crucial for maternal and infant survival and health. This new effort will focus on increasing the number and improving the capacity of trained village-based midwives to provide better and more convenient services to mothers and children in rural areas. The strategy offers a wider range of integrated family planning and health services to mothers near their home and will improve both maternal and child survival through the provision of ante-natal, delivery and post-natal care.

TOWARDS SUSTAINABILITY—*KB MANDIRI*

To further ensure the sustainability of the national programme, private-sector contraceptive supplies are becoming available at discounted prices through a social-marketing programme called the 'Blue Circle' or *KB Mandiri*, the self-reliant family planning programme. The gradual transfer of responsibility for family planning from the government to the people will focus initially on improved services provided through the private sector. Convenient, high quality, personalized family planning counselling and services with the widest possible mix of modern options will be self-financing. This cost-recovery scheme makes the Indonesian family planning programme yet more multi-sectoral and community-based. Initially *KB Mandiri* was confined to major cities where adequate economic capacity exists. The number of acceptors currently paying for their own contraceptive supplies has increased rapidly. While in the past commercially-purchased contraceptives accounted for less than 5 per cent of the total used, by 1991 that share had risen to 15 per cent. This year the programme will expand to all Indonesian cities and villages ready to take on their own initiative to become self-sufficient. By the year 2000 Indonesia expects that 30 to 40 per cent of current users will be paying for their own supplies and services.

While in the early years *BKKBN* appealed to the people's civic consciousness and sense of community spirit to develop a village-based family planning movement, they now appeal to individuals using a variety of ap-

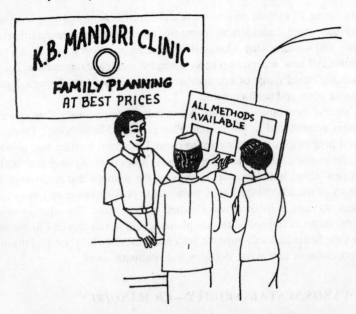

*The Blue Circle identifies private clinics where patients pay for
personalized family planning services.*

proaches. For instance they advocate that an individual who is self-reliant
is making a valuable contribution to the development of a strong and completely independent nation, thereby evoking a sense of national pride. They
point to the personalized nature of professional services marked by convenience and high quality. A Family Planning Insurance Scheme started in
1991 offers life-time indemnity against unwanted pregnancy or medical
complications of IUDs, injectables or implants for a single low premium.
Family planning insurance is seen as a guarantee of prosperity.

However, the sustainability of family planning requires more than finance—it calls for a national 'frame of mind'. Population planning has always had an important role in national development. Indonesia has made
planning of the individual family a critical path to prosperity and happiness,
much beyond quantitative demography and clinical issues. True family
planning is both vital for bringing about changes in the nation's value systems and norms which are essential to development, and has broader socio-
economic implications.

For instance, education has been important both in family planning and national development. In a very real sense, the development of Indonesia's primary and secondary education system over the past 20 years has been a part of the family planning strategy. Surveys show that education contributes to couples postponing marriage and allows more women to participate in the work-force to improve family economic status. Education has also increased awareness that several children spaced closely can increase health problems for both mothers and their children. Better education has increased people's awareness of their responsibility to plan their families.

It must be remembered that Indonesia started with many disadvantages; an extremely large population base, a relatively low GNP per capita, low literacy, high infant mortality. Today population growth is slowing and is expected to stabilize by the year 2060 at 300 or 350 million. GNP has risen to US $525 per capita (1989). In 1985 literacy was 87.8 per cent among males over ten years of age and 74.3 per cent among females over ten. Infant mortality which was 140 in 1971 declined to 58 by 1990 and is expected to decline to at least 40 in the next decade. Life expectancy increased from 47 years in 1971 to 60 years in 1985.

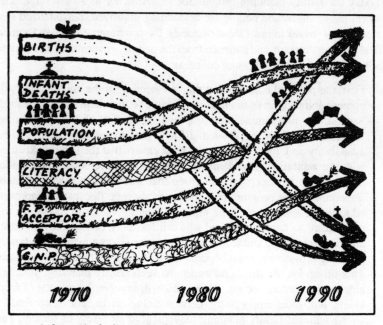

A dramatic decline in births has accompanied the fall in deaths, rising literacy, family income and acceptance of family planning.

Indonesia's total fertility rate has fallen from 5.6 in the 1970s to 3.3 in the 1984–87 period and the crude birth rate has declined from 46 to 28 births per thousand population (1985) and is expected to reach 25 by 1995. From 50 000 family planning acceptors in 1970, there are 18 million today. The family planning programme has 70 000 volunteer family planning workers and 27 000 full-time *PLKB*.

Over 65 per cent of currently married women have used a contraceptive method at some time and approximately half are currently using a modern method. The pill is the most common, used by 41 per cent of all acceptors, followed by the IUD (27 per cent), injectables (20 per cent), condoms (3 per cent), and female and male sterilization (9 per cent). Women users are higher among urban women (54 per cent) than rural women (45 per cent). The higher the level of education, the higher the proportion of women practising family planning.

THE CHALLENGES AHEAD

Today the family planning programme is advancing to a new stage. The world has changed and people are demanding improved, personalized services. As it strives to meet these demands, the programme will need a great deal of moral support and patience from the people, government and donors alike. There are four important concerns:

— First, the political commitment that is essential for the continued development and support of the movement must be maintained and refreshed.
— Second, the programme must improve the quality of family planning services that are being offered. *BKKBN* has to improve accessibility, availability and, most importantly, must ensure that the services keep up with the aspirations and demands of younger, more educated potential family planning acceptors, the group that will become more and more important for the programme's continued success. Because of improved educational opportunities and rapidly changing values in Indonesia, the programme's 'target audience' will call for more considered responses and more complete and technical information. Consequently, the family planning programme must become more professional and sophisticated.
— This brings on the third challenge—to keep family planning 'fashionable' in Indonesian society. Again, this will involve the science of marketing but, more importantly, deep sociological insight to continue a strong national family planning movement at all levels of society. The family planning concept and methods must continue to be seen as modern and sophisticated, something people need and want. 'The Small

Happy Prosperous Family' slogan must continue to evoke a response from Indonesians.
— Fourth, the family planning programme must show more specifically how it supports the goals of national development. When the programme was developing, it was enough to look only at the numbers of couples accepting family planning. The *BKKBN* was introducing an innovation to a traditional society, so achieving awareness, understanding and acceptance was the main goal. Now as the programme comes under more scrutiny from government planners and policy-makers, it is important to show its impact on fertility. The *BKKBN* must show what are the real qualitative goals of the national effort, and discuss how they can be assessed and measured. In addition to the health and humanitarian grounds that guided the programme in its first 20 years, its socio-economic impact on the nation, the family and the individual must be shown.

In this day and age, governments everywhere are experiencing difficulty financing social welfare programmes. Indonesia is attempting to reinvigorate a sense of individual responsibility among its people. By doing so, the government's limited resources, previously spent on providing basic welfare services such as family planning, could and eventually should be redirected towards the full and equal development of other segments of the economy. This is essential to attain a healthy economic base which, in the long run, will make nationally-sponsored government family planning programmes obsolete. It is crucial for the family planners strategy to retain an understanding of the people's psychology, their needs, their aspirations, and their sense of ownership and national pride. In so doing, family planning will remain a powerful tool for the welfare of the Indonesian peoples.

SOME LESSONS FOR OTHER COUNTRIES

Several elements of the Indonesian experience are of broad relevance and applicability.

A Relevant and Flexible Organization

The role of the *BKKBN* has been central to making family planning a truly integrated national effort. Its structure has ensured not only the provision of services, effective communication and up-to-date information, but has also monitored and predicted the impact on Indonesia's population and economy. A dynamic R&D programme ensured that family planning activities did not stagnate but evolved with—even led—changes of interest in and demands for family planning. By answering directly to the President, the *BKKBN* was able to mobilize consistent and unwavering political support, and its own leadership has been constant and committed for over 20 years. While *BKKBN* is not primarily a service delivery organization, its field personnel (the 27 000 family planning workers recruited in the villages), are supervised and directed by staff at every government level, right up to a self-contained, well-funded office at the centre. A well-defined career track exists for *BKKBN* staff, as well as the possibility of lateral entry. Coupled with the entrepreneurial spirit of the *BKKBN* leadership, the availability of adequate financial resources has helped the organization to perform as a dynamic social development agency rather than as a typical government bureaucracy. The budget of US $200 million for 1991, just over $1 per capita, is managed flexibly and to a large extent is delegated to peripheral levels. The *BKKBN* is responsive to new ideas and innovations, and has a close partnership with various community and religious organizations, NGOs, academic institutions and professional organizations.

The *BKKBN* has run its own training centres at national and provincial levels and in selected districts. The centres provide pre-service and in-service training for the family planning field workers and their supervisors. Through a series of orientation programmes, these centres perform other important tasks in providing forums for communication with local leaders, NGOs and professional groups, which has been critical to creating positive broad-based support for family planning. Inter-sectoral discussions and reviews of programme performance at district and provincial levels are usually done in workshops organized by these *BKKBN* training centres.

The *BKKBN* is unique in its approach to decentralization. Its keen understanding of the value of local government as a strategic ally to achieve programme objectives has led to a fruitful cooperation between *BKKBN* and government at all levels. The programme has managed to achieve a happy mix of centrally-developed policy and overall direction and locally-initiated and sustained implementation. It thus enjoys strong support from local government—achieved by few centrally-managed programmes. The key to this success is *BKKBN*'s ability to create a high degree of ownership of the programme—a major prerequisite for real community participation.

Effective Communication

From the outset *BKKBN* has seen its mission as 'the introduction of broader and more lasting change in societal values, towards the ideal number of children in a family' rather than just popularizing contraceptive practice.

Thus, communication in the programme has gone far beyond the 'sloga-neering' through family planning posters and radio jingles. In fact, the en-tire programme can be viewed as a communication exercise. Key compo-nents of this comprehensive strategy have been:

— *securing support from key community leaders, especially religious leaders, at the very beginning of the programme.* This consensus-build-ing effort was given top priority during the first few years. This is also the reason why abortion and sterilization were not entertained by the programme in its early phases.

— *creating a community movement for family planning by actively invol-ving women's groups and other community organizations.* They were given responsibility for programme implementation as motivators, dis-tributors of contraceptives, enumerators of eligible couples and monthly reporters.

— *supporting thousands of village acceptor clubs to conduct a variety of activities beyond family planning* such as credit schemes, income-gener-ating activities, literacy classes, even traditional dance and music events. This strategy was intended to convey that family planning is an integral part of social and economic life. It also showed that the government appreciated people's support of the country's development effort through their participation in the programme. It helped to project the programme as one that cared about the well-being of the family and the community, not just as a government scheme to achieve targets unrelated to the people's lives.

— *integrating family planning with an array of relevant community-based mother and child health and nutrition activities* including immunization, oral rehydration, distribution of vitamin A and iron-folic acid tablets, ante-natal care and monthly growth monitoring. In this way family plan-ning also formed the basis of a nation-wide, integrated community-based primary health care effort.

— *facilitating people's choice of contraceptives through a communication strategy rather than on the basis of an assessment of demographic im-pact of various family planning methods.* Thus, temporary contracep-tives (pills, condoms and IUDs) were offered initially and only later were injectables and sterilization added to build a true cafeteria ap-proach. Offered as one amongst several contraceptives of equal respect-ability, the pill was by far (and still is) the contraceptive of choice, used by about 65 per cent of all acceptors. This 'low commitment' method is very popular among the younger low-parity groups, the most strategic segment to be reached in marketing the idea of family planning. Even exclusive breast-feeding is promoted for its spacing effect as well as for the health of mother and child. The programme encourages couples to choose the contraceptive appropriate to the decisions they make from marriage onward regarding when to start having children, how far apart to space them, and how many to have. If a young couple accepts the idea of planning a family, and after their two children are born properly spaced, they are encouraged to 'move up' to a more dependable method, such as the IUD, implant or injectable and eventually to sterilization. Thus, sterilization tends to reach only older couples who have achieved, or even surpassed, their ideal family size and would like to end reproduction.

— *carefully choosing terminology to convey the positive attributes of family planning and allay fears.* 'Traditional' methods refers to *coitus interruptus*, rhythm or breast-feeding; 'modern' methods are the pill or condom; 'selected' methods are the IUD and injectables; and 'firm' methods describes the longer-term implant or sterilization. This last term is almost never used in *BKKBN* promotional literature but accounts for some 8 per cent of protection. The shift to more permanent methods resulted from demand by experienced family planning users for a more reliable and convenient method and not from the wish of programme managers to push more cost-effective or permanent contraception. Thus, compatibility with the community-based strategy and individual health needs, rather than clinical and cost-effectiveness, have been the primary factors determining the contraceptive mix.

Meaningful Target-setting and Information Systems

Target-setting has undeniably been a critical management tool as it is for any undertaking with a set of goals and objectives. The challenge has been to use this tool without negative 'fall-out'. The Indonesian family planning programme initially allocated targets to administrative units, and some overzealous workers created a backlash in the community by pushing IUDs too strongly. However, the problem diminished with community participation and management of the programme. Several lessons emerge:

— It is important that the community set its own targets after knowing who are the eligible couples and what are the choices or methods. Open discussions make family planning everybody's business.
— Assigning targets to administrative areas rather than to individual workers makes the entire government team responsible and encourages them to strive for broad-based community support.
— A broad range of targets rather than a 'body-count' system is helpful. These may change as the programme evolves. New acceptors by

method, current users, new family planning groups formed, children participating in growth monitoring, percentage of self-reliant acceptors, the community birth rate, individual fertility rates, average spacing between children are all examples of programme targets which both encourage and monitor a wide range of desired behaviours.

— A simple feedback mechanism which provides managers at all levels with up-to-date information on their own programme performance and that of their neighbours is a critical motivational and management tool. The information includes child nutrition and health parameters beyond acceptors and current users. These parameters have become part of a broader village evaluation procedure carried out annually by the Ministry of Home Affairs to determine the level of development of each village. Periodic independent checks of the validity of the information are part of the system.

— Programme reviews start with each district and progress upwards to the national level. They are not centred around discussions of target achievements, but are a broader performance-analysis and problem-solving exercise in which targets are used as a productive management tool to uncover and solve problems rather than as an end in themselves.

The Programme Management Information System has become a strategic management and coordination tool, completely designed and run by *BKKBN*. Each acceptor is recorded on a computer-coded post-card. The monthly report—one page submitted by health centre doctors—contains key information on the number and characteristics of acceptors, type of contraceptives and continuation rates. The data is analysed centrally and feedback is provided to district managers on a given month's performance before the 25th of the following month. Ninety-seven per cent of the 10 000 health centres send their monthly reports regularly. The short, simple and convenient format—only 18 items to fill—and the immediate feedback are key factors which make the system work well. The data are scrutinized at the provincial, district and sub-district levels, not only by health and family planning personnel but also by civil authorities.

Doing without Incentives

As a late-comer to the world of family planning, Indonesia benefited from the experience of other countries. It was clear to policy-makers that they should avoid the incentive trap. Strategically it was not compatible with the underlying philosophy of the programme that practising family planning is in the best interest of the individual, of the community and of the country (in that order). An incentive always carries a message that the giver is grateful for something done by the receiver. Thus, offering incentives would imply that the government was the recipient of the primary benefit and not the acceptor, which would undermine the central message that family planning is desirable and beneficial to the family. Therefore, it was decided early in the programme that no material incentives would be given either to acceptors or service-providers. Instead, those practising family planning are recognized for their contribution to the national development effort. Long-term acceptors, chosen by their local acceptor club, are invited to Jakarta to meet the President. Those who have used family planning for ten years or more receive a plastic credit card identifying them as eligible for a special 'family planning' discount at participating restaurants and retail outlets. Family planning users are proud of their status and often announce it with bumper stickers, labels on houses, or even T-shirts. Billboards remind commuters 'Have you taken your pill this morning?' and the family planning logo is found on stamps, coins, vehicles, public buildings, banners, and clothing. Family planning has become the centre-piece not only of health services for mothers and children but of a wide range of social and development services including consumer cooperatives, agricultural extension and youth clubs. It is truly at the centre of the Indonesian development agenda.

In Indonesia, family planning is indeed everyone's business. The programme is evolving constantly. We are always looking for new ideas, not only within Indonesia but also abroad. We read about other programmes and invite consultants with knowledge of other countries to work for a time with us. We listen very carefully to visitors for we know from long experience that many visitors will describe something which their country is doing, which we might adapt, or provide us with a new insight into an element of our own programme which will assist us to understand it better. We have found this an effective way of improving our programme. We are convinced that Indonesia's quest for 'Health for All by the Year 2000' and indeed its continued development is related integrally to continuing commitment to a strong family planning effort.

Reaching Health for All

Throughout *Reaching Health for All* the reader has been encouraged to seek lessons which apply broadly and have general value to the planning and practice of health. Surely each of us will derive ideas and modify them to suit the situation in which we live and work. Their relevance is highly conditioned by our own experience and context. Even considerations of contradictions, dilemmas and unanswered questions lead us to examine more carefully our own 'truths' and principles in order to strengthen our approaches and actions. But amidst this medley of studies lie some common threads, some elements of principle that seem to transcend social, political and economic differences. These lessons provide the foundation for progress. In this concluding section we, the editors, would like to share our views of these lessons and point to their uses in the decade ahead.

SUCCESS AND COMMUNITY CONTROL

The first lesson has to do with the definition of 'success'. A decline in mortality is readily accepted as an indicator of success in health, leading programmes which are planned and driven by careful epidemiological analysis and cost-effectiveness to be considered the most successful. But some of the stories told here—such as those of Zimbabwe or Nicaragua—suggest that success by this definition may be transient or even illusory at times, regressing in the face of adverse conditions such as financial constraints. Thus, sustainability is an important criterion of success.

The experiences related in this book have revealed a number of other, less obvious definitions of 'success'. A broad consensus suggests that success can be equated with a level of confidence among people to deal with their own health problems, with positive feelings about their own health and the health systems that serve them. This is seen clearly in the experience with *mawas diri* in Indonesia and community health committees in Zaire and Villa el Salvador, Peru. Community control, self-reliance, involvement and pride characterize these programmes, demonstrating both health impact and sustainability in the face of resource constraints. Community ownership is also characteristic of the successful elements of large projects such as the Indonesian *posyandus* or Iringa in Tanzania. And it can persist even through national efforts, as it has in the socialist societies of Zimbabwe, Nicaragua and Costa Rica, and in Indonesia's family planning programme.

Each of the experiences deemed 'successful' involved communities to a substantial degree in the planning and/or implementation of health acti-

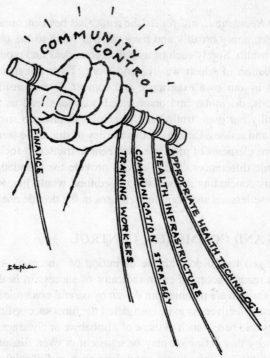

Community control over health activities is a common thread in stories of success.

vities. However, this does not mean necessarily that paramedic or village volunteer-delivered health services automatically work well. In India, although the village-level Health Guides came from the communities they served, they were inadequately responsive to those communities. They were also ineffectively connected to the public health system which was responsible for their continuing supervision and support. The absence of accountability to the community among these volunteers as well as to the health system led to the eventual failure of this programme.

In addition to inadequate attention to community control the Health Guides' scheme weakened considerably when a change in the ruling political party resulted in the withdrawal of necessary central political support. This situation is almost analogous to that of the barefoot doctors in China, who were initially 'managed' and rewarded by their communes and hence worked effectively. But recent developments have demonstrated the dependence of this system on strong direction from the top. With the demise of stringent central controls the same doctors have opened themselves up to 'serve' market forces.

Both China's decentralized, people-controlled health care system and Vietnam's which were centrally-mandated have experienced set-backs with political changes and economic hardships. In Vietnam, where there was little real control by communities of the centralized model of universal primary health care, the decline in resources and power of the Centre resulted in the decay of the system itself, and a chaotic turn to the private sector with substantial losses in public health objectives.

In those Indonesian *posyandus* where community control was strong, nutrition and family planning activities persisted even when the Health Department took a strong, directive role. In contrast, where community involvement in decision-making had been weak and participation had been more a matter of 'following instructions', programme coverage and accomplishments often diminished substantially with the rise of health department control. In many countries where immunization programmes were organized by communities and supported by health systems, service delivery has been maintained and strengthened. But in countries where universal immunization goals were accomplished solely through national campaigns in largely passive populations, sustainability has become a grave problem for the 1990s.

Even comprehensive health care systems which have failed to involve communities have not performed well. India has invested extensively in infrastructure and manpower for its national health care system. But this remains, to a large degree, under-utilized and poorly responsive to people.

In contrast, within India, both the Tamil Nadu Nutrition Programme and non-governmental health organizations have shown that health care delivery and communication strategies carefully tailored to people can involve communities and improve health effectively.

These and other experiences have shown the critical importance of properly trained and motivated health 'person-power', responsive to people's felt needs and able to work simultaneously with poor individuals, families and communities and 'bureaucratic' support systems. The major experiment carried out by the Institute of Health Sciences in the Philippines to systematically develop such workers has put actions to rhetoric voiced in many parts of the world and provided important lessons. The 'production' of appropriate workers can only be achieved through a three-way partnership between the community to be served, the trainee and the health system.

HEALTH, POLITICS AND DEVELOPMENT

The provision of health services responsive to public need has come increasingly onto the political agendas of nations. Among 'new' governments such as those of Zimbabwe or Nicaragua health care issues have characterized both the struggle for power as well as the visible results of a new polity. Established governments have built strength at the community-level through responsive innovation in health. Some have even diverted resources towards community health such as in the Indonesian *posyandus* or in the immunization campaigns led by political leaders in many countries.

However, excess political visibility can be detrimental. Over-politicization of the community Health Guides was a factor cited by the Government in India which withdrew support to them. The strong participatory nature of primary health care may be seen as a threat by existing power systems, leading to inhumane and disastrous suppression of peoples as witnessed through the decade in various parts of Latin America.

In most settings, however, health is increasingly seen as an entry-point for broader community development activities. Communities have been mobilized first to meet their health needs and later into a wide range of self-help efforts. In Tanzania, a community focus on child nutrition led to a national strategy for village development in child care, education, agriculture and small business in addition to primary health care. In Bangladesh, an NGO demonstrated the possibility of integrating health and nutrition care with education, especially for girls, and rural credit in order to address a wide spectrum of health determinants. Almost all the case studies in this collection testify to the strong linkages between health, development and politics!

INFLUENCERS IN PRIMARY HEALTH CARE

Our review of the case studies in this collection brought out a perplexing fact: despite the strong thread of community involvement and control in many of the studies there were no examples of true self-generated, 'spontaneous' community programmes. From David Werner's work with the disabled in Mexico to the Chinese communes of the 1970s, all health programmes involved a catalyst from outside the community at least initially. This may have been a leader, a vision, a directive or a community member returned from 'outside'. This appears true more broadly of primary health care efforts throughout the world. The type of outside influence—i.e. the role played by 'outsiders' in a community and the nature of their programme inputs—determines in large measure the type of primary health care 'model' that emerges. We have identified four levels of 'influencers',

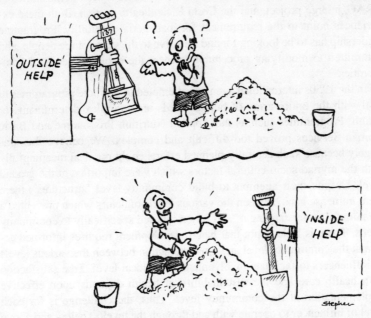

Leadership from within tends to be more socially acceptable even if the technology adopted is less sophisticated.

coincidentally analogous to the four sections of this book: community 'insiders' trained 'outside', outside professional individuals or groups or NGOs, government agencies, and international organizations. The closer an influencer is to the community, the more immersed in the socio-cultural particuliarities of that community is the health care model which develops. It is more likely to be flexible, uniquely-attuned to the character and composition of the community served and 'comprehensive', tackling a wide array of community problems and their underlying causes. Conversely, the further away an influence comes from, the more likely is the programme to be a standardized, 'generic' and 'selective' form of health care.

This makes it obvious why global efforts catalysed by international agencies are more technologically- and less sociologically-oriented. The complexity of social issues requires a degree of contact and knowledge of communities that makes it difficult if not impossible to build socially-sensitive international (and sometimes even national) programmes. Put another way, technologies which are aimed at large, diverse populations must be socially neutral. This does not mean that they cannot be adapted to suit community norms. That such adaptation is possible is seen in the stories of BRAC, a large project, and the Costa Rican health system. Both these experiences point to the requirement for managerial flexibility. Programme leadership has to be looking for and sensitive to the voice of the people, and committed to modifying procedures to meet the evolving needs of communities.

In the 1950s international agencies attempted to promote programmes to deal with the entire array of human needs and complex determinants of health. Programmes such as the Applied Nutrition Programme and Basic Human Services proved too difficult and complex. We believe this was largely because such centrally-planned efforts could not deal meaningfully with the myriad socio-cultural factors which were important at the ground level. Despite their attempts to build community-level 'structures', there were immense gaps between the various levels of actors which prevented a meaningful understanding of and action tailored specifically to community needs. There is little doubt that health development requires informed action at the community level and thus interaction between the various levels of influencers to facilitate involvement at the local level. True satisfaction with health care and the sustainability of health depends upon effective implementation at the community level. Thus, the challenge is for each level of influencer to operate with and through the level(s) below and above to support a concerted approach to health care. In this way appropriate decentralization of activities and resources throughout the system could be achieved.

'SELECTIVE' OR 'COMPREHENSIVE' PRIMARY HEALTH CARE?

A major debate occurred during the 1980s on the issue of 'selective versus comprehensive' primary health care. One side favoured technological responses to the most prevalent and important epidemiologically-demonstrated health needs, incorporating the highest levels of economic efficiency. The other placed maximum emphasis on tackling the roots of ill-health through broad-based programmes, on the involvement of communities, on their right to choice, on self-reliance and cultural uniqueness in health care. However, the experiences reported here suggest that such polarization has not in fact occurred at the level of programme implementation. Few efforts have been either entirely selective, focusing on a single intervention to the exclusion of all others, or comprehensive in their ability to meet all the health needs of the population at once. All have had to make choices and compromises.

For example, while apparently 'comprehensive', the *mawas diri* effort in Indonesia and community health and development in Zaire had only a limited set of health interventions. Their essence lay in being flexible in the identification of problems and admitting a diversity of approaches to their solution. At the other end of the spectrum is EPI, allegedly a 'selective' PHC strategy. This focused approach aimed to establish an effective system to provide an essential service. Global experience has shown that once such a system is in place its activities can be diversified to meet an array of

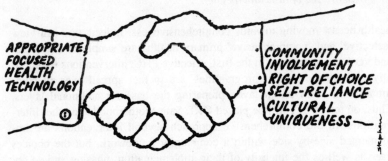

Primary Health Care: A matter of choice and compromises.

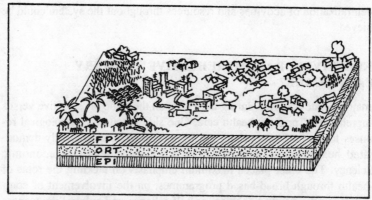

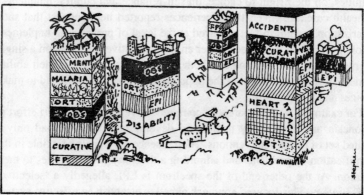

*So-called 'vertical' programmes spread horizontally to cover the
entire population (above), while more limited population receiving
'comprehensive' programmes are like small islands—vertically rising
above sea of ill-health (below).*

health needs, moving towards comprehensiveness. Indeed, one can view
'selective' and 'comprehensive' primary health care simply as horizontal
and vertical approaches. In the first, selective PHC, interventions traditionally viewed as 'vertical programmes' are in fact spread over all communities in a *horizontal* layer, preparing the base for additional layers.
Thus, on top of EPI will be placed ORT, Safe Motherhood and other interventions. In the comprehensive approach several interventions are implemented side-by-side within a community framework, but the choices
vary as well as the intensity of their implementation, phasing and so on.
This gives a picture of upright (*vertical*) stakes of varied health activities in

different communities. Eventually, both approaches provide a fairly standard array of health services to all communities.

We conclude that all programmes need both appropriate, focused health
technology and community control. Programmes differ markedly in the mix
of these two elements. Those emphasizing community participation, flexibility and demand still make a choice between interventions, unable to afford everything, especially at the outset. Those with an over-riding service
delivery design emphasizing 'management' and 'efficiency', such as the
EPI and ORT programmes, have discovered the critical importance of informing the public and encouraging people to share responsibility for implementing even these 'technical' interventions.

TECHNOLOGY OR PROCESS

These differing experiences demonstrate that it is the *process* of intervening
for health that is critical, not the particular service that is delivered. Technology may be seen as providing a starting point—and can be of vastly
differing types. For example, in *mawas diri* the technology is a self-survey,
a means of assessing community needs and assigning priorities. In *posyandus* it is the community weighing-post and the community nutrition scoring

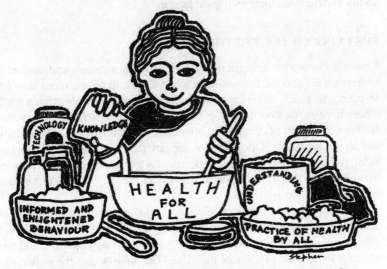

*Many ingredients are necessary for Health for All—but it is the
recipe, the process by which they are mixed, that determines the
outcome.*

system. In EPI it is the provision of safe, effective vaccines delivered in a timely and reliable way to all infants. All programmes are 'selective' to begin with. All aim towards an increasingly complex series of interventions to meet the entire range of community health needs. In both the delivery system and in the community of users, it is the *process of reaching health* that is the important contribution to health.

Perhaps nothing of the 1980s will make medical history more forcefully than the emergence of AIDS. Although the most sophisticated and costly biomedical technologies available have been mobilized against it, this pandemic threatens to bring bankruptcy to health services as it continues its relentless spread around the world. While it is recognized as a global and national problem, its resolution really lies in the modification of individual and community behaviours. AIDS is perhaps the ultimate test of the principle that 'Health for All' rests on informed and enlightened behaviour, on knowledge, understanding and the practice of health by each member of society. Today the major part of the global health dollar is spent on treating the results of unhealthy practices: bottle-feeding, poor hygiene, inappropriate food allocations, high fertility, sexual practices, smoking, and so on. A major challenge for the 1990s is to reorient health investments in order to inculcate in each individual, family and community both the desire and the ability to determine their own good health.

SUSTAINABILITY THROUGH CRISES

Resource constraints necessitate choices between options—and such constraints are ubiquitous. Interestingly, while almost all programmes have felt an economic pinch, some have seen a decline in the services offered while others have carried on despite cut-backs. There is a definite relationship between the extent of community involvement and control of a programme and its sustainability. Once again it appears that the nature of the service being provided or activity being undertaken is less important to determining its viability in times of economic stress than the way in which the community came to 'own' it.

As countries are forced to reallocate internal resources, the pressures to abandon preventive and promotive primary health care will be considerable, especially where political systems support private enterprise and particularly the private practice of medicine. This underscores the importance of developing societal 'safety nets' for the most critical programmes, especially for the poor. The emergence of the private sector is seen by many as a mixed blessing. While a shift away from state-provided services gives

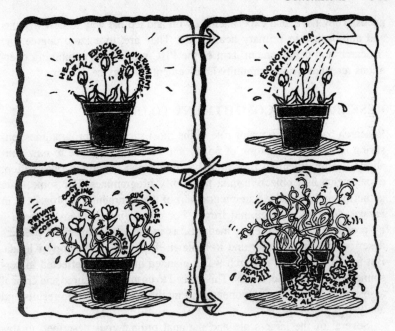

*While economic liberalization is seen by some as the solution to
social problems, resulting proliferation of free market activities could
stifle the most essential services.*

relief to strained budgets, the private sector tends to reverse priorities, excluding the poor. In Nicaragua and China the decline of public protection
has been accompanied by the emergence of harmful medical practices related to polypharmacy and excessive use of laboratory tests, hospitalization,
curative and 'interventionist' medicine. While the private sector can readily
be expected to handle an increasing proportion of the needs of the better-off
in society, it is unlikely to meet the needs of the poor or protect the health
of the public, activities for which social health care systems have been
particularly tailored. In the decade ahead programmes are needed to guide,
channel and encourage the private sector into responsible, cost-effective
and efficacious medical practice.

Amidst the public–private dichotomy, non-governmental organizations
have emerged as important, particularly those indigenous organizations
dedicated to participatory self-reliance. BRAC is one of the largest extant
NGOs but hundreds, even thousands, of organizations throughout the developing world serve to protect the rights of the poor and cater to their

needs. They have also experimented with and led the way to new insights and approaches in primary health care. They are, to a large degree, the 'research and development' arm of the PHC movement, combining operations research with community involvement and service delivery.

RESEARCH AND COMMITMENT TO CHANGE

Research has played a major role in the most successful programmes, ensuring an ordered evolution of policy and action in response to new situations. Commitment to flexibility has built upon structured observation, experiments and objective data to modify programmes. For some, data gathering and analysis is an integral part of the community approach, as in *mawas diri* and at Boga and Iringa. For others, information has been a by-product of trial and error methods, as in the Latin American projects described by Frits Muller and in Malawi, discussed by Anthony Klouda. But for most, built-in research was a planned investment reflected in personnel and budget allocations. This served to ensure a measured and critical assessment of project components and modifications based on results and analysis.

Several of the large-scale and national programmes described in this book have had research as a major feature. In TINP a research cell conducted over 60 independent studies to compare feeding regimens, educational approaches and training strategies and to determine the impact of various project components. BRAC's research and development wing has been responsible for the changes in specific field approaches used by oral rehydration trainers and for many features of the health and development activities undertaken subsequently. The ICDS programme in India has involved over 60 medical colleges in its on-going evaluation and even more in research studies. However, this programme has been slow to absorb these extensive research findings into operational changes. The Indonesian Family Planning Board (*BKKBN*) has a large research division charged with testing new contraceptives, information and logistics systems. It has helped to strengthen the field programme through the development of strategies such as community distribution posts, integration with *posyandus* and privatization through the Blue Circle initiative.

Research has clearly also driven the global efforts for immunization, oral rehydration, vitamin A and family planning as these technology-based programmes have sought to adapt to local situations. Many incorporate a special research division into programme design. The recommendation of the International Commission on Health Research to allocate five per cent of all project costs to research is reflected in the changing designs of these internationally-sponsored efforts. Research and commitment to utilize relevant insights for programme modifications are a key element of success. They will become even more important in the decade ahead as the complexity of programmes increases and financial constraints demand even greater cost-effectiveness.

THE HEALTH TRANSITION

As health services and economic development improve the health conditions of substantial portions of society, mortality rates decline pushing up life expectancy, and fertility rates fall, leading to the 'ageing' of societies. This 'demographic transition' is invariably accompanied by an 'epidemiological transition' characterized by a declining proportion of deaths among the young while the diseases of ageing become predominant over the communicable diseases and malnutrition. This 'health transition' has led some planners to propose a shift in public health expenditures from programmes affecting the young and controlling infection to programmes caring for chronic illnesses and degeneration in the elderly.

But dynamic situations so often distract attention from the unchanging, and averages so often obscure the skewedness of reality. In general, populations do not undergo transformation all at once. Rather, they have experienced increasing epidemiological polarization associated with economic development and the frequently-accompanying economic and social disparities. Small but growing segments of societies have become more wealthy, are encountering infection and malnutrition less and experiencing fertility decline. At the same time substantial proportions of the population—notably the poor—are left behind with demographic and epidemiological characteristics that can easily be described as a 'pre-health transition society'.

Continued allocation of public resources to the young and to the control of infectious diseases and malnutrition will favour this neglected portion of society and therefore be inherently more equitable. Conversely, any effort to re-programme public resources to the enlarging well-to-do class will be inherently regressive and increase inequality between social groups. Thus, until the health transition can be shown to be occurring even amongst the poorest segments of society, public resources should continue to be invested to combat infection and malnutrition among the young. Such a strategy serves maximally the principles of efficacy and efficiency as well as equity.

The 1980s saw increasing recognition of the role of communities in both demanding and creating the conditions for improved health. Side by side, it was demonstrated that key modern health technologies can be managed to reach even the most deprived and isolated communities and families. At the same time, financial constraints forced increasing efforts at efficiency, encouraged payment by those who can afford health services while seeking to ensure free care to those who cannot. Over the next decade even greater efforts will be needed to avoid duplication, to integrate service function, and to mobilize the resources of communities to take action to ensure the health of all. A critical element will be the extent to which individuals are informed and convinced to take health actions in their own interest—from diet to hygiene to early home care of illness to family planning. For this to occur, political enfranchisement and universal education are critical enabling factors.

ADDRESSING INEQUALITIES

While the programmes described in this book—indeed, health programmes in general—predominantly address the manifestations and proximal causes of morbidity and premature mortality, increasing recognition of the underlying causes of ill-health has characterized development in the 1980s. Strategies to address these underlying causes will become increasingly important in the decade ahead. Among these, education, particularly of young girls, has been shown as a major determinant of health and survival across all societies.

The lack of education and even of health care is intimately linked to issues of gender disparity. In societies where females experience discrimination, often from birth, higher overall rates of infant and child death and malnourishment, low schooling levels, and poor inter-generational health is seen. Redressing gender bias in these societies will make a major contribution to health improvement not only among women but in the society as a whole. Universal education is a prime strategy to address this bias. Indeed, it is gender equality, particularly evidenced in high female literacy rates, which led the demographic transition of Kerala, economically one of the poorest states in India. Investment in education will be seen over the next decade to offer a major strategy not only for improved health but as the driving force for all development efforts.

NEW PARADIGMS FOR LIFE ON EARTH

At an even more basic level, poverty, economic deprivation, unemployment, debt and political disenfranchisement underlie much of the ill-health that is seen in the Third World today. To redress these problems an entire revision of the world economic and political order is called for, a revision which *is* increasingly possible in the rapidly-changing world of the early 1990s. With the dissolution of the Cold War and the rise of democratic movements and ethnic identities across the world, the possibility of a major restructuring of political systems and a new world economic order is emerging. Such a new order must be more just and provide greater opportunities for human endeavour to be rewarded with at least the *minimal basic needs for healthy living.*

Most analysts admit that this must begin with the elimination of Third World debt and a reversal of the present situation in which resources are transferred from the Third World to the First. Eliminating debt repayments and interest schedules, more equitable pricing and market structures in which primary materials and human production are valued as highly as manufactured products and services generated in technically-sophisticated societies are some of the steps which need to be taken. Such changes are required for a truly healthy and just planet, and appear increasingly possible. The emergence of equitable and efficient health systems will contribute substantially in turn to progress toward an equitable and just world society.

During the past three decades world population growth has been sustained at an unprecedented rate of over two per cent, resulting in a doubling over 30 to 35 years. At current rates a billion persons are added to the world each decade, an addition which stresses health systems and the very ecology which sustains life on earth. Entire books and numerous conferences have addressed the population, ecology and environmental issues which are so pressing in our times. To some analysts this rapid population growth is a direct result of the success of public health efforts over the past century or so, and it has been seriously suggested that a 'solution' to the strain on our ecosystems is to withdraw these health measures and allow death rates to rise. The case studies in this book are adequate evidence that humane solutions do exist to bring about a reduction in fertility coincident with an improvement in life expectation and quality of health and nutrition. China's is the best known case, but Costa Rica, Kerala in India, and Indonesia have demonstrated the ability of societies to achieve ecologically-sound population stabilization with good health for all.

Importantly, 'Health for All' must include the West, whose population and living patterns contribute substantially to our deteriorating ecosystem. Its relatively smaller population consumes the vast majority of the world's resources and contributes by far the greatest amount of pollution. The economic system of the West, dependent on growth, future discounting, high consumption, competition and an inherently inequitable economy, is a predominant threat to the global ecosystem. There is a move towards a new paradigm for living, a move which will contribute immensely to reaching Health for All. Efforts to live in voluntary simplicity, in environmentally-neutral life-styles, espousing Gandhian values of self-reliance based on simple technology and human caring, all support the emergence of a new global ethic.

Gaia, the living planet, is at a critical juncture poised between the threat of over-population and eco-destruction and the hope of a sustainable global society. The case studies in this book describe health contributions to a new development based on humane values, dignity, equality and sustainable systems. This is indeed the only route to world peace, and the only way to eliminate ill-health, malnutrition and the ultimate violence of poverty. One decade is but a passing moment in the eyes of history, but the coming decade may well determine the very fate of this planet and our species. Achieving an effective equitable system that will lead to a decent quality of life for every individual in the world will convince and enable families to limit their fertility to replacement levels. It will assure future generations that the quest for 'Health for All by the Year 2000' was dramatic testimony of the conviction of people of the second millennium that humane systems can prevail to sustain the well-being of humans throughout the planet Earth for all time.

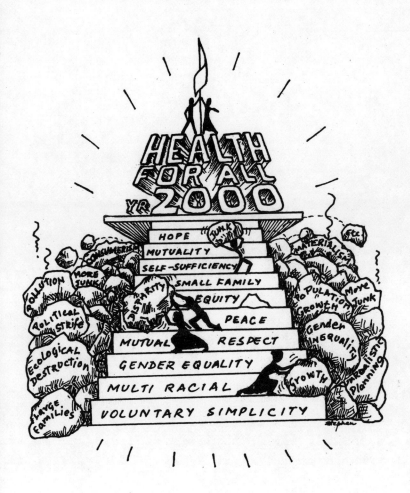

Make the best use of this book

The editors of this book are pleased to find that in a world in which there is so much gloom, there are also so many promising changes and new ideas. We know that the best use of all this information will only come when health workers and colleagues from other development disciplines sit down and discuss the problems communities and countries have run into and the approaches they have taken to overcome them. This discussion is important amongst staff in health programmes, but it is particularly important for those in postgraduate courses, medical students, nursing students and other health workers for whom discussion itself will become a sharing exercise drawing on their own varied experience.

Just as this book shows the tremendous changes that have and are occurring in health care, so have there been similar changes in teaching methods world-wide. Fortunately, in most countries lectures have given way to more discussion and student participation. The questions which have been suggested for the various chapters are merely a starting point, and the teacher will think of many other appropriate questions to raise, based on the local situation. These questions can be used for students to present the contents of a chapter to others or to project the lessons of the chapter into a local context. The teacher's role is to encourage this discussion and to see that it remains relevant. The questions can also be adjusted to create a debating situation in which the class is divided into two groups which take different positions and try to persuade the other group of the correctness of their view. Diagrams from this and other books can be given to the students to discuss in pairs, or the teacher may project a diagram and encourage the students to speak concisely on what they think are its intentions.

As editors we hope that this book will not be read and put away on a shelf, but lent to others and used in many ways to stimulate discussion. If this happens we will be satisfied that our task has been really worthwhile.

1. Prevention is *Still* More Costly than Cure / KLOUDA

After reading this chapter, list the means suggested to help health workers fully understand local health problems. What are the non-health factors that most influence the health of communities?

2. Community Participation through Self-introspection /
JOHNSTON

Can you identify from this chapter why *mawas diri* (self-introspection) became such an important force in the Indonesian programmes? What questions would be most relevant to raise health awareness and stimulate community action in your community?

3. Community-determined Health Development in Zaire /
NICKSON

In the initial stages of the work in Zaire a story was used. Why are stories (case studies) so useful and how can they best be used? What stories are used in your culture that (can) stimulate community dialogue on health matters?

4. Training Appropriate Health Workers in the Philippines /
BORRINAGA AND TANTUICO-KOH

During its 14-year existence the Institute of Health Sciences narrowly survived three morale-shattering threats of closure instigated by influential reactionary officials or vested interest groups. Describe the possible reasons behind the actions of these groups and whether there would be similar groups in your own country/community. How would you handle such threats to an innovative programme?

5. Enabling Primary Health Care through Disabled People /
WERNER

Should individuals with disabilities be encouraged to become local health workers? And be involved in setting up services for other disabled individuals? Suggest the advantages and disadvantages of these two measures in your community setting.

6. Participation, Poverty and Violence: Health and Survival in Latin America / MULLER

From this discussion of Latin American countries, identify the relationships between the village health workers and communities, professional health workers and those in power. How and why may their relationships change? How can communities and especially health workers be sheltered from outside political pressures in your society?

7. Indonesia's *Posyandus*: Accomplishments and Future Challenges / ROHDE

The *Posyandus* spread to 68 000 villages. Discuss the political and cultural background that made this possible. What compromises are necessary in a community-based primary health care design to enable expansion at this pace and to this extent?

8. Tamil Nadu's Successful Nutrition Effort / BALACHANDER

Most food supplementation programmes are a failure. Is TINP a success? If so, why? What is the role of measuring weight (growth monitoring) in the overall achievements of TINP? Could similar results be achieved without measuring growth?

9. Mobilization for Nutrition in Tanzania / JONSSON, LJUNGQVIST AND YAMBI

Describe the Triple A Cycle of this programme at local, district and national levels. What difficulties had to be surmounted? Identify triple A cycles already at work in your home community or work place. What problems in your community could be solved in this way?

10. Scaling-up in Health: Two Decades of Learning in Bangladesh / LOVELL AND ABED

Read this chapter carefully and try to identify the changes that occurred as BRAC developed into one of the largest indigenous NGOs. Aside from adequate outside financial support, what factors are required to enable an NGO to expand to this degree? Could this occur in your country and, if so, how would the process compare with the experience of BRAC?

11. The Potential and Limits of Health Sector Reforms in Zimbabwe / SANDERS

Analysis of feeding programmes world-wide usually shows they are ineffective. The one developed in Zimbabwe may have been more effective than most. Can you suggest reasons? How might Zimbabwe maintain its commitment to equitable high coverage health services in the face of severe fiscal constraints?

12. Nicaragua: Health under Three Regimes / GARFIELD

From this account identify the disadvantages of each regime. What can planners do to ameliorate the effects of such disadvantages? Try to define each of the three regimes in less than 20 words and then identify the health policy of each, and who gained and who lost as a result of this policy in terms of overall health.

13. The Dynamics of China's Health Care Model / RIFKIN

In Table 3 in this chapter, health care is related to political change. How relevant are these to health development in other countries? What important changes could be made in your own country even without major political change?

14. Transitions in Health Care in China / TAYLOR

Try and identify what changes have occurred in China. How are these likely to affect the less privileged members of a Chinese village? How would you propose to protect this group and still allow the trend to privatization?

15. Primary Health Care in Vietnam / ALLMAN

Initially, the health care developed by the socialist government of the north was excellent and successful. Why did it deteriorate over the years and the south apparently catch up? How might the entire country benefit from these two experiences and what actions would you suggest in the future?

16. Health for Too Many: India's Experiments with Truth /
CHATTERJEE

What were the critical differences accounting for the demise of the village Health Guides' scheme and the sustainability of the Integrated Child Development Services? Discuss the role of health services and other social sector advances in the success of Kerala. What implications do you see for health planners in India?

17. Changing Health Paradigms in Costa Rica / MOHS

Development of health care in Costa Rica was considered under three paradigms. How relevant are these in planning of health care in other countries such as your own?

18. Expanded Programme on Immunization: A Goal Achieved Towards Health for All / HILL, KIM-FARLEY AND ROHDE

The EPI has been considered the most successful of all the mass programmes. Try and identify from this chapter ten reasons for its success. Then, if possible from your own experience, discuss where problems have arisen. How can EPI success be sustained and extended to achieve the new goals related to immunization?

19. Oral Rehydration Therapy: From Principle to Practice / NORTHRUP

In oral rehydration there is a division between countries who depend largely on ORS packages and those which try to develop preparations prepared in the home using local ingredients. List the advantages and problems in both systems. (You may also want to read the chapter on the BRAC programme in Bangladesh.) What elements of EPI could be applied to ORT programmes?

20. Vitamin A for Child Survival: Science and Politics / SOMMER

What findings suggest that vitamin A is likely to reduce mortality? From this study and other studies you may know of, identify ethical problems which may arise in large community studies.

21. Family Planning can Contribute to Health for All /
ROWLEY AND MAHLER

List reasons why some nations, some races and some religions may be against family planning. How can we react to these arguments?

22. The Family Planning Movement in Indonesia /
SUYONO, HENDRATA AND ROHDE

This programme went through a number of stages. Can you identify these and suggest why the changes were made? Which of these elements could be readily incorporated into the family planning activities of your own country?